D1731628

Guidelines
for Occupational Medical
Examinations

Guidelines
for Occupational Medical
Examinations

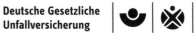

Gentner Verlag

Deutsche Gesetzliche
Unfallversicherung

Impressum

Publisher:
Deutsche Gesetzliche Unfallversicherung DGUV (German Social Accident Insurance)

Editor:
Priv.-Doz. Dr. Jürgen J. Milde, Ausschuss Arbeitsmedizin (Committee for occupational medicine of the DGUV)

Translator:
Dr. Ann E. Wild

Copy-Deadline: September 2007

Deutsche Bibliothek Cataloguing in Publication Data see: http://dnb.ddb.de

ISBN 978-3-87247-691-3
© 2007 Gentner Verlag, Stuttgart, Germany
Cover: GreenTomato GmbH, Bielefeld/Stuttgart
Production: Druckerei Marquart GmbH, Aulendorf
Printed in Germany
All rights reserved

Contents

Preface

In its Centennial Declaration in Milan on the 11th of June 2006 the International Commission on Occupational Health, ICOH, called for the following global actions: "provision of competent occupational health services for every working individual and every workplace in the world, ensuring services for prevention and protection as well as competent diagnosis and recognition ...".

The present standard work on occupational medicine makes a contribution to this global target of the ICOH. It describes the fundamentals of quality-controlled occupational medical prophylaxis, which are in line with the stipulations for health surveillance found in the European Council Directive for improving the safety and health of workers at work.

In some European countries the Guidelines for occupational medical examinations are already known as established procedures for the medical care of persons exposed to certain specific work-related health risks, especially hazardous substances, noise, airway disorders, risk of infection, skin disorders, but also work at VDU workplaces and work involving strain on the musculoskeletal system.

For decades, specialists in occupational medicine have been working on the basis of these guidelines which are generally accepted to provide a good basis for qualitatively consistent procedures in occupational medical prophylaxis. The Guidelines are elaborated, kept up to date and further developed by teams of experts from all relevant fields under the auspices of the German Social Accident Insurance (Deutsche Gesetzliche Unfallversicherung, DGUV). The Guidelines recommend methods of examination to be used and apparatus required, they include information about exposures, symptoms and syndromes, and give the physician support in advising the patient and assessing the examination results.

This standard work on occupational medicine is organized according to a universal concept and the resulting clear structure makes it easy to use in occupational medical practice. The German Social Accident Insurance, DGUV, which since its institution in 1884 has committed itself not only to compensation but also to the prevention of workplace accidents and occupational disease and to the rehabilitation of employees, welcomes suggestions and comments for the improvement of the Guidelines.

Sankt Augustin, September 2007
Deutsche Gesetzliche Unfallversicherung

Introduction: Guidelines for occupational medical examinations

1

1

Introduction:
Guidelines for occupational
medical examinations

1 Introduction: Guidelines for occupational medical examinations

J. J. Milde, German Social Accident Insurance (DGUV), Sankt Augustin

1.1 Occupational medical care

Globalization and the increase in competition resulting from international trading have led to increasing expectations of workforce productivity in enterprises everywhere in Europe. In addition, demographic developments are increasing the average age of workers (the ageing workforce). The economic success of an enterprise depends on the abilities of well-trained and experienced employees. Thus, the maintenance and promotion of health of employees is becoming increasingly important from both the social and economic points of view, to do justice to the demands of society for appropriate quality of work and also to provide a basis for economic success. A healthier work environment does not only provide competitive advantages, it becomes an indicator of the social acceptability of successful commerce.

In the European Union, employers are required as part of their statutory "duty of care" to provide adequately for the health and safety of their employees. Although there are considerable differences between the relevant regulations in the various member states of the EU, there is a common basis which is described in the Council Directive 89/391/EEC and the associated individual directives. Occupational medical care, which is concerned with the interaction between work, profession and health, is covered by these directives. Its particular aims include:

- assessment of working conditions (risk assessment)
- provision of recommendations for improvement of working conditions
- informing and advising the employees about work-related risks
- early recognition and prevention of occupational diseases and work-related illnesses
- improving our knowledge of exposures and risks.

Thus occupational medical care does not only aim to keep employees healthy but also to bring about improvements in health protection at the workplace. By means of occupational medical care, the employer can demonstrate that he is meeting his "duty of care" responsibilities, provided that the medical care is provided by qualified specialists under quality-controlled conditions and the results are appropriately documented.

1.2 Risk assessment and health surveillance

Fundamental to health and safety protection at the workplace is the risk assessment. For this purpose the employer assesses (before a person starts work and at certain intervals afterwards) whether and to what extent health and safety hazards for the employee are associated with the work. In this process he can use the support of health and safety experts and the works physician or an occupational health professional. In principle, the employer is required to reduce any risks to a minimum and to institute any necessary general and individual protective measures. The risk assessment must be appropriately documented.

If the results of the risk assessment suggest that in spite of all protective measures a significant risk for the health of an employee remains, occupational medical examinations carried out by a doctor or an appropriately qualified person should be considered. The conditions under which occupational medical examinations are required before an employee may begin or continue a job are stipulated by law. These examinations are therefore quite different from health check-ups or general examinations to establish whether a person is fit for work, which are not regulated by law nor associated with specific workplace exposures. Nonetheless, such medical examinations can also be a starting point for a general improvement of the health of a workforce and the maintenance of fitness for work; they are not the subject of the Guidelines but can supplement them usefully. If an employee is obliged to go to an occupational medical examination, it remains his own decision whether he allows himself to be examined and whether he answers the physician's questions adequately. If he does not, the occupational health professional must inform the employer that no statement can be made about the person's state of health or fitness to begin or continue work.

Unlike group preventive measures offered by the works physician, e.g., in the form of general occupational medical toxicological advice for employees in training sessions, occupational medical examinations are preventive measures for the individual: the observation of the state of health of an employee exposed to specific health risks during the course of his work. The object is the early diagnosis of work-related health disorders and the establishment of whether or not a particular job is associated with an increased individual health risk. At the same time, the medical examination can serve to check whether preventive measures have been effective and can document any evidence of occupational diseases. Such occupational medical examinations carried out on the basis of a risk assessment include the following procedures:

- work anamnesis and anamnesis
- physical examination
- assessment of state of health in view of the job to be carried out
- individual occupational medical advice
- documentation of the results of the examination.

1.2.1   Responsibilities of the occupational health professional

The occupational medical examination is from its very nature a medical examination and so should be carried out by a doctor. That does not mean that, depending on local practice and the national health system, the examination or parts of it cannot be carried out by other qualified specialists. In such cases the national regulations are binding. Nonetheless, medical procedures which are not carried out by a physician himself should at least be carried out under his supervision and on his responsibility and be subject to strict quality control. Fundamentally, the carrying out of occupational medical examinations is associated with a series of responsibilities.

First, the person carrying out the examination must have access to the necessary apparatus and other requirements and have the appropriate qualifications. This includes knowledge of the individual workplace, in the ideal case knowledge obtained by personal inspection of the place of work. Before the examination the employee must be informed of the planned procedures. The examination itself must meet quality control criteria and be in line with the latest developments in occupational medicine.

Of particular importance is the advice given to the employee. This should take into account the individual disposition of the person and should concentrate on any concrete health risks but should also involve general advice as to occupational hygiene and healthy behaviour. Convalescents may also be advised as to their possibilities for returning to work. Thus, the Guidelines include suggestions for the content of such advisory sessions as well as sources of information.

Regulations for occupational medical examinations must include clear instructions for the method of communication of the results to the employee being examined and his or her employer. The results of the examination and the assessment are to be recorded in writing; the employee is to be informed. As with any medical examination, the results are subject to the rules of medical discretion. Therefore the communication of the results to the employer must be limited to the date of the examination, a simple statement as to whether there is cause for concern about the person's health, and details of any conditions to be observed in the job in question.

If the results of the occupational medical examination yield evidence of critical conditions in the enterprise, the occupational health professional, while observing medical confidentiality, is to inform and advise the employer.

1.3 Guidelines for occupational medical examinations

In view of the multiplicity of national health systems and the differences in legal duties stipulated in the different European countries, at first glance it seems pointless to try to present a system shown to be worthwhile in a single national system at an international level. Nonetheless we have made the attempt, in the firm conviction that once the legal regulations and the different occupational health system of the single country have been removed from the Guidelines, what is left is the essence of occupational medical procedure, in line with the latest developments in occupational medicine and thus, incorporating generally accepted rules of the profession, oriented on international standards. This means that a certain minimum of diagnostic methods and knowledge is necessary if a sound assessment of the state of health is to be made and a firm basis for deciding on further measures obtained. The description of just this minimum standard is the essential core of the Guidelines. On the basis of the Guidelines, the occupational physician carries out the occupational medical examination to obtain the data necessary to assess the risk and to advise the employee.

That the Guidelines are used so widely ensures that the occupational medical examinations – independent of regional features or conditions in a single branch of industry – are carried out uniformly and the results assessed and evaluated according to the one set of criteria. Only then is it possible to use the information yielded by the examinations for universal improvement of health and safety at work.

The Guidelines are procedures for occupational medical examinations which fulfil the legal requirements for "health surveillance". They are to be understood as a recommendation in the sense of "best practice". Unlike the guidelines of the medical societies, they do not reflect the opinions of a single professional group. Rather they are the combined results of a dialogue between members of the occupational medical profession, social workers, experts in occupational health and safety, and government representatives. In this process the medically desirable is brought into line with the medically possible, taking into account legal stipulations and the situation at the workplaces, and the result is guidelines which are oriented on day-to-day procedures for ensuring health and safety at work.

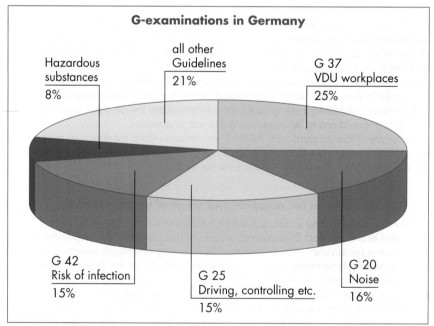

Figure 1: Frequency distribution of the occupational medical examinations carried out according to the Guidelines in the year 2002, in all 5,085,572 examinations.
G 37 "VDU workplaces"; G 20 "Noise"; G 25 "Driving, controlling and monitoring work"; G 42 "Activities with a risk of infection"; total of all Guidelines dealing with hazardous substances; total of all other Guidelines.
Note: G 46 "Strain on the musculoskeletal system (including vibration)" exists only since 2005 and so was not included in the above statistics.

Another characteristic feature of the concept is its systematics. The clear and consistent structure of the Guidelines ensure that every occupational medical examination, no matter which exposure is the reason for carrying it out, follows the same principles. The Guidelines provide the medical examiner with an instrument for carrying out quality-controlled health surveillance without limiting freedom of medical procedure in the individual case. The viability of the concept has been demonstrated in Germany where the Guidelines have been a success for decades.

Apparently it does not play an important role whether the occupational medical examination is to be carried out because of statutory requirements, because an employee wishes it or because of the voluntary commitment of an employer. It is certainly not the legal requirements which decide how often an occupational medical examination is carried out in practice. As shown in Figure 1 for the examples G 37 and G 25, these two occupational medical examinations are among those carried out most frequently, although their implementation is not at present required by law.

1.3.1   Which Guidelines exist?

The Guidelines cover a wide spectrum of workplace health risks. They deal with work with hazardous substances (dusts, fumes, chemicals), biological working materials and physical agents (heat, cold, noise, vibration, hyperbaric pressure). Other topics are strain on the musculoskeletal system, skin disorders, skin cancer, obstructive airway disorders, VDU work, respiratory protective equipment and working abroad. Two other Guidelines ("Driving, controlling and monitoring work" and "Work involving a danger of falling") describe examinations to determine whether a person is fit for or capable of doing that kind of work. The numbering of the Guidelines serves only for identification purposes; there is no special system involved.

At present there are 44 Guidelines and four appendices on special topics. Of these, those contained in the present book are listed below.

List of Guidelines
1.1   Mineral Dust, Part 1: Respirable crystalline silica dust
1.2   Mineral Dust, Part 2: Dust containing asbestos fibres
1.3   Mineral Dust, Part 3: Man-made mineral fibres (aluminium silicate wool)
1.4   Exposure to dust
2   Lead and lead compounds (with the exception of alkyllead compounds)
3   Alkyllead compounds
4   Substances which cause skin cancer or skin alterations
        which tend to become cancerous
5   Ethylene glycol dinitrate and glycerol trinitrate
        (glycol dinitrate and nitroglycerin)
6   Carbon disulfide
7   Carbon monoxide
8   Benzene
9   Mercury and mercury compounds
10   Methanol

Appendix 1 "Biomonitoring" contains supplementary information as to the situations in which this kind of analytical procedure may be used as part of an occupational medical examination. Appendix 2 describes the methods and procedures for diagnosing musculoskeletal disorders within the time frame and cost limits of an occupational medical examination.

1.3.2 Browsing the Guidelines

Each Guideline is structured systematically; the universal basic structure is made visible by graphic elements. The table below shows the structure of the Guidelines using the contents of G 14 as an example.

G 14 Trichloroethene (trichloroethylene) and other chlorinated hydrocarbon solvents
Preliminary remarks
Schedule
1 Medical examinations
   1.1 Examinations, intervals between examinations
   1.2 Medical examination schedule
       1.2.1 General medical examination
       1.2.2 Special medical examination
       1.2.3 Supplementary examination
   1.3 Requirements for the medical examinations
2 Occupational medical assessment and advice
   2.1 Assessment criteria
       2.1.1 Long-term concern about health
       2.1.2 Short-term concern about health
       2.1.3 No concern about health under certain conditions
       2.1.4 No concern about health
   2.2 Medical advice
3 Supplementary notes
   3.1 External and internal exposure
       3.1.1 Occurrence, sources of hazards
       3.1.2 Physicochemical properties and classification
       3.1.3 Uptake
       3.1.4 Biomonitoring
   3.2 Functional disorders, symptoms
       3.2.1 Mode of action
       3.2.2 Acute and subacute effects on health
       3.2.3 Chronic effects on health
4 References

Under the title of each Guideline, the responsible working group of the Committee for occupational medicine is given (see Supplementary notes at the end of this chapter for contact address). This makes it possible for the user to contact the authors, to ask questions and to point out any problems. Such feedback makes it possible to recognize difficulties in the practical use of the Guidelines which can then be cleared up cooperatively.

Under **Preliminary remarks** the objects of the examination are described.

The **Schedule** which follows shows graphically the parts of the examination and their order. Here the essential features of the examination according to a given Guideline may be seen at a glance.

Schedule

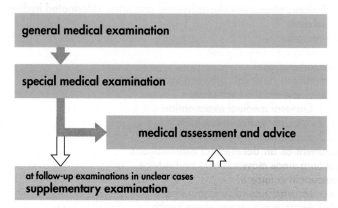

The Guidelines G 20 "Noise", G 37 "VDU workplaces" and G 46 "Musculo-skeletal system" include additional schedules and assessment schemes which are intended to provide a clear picture of the procedures.

Under **Medical examinations** the text describes first the group of people for whom this occupational medical examination may be used, e.g., for those exposed to a hazardous substance at concentrations in excess of the occupational exposure limit. If binding European regulations exist, they are referred to in the Guidelines. Otherwise, for hazardous substances the reader is referred to the recommendations of the German Commission for the Investigation of Health Hazards of Chemical Compounds in the Work Area (MAK Commission) which are recognized and available internationally. In a few cases the suggestions are based on the situation in Germany and then this is pointed out expressly. All such data serves only for orientation purposes. Decisive is only the result of the risk assessment in terms of the national law in the country concerned.

In the Guidelines two kinds of medical examination are distinguished and marked in the text with a coloured bar.

Initial examination

The purpose of the **Initial examination** is to establish, before the beginning of exposure, whether the person already has any defects (inherited or acquired) which could lead to health risks in the job in question. In addition, the documentation of the results of this examination can be of importance in any later claims for compensation because of adverse effects on health.

Follow-up examination

At the **Follow-up examination** it is the task of the physician to establish whether the person's state of health has altered. The follow-up examinations include also a final examination when a person finishes work in a certain job; this can be useful especially for any later occupational disease litigation.

If the procedures to be carried out (or the assessment criteria) are identical for the two kinds of examination, they are listed under a single bar:

| Initial examination | Follow-up examination |

Note: in Germany there is also a third kind of examination, the **Nachgehende Untersuchung** (long-term follow-up examination), which is also carried out on the basis of the Guidelines. These examinations serve to detect adverse effects on health which have a long latency. Many years can pass between the work in a hazardous job and the development of an occupational disease (e.g. cancer). Often the affected employee has long since moved to a different area of work or has retired. The German Social Accident Insurance has therefore set up a central service to ensure that affected persons can also have an occupational medical examination after they have stopped working in a job. Such examinations are offered to persons who have been exposed to carcinogenic substances such as asbestos or benzene.

The kinds of examination covered by a Guideline are summarized in a table together with the intervals between the examinations (example from G 14).

1.1   Examinations, intervals between examinations

initial examination	before taking up the job
first follow-up examination	after 12–24 months
further follow-up examinations	after 12–24 months and when leaving the job
premature follow-up examination	• after an illness lasting for several weeks or when a physical handicap gives cause for concern about whether the work should be continued • in individual cases when the physician considers it necessary, e.g. when there is short-term concern about the person's health • when requested by an employee who suspects a causal association between his or her illness and work

The suggested intervals are intended to provide for continual, regular health surveillance. At the discretion of the occupational health professional, given reason in individual cases, a premature follow-up examination may be carried out. An examination carried out at the request of an employee should be medically justifiable on the basis of concrete work-related health risks deducible from the risk assessment.

In the section **Medical examination schedule** the examination procedures are described. They begin with a **General medical examination** which consists of anamnesis and work anamnesis with a general examination. The subsequent **Special medical examination** targets effects of the specific exposure and provides information about the necessary diagnostic methods. When indicated, or when the examination results are unclear, a specific **Supplementary examination** can be necessary. At this point, the works physician may require consultation with other medical specialists, e.g., in the form of a recommendation that the person sees a specialist to clarify the findings or in the form of a referral.

Under **Requirements for the medical examinations** the qualifications necessary to carry out the examinations are specified (in Germany always a specialist in occupational medicine ("Arbeitsmedizin") or a doctor with the additional title "Betriebsmedizin"), as are requirements for further education and apparatus.

Health surveillance is an effective instrument only if its results are evaluated and used to improve health and safety at the workplace. An important aspect of the Guidelines is therefore the aids to interpretation and assessment of the findings and the resulting advice for the employee. The section **Occupational medical assessment and advice** begins with the reminder that, as stipulated in the EU Council Directive and the associated individual directives, a risk assessment is necessary. If the occupational health professional was not involved in making this assessment himself, he must at least have access to its results. Only if the situation at the workplace and the exposure of the individual are known is it possible to assess the medical findings and give the employee appropriate advice.

For standardization of the assessment of whether and to what extent the carrying out of certain jobs is associated with concern about the health of an individual, a stepwise process based on **assessment criteria** is described. With the assessment **"no concern about health"**, the physician states that there is no increased health risk for the individual.
If the physician wishes to defer concern about health for a time (e.g. with shorter intervals between follow-up examinations) or to make it dependent on the implementation of protective measures for the individual, he selects the assessment **"no concern about health under certain conditions"**.
"Short-term concern about health" is an assessment which applies for a limited period because of transient symptoms (e.g. use of hearing protectors not possible because of acute inflammation of the auditory canal or outer ear) which can regress after medical treatment.

The assessment **"long-term concern about health"** is only possible if no way can be found by workplace-related measures, conditions or limitations to counteract a health risk for the employee which can be associated with grave consequences. For the person being examined, this means that from the medical point of view there is no way that he can continue working in the current job. This assessment can result in his being transferred to another workplace or even in the loss of his job. Of course, the occupational health professional will make use of this assessment only after careful consideration of its consequences (the weighing up of the risks for health against the risk of job loss). In Germany this assessment is also associated with serious consequences for the employer. He has to arrange occupational medical examinations for all persons he employs at similar workplaces and also to prove that the workplace is safe or document the measures he has taken to improve its occupational hygiene.

In practice, whenever it is medically defensible, the physician will prefer to produce the assessment "short-term concern about health" or "no concern about health under certain conditions". The medical findings on which the assessment criteria are based are given in detail in each Guideline.

The personal contact between the occupational health professional and the employee during the occupational medical examination makes it possible to offer the employee individual advice, an essential measure for effective health and safety at the workplace. The advice should be commensurate with the workplace situation and the results of the medical examinations and should include explanations of the risks associated with the job and medical recommendations for dealing with the risk. On this point, under the title **Medical advice**, the Guidelines offer further information for the occupational health professional including topics such as general hygienic measures, use of personal protective equipment, carcinogenicity of substances, alcohol consumption, smoking and also specific information for pregnant women.

Section 3 of each Guideline provides the background information necessary for an occupational medical examination. Here not only **occurrence** and **sources of hazards** are discussed but also **functional disorders** and **symptoms**. In addition, this chapter lists additional properties of hazardous substances and of freely available sources of further information in the English language (GESTIS databases, see Supplementary notes) from which details of threshold limit values, substance classification and evaluation and other substance-specific information may be obtained. In cases for which soundly based biomonitoring data is available (see also Appendix 1), the internationally recognized reference values for occupational exposures published by the DFG Commission for the Investigation of Health Hazards of Chemical Compounds in the Work Area (MAK Commission) are given for orientation purposes.

Under **References** the directives and recommendations of the European Union, international standards and other generally available literature and information sources are listed.

Practical experience has shown that printed forms are a help in the proper carrying out and documentation of medical examinations and that they reduce the amount of work involved. Because of the different situations in different countries, it is difficult to design such forms for universal use. For the Guidelines listed below, an attempt has been made:

Guideline	Form
G 1.1-1.3 "Mineral dust"	Protocol sheet for anamnesis
G 20 "Noise"	Screening test NOISE I, Supplementary examination NOISE II, Extended supplementary examination NOISE III
G 37 "VDU workplaces"	Examination form G 37 "VDU workplaces"
G 46 "Strain on the musculoskeletal system (including vibration)"	Anamnesis questionnaires: 1 Self-reported musculoskeletal disorders 2 Medical anamnesis of musculoskeletal disorders and hand-arm vibration exposure Questionnaire for the supplementary examination of persons exposed to hand-arm vibration

If the forms should not meet the specific local requirements, they can nonetheless serve for orientation purposes and can be modified as necessary. The forms are to be found in the internet at www.dguv.de/guidelines and may be downloaded.

1.4   Supplementary Notes

The Committee for occupational medicine of the German Social Accident Insurance (Ausschuss Arbeitsmedizin der DGUV) was set up in 1971. Together with the associated specialized working groups, it develops recommendations for applying occupational medical findings for the protection of employees from work-related health risks, accidents and occupational diseases. The fact that representatives from all the relevant institutions are involved in this process has the effect that the recommendations of the Committee for occupational medicine achieve a high level of acceptance and set the pattern for occupational medical health protection in Germany.

Contact address: Ausschuss Arbeitsmedizin der DGUV
                  Alte Heerstrasse 111
                  53757 Sankt Augustin, Germany
                  Tel.:   +49 2241 231 1469
                  e-mail: juergen.milde@dguv.de
                  Internet: www.dguv.de

The **GESTIS-Substance Database** contains information for the safe handling of chemical substances at work, e.g. health effects, necessary protective measures and such in case of danger (incl. First Aid). Furthermore the user is offered information about important physical and chemical properties of these substances as well as any special regulations. The available information relates to about 8,000 substances. Data are updated immediately after publication of new official regulations or after the issue of new scientific results.
Internet: www.dguv.de/bgia/gestis-database
GESTIS International limit values for chemical agents. This database contains a collection of occupational limit values for hazardous substances gathered from various EU member states, Canada (Quebec), Japan, Switzerland, and the United States. Limit values for more than 1,000 substances are listed.
Internet: www.dguv.de/bgia/gestis-limit-values
The GESTIS-Databases are maintained by the BGIA – Institute for Occupational Health and Safety of the German Social Accident Insurance.

Guidelines
for occupational medical
examinations

2

2

Guidelines
for occupational medical
examinations

G 1.1   Mineral Dust, Part 1: Respirable crystalline silica dust

G 1.1

Committee for occupational medicine, working group "Occupational risks for the lungs", Bergbau-Berufsgenossenschaft, Bochum

Preliminary remarks

The present guideline describes a scheme for occupational medical prophylaxis which aims to prevent or ensure early diagnosis of disorders which can be caused by inhalation of respirable crystalline silica (including cristobalite and tridymite).

Schedule

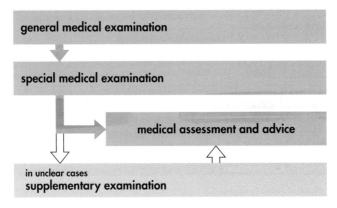

general medical examination

special medical examination

medical assessment and advice

in unclear cases
supplementary examination

1   Medical examinations

Occupational medical examinations are to be carried out for persons at whose work-places exposure to respirable crystalline silica could endanger health (e.g. the occupational exposure limit value is exceeded).

1.1   Examinations, intervals between examinations

initial examination	before taking up the job
first follow-up examination	after 36 months
further follow-up examinations	after 36 months and when leaving the job
premature follow-up examination	• after an illness lasting for several weeks or when a physical handicap gives cause for concern about whether the work should be continued • in individual cases when the physician considers it necessary, e.g. when there is short-term concern about the person's health • when requested by an employee who suspects a causal association between his or her illness and work

1.2   Medical examination schedule

1.2.1   General medical examination

Initial examination

• Review of past history (general anamnesis, differentiated work anamnesis), detailed smoking anamnesis[1]
  • non-smokers, smokers, ex-smokers
  • cigarettes, cigars, pipes (number per day)
  • year of starting and, if applicable, ending tobacco consumption (number of cigarette pack years)

Follow-up examination

• interim anamnesis (including differentiated work anamnesis)

---

[1] See protocol sheet for anamnesis ("Mineral Dust", G 1.1, G 1.2, G 1.3) and remarks concerning tobacco consumption in Section 5.

1.2.2   Special medical examination

Initial examination   **Follow-up examination**

- examination of the respiratory and cardiocirculatory organs
- spirometry
- large format posterior-anterior thorax radiograph taken with high kilovolt technique unless results are available from such an x-ray examination which has been carried out within the previous year (or previous half-year for follow-up examinations)

1.2.3   Supplementary examination

Initial examination   **Follow-up examination**

When indicated, e.g. if 140 > Broca's index > 130, supplementary lung function tests.

1.3   Requirements for the medical examinations

- competent doctor or occupational health professional
- continual medical education in reading and classification of radiograms according to the international pneumoconiosis classification ILO 2000, specific x-ray diagnostic experience
- apparative and other requirements for the examinations: x-ray examination, lung function tests, ILO standard x-ray images

2   Occupational medical assessment and advice

An assessment is only possible when the workplace situation and the exposure of the individual are known. For this purpose a risk assessment as defined in Article 9 Council directive 89/391/EEC must have been carried out; it must specify which technical, organizational and individual protective measures have been applied.

2.1   Assessment criteria

2.1.1   Long-term concern about health

Initial examination

Persons with existing disorders and/or functional defects especially of the cardiopulmonary system for whom the exposure to respirable crystalline silica would be expected to result in a clinically relevant worsening of their state of health.
As examples are mentioned here especially:
- severe disorders of lung function and of the cardiocirculatory system
- chronic bronchitis, bronchial asthma, pulmonary emphysema
- pleuritis, chronic or recurrent
- radiographically detectable dust lung or other fibrotic or granulotamous lung alterations
- malformations, tumours, chronic inflammation, pleural fibrosis or other damage which significantly impairs the function of the airways or lungs or which favours the development of bronchopulmonary disorders
- deformities of the thorax or spine which have adverse effects on breathing
- condition following lung resection or injury with functional impairment of the thoracic organs
- active, also latent tuberculosis, extensive inactive tuberculosis
- reduced nutritional status, weakness, body weight more than 30 % above the optimum weight determined by Broca's formula (height in cm minus 100 = optimum weight in kg), constitutional defects and weaknesses
- manifest or expected premature cardiac insufficiency, such as is found with cardiac valve defects, other organic cardiac damage or recent disorders which are known to result frequently in premature cardiac insufficiency
- high blood pressure especially when this does not respond to therapy
- other chronic disorders which reduce general resistance

Follow-up examination

As for the initial examination and for persons with clear silicotic alterations in the lungs of the p, r, q form and profusion $\geq 1/1$ and/or hilar lymph node calcification (es)
- before the age of 30 years and after less than 10 years of work involving exposure to silicogenic dust
- before the age of 40 years and after less than 15 years of work involving exposure to silicogenic dust
- before the age of 50 years and after less than 20 years of work involving exposure to silicogenic dust

2.1.2   Short-term concern about health

Initial examination	Follow-up examination

Persons like those described in Section 2.1.1 but who are expected to recover.

2.1.3   No concern about health under certain conditions

Initial examination	Follow-up examination

If the illnesses or physical deficits mentioned in Section 2.1.1 are less severe, the doctor should establish whether or not it is possible for the person to start work or go on working under certain conditions. Such conditions could include transfer to workplaces known to have lower concentrations of respirable crystalline silica, shorter intervals between follow-up examinations, etc.

2.1.4   No concern about health

Initial examination	Follow-up examination

All other persons, provided there are no restrictions on their employment.

2.2   Medical advice

The advice in an individual case should be commensurate with the workplace situation and the results of the medical examinations.

Cigarette smoking is the main cause of lung cancer and of the development of chronic obstructive airway diseases. Stopping inhalative tobacco consumption has been shown to result in an improvement of lung function and in a reduction of the overall risk of developing cancer, especially lung cancer. The physician is to inform the smoker of these facts and that treatment can be successful in helping him or her to stop smoking.

3   Supplementary notes

3.1   Exposure

3.1.1   Occurrence, sources of hazards

A large number of mineral substances, additives and industrial products contain free crystalline silica, especially quartz. During extraction and processing of the raw materials and during the industrial processes involved in making the products, crystalline silica dust can be produced. Sectors of industry with this kind of exposure include mining and tunnel building (excavation, mining, transport), the rock and building stone industry (drilling, extraction, crushing, cutting, polishing, sandblasting, building work underground), ceramics industry (production of porcelain, earthenware, stoneware, fireproof products), foundries (degating, casting, blasting).

If AES (alkaline earth silicate) wool is used at temperatures above 900°C the material recrystallizes to form cristobalite.

3.1.2   Physicochemical properties and classification

The crystalline SiO_2 modifications quartz, cristobalite and tridymite are called crystalline silica. Respirable dust containing free crystalline silica has silicogenic effects. The information system on hazardous substances (GESTIS) provides details of classification, evaluation and other substance-specific information (see Section 4).

	CAS number
Quartz	14808-60-7
Cristobalite	14464-46-1
Tridymite	15468-32-3

3.1.3   Uptake

The dust is taken up via the airways.

3.2   Functional disorders, symptoms

3.2.1   Mode of action

The effects of crystalline silica dust (including cristobalite and tridymite) are determined by the level of free silica in the dust which enters the respiratory tract, the doses and the pattern of exposure as well as by the disposition of the individual. In the alveolar region of the lungs the SiO_2 particles come into contact with alveolar macrophages. The particles are phagocytosed and then cause destruction of the macrophages. The particles released from the macrophages are phagocytosed again and can repeat the cycle of cell damage. Macrophage destruction is considered to be a prerequisite for the formation of new reticular and collagenous connective tissue. The growth of connective tissue in the pulmonary interstitium is mostly nodular. The hilar lymph nodes are also often affected. Characteristic is the tendency of the silicosis nodules to shrink; this leads to the development of so-called perifocal emphysema. Increase in the size of and confluence of neighbouring nodules causes callous formation and deformation of airways, pulmonary vessels and lymph ducts.

3.2.2   Acute and subacute effects on health

not applicable

3.2.3   Chronic effects on health

The symptoms of quartz dust lung depend on the kind and extent of the structural and functional changes.

In practice, apart from lung tuberculosis, chronic unspecific respiratory syndrome (CURS)[2] and, in the late stages, chronic cor pulmonale are the most important sequelae of quartz dust lung. In patients with silicosis the triad of symptoms – shortness of breath, coughing and expectoration – are generally determined essentially by the severity of the CURS. The same applies to the results of the physical examination, e.g. to breathing noises and vesiculotympanic resonance. CURS can have other causes apart from silicosis. Severe advanced silicosis can, in rare cases, cause shortness of breath and chronic cor pulmonale simply because of restrictive ventilation disorders.

Diagnosis of quartz dust lung is made on the basis of the radiogram, given the appropriate work history.

During the course of the disorder, the nodular fibrosis is seen in the radiograph as roundish opacities in the sizes p, q and r. They affect mainly the two lung mantles. Radiographically characteristic of the late stages are callouses (A, B, C) mainly in the superior lung lobes. There is not unusually a considerable discrepancy between the severity of the silicotic changes, the subjective feeling of illness, the results of the physical examination and the detectable impairment of lung function.

The radiograph is categorized according to the ILO system for dust lung classification (ILO 2000).

Of pathophysiological interest in silicosis cases is especially the demonstration of a restrictive and/or obstructive ventilation disorder, disorders of ventilation distribution, pulmonary emphysema, disorders of respiratory gas exchange and/or increased pressure in the pulmonary circulation.

Quartz dust lung generally progresses slowly.

---

[2] CURS is understood to include chronic bronchitis, unspecific bronchial respiratory disorders, pulmonary emphysema and combinations of these.

The duration of exposure to silicogenic dust before silicosis develops is presently of the order of 15 years or more. There are also cases of so-called acute silicosis, which develops after exposure periods of only a few years. The alterations associated with quartz dust lung can also appear or progress after the end of exposure. Lung tuberculosis which develops simultaneously with silicosis is generally relatively severe and more resistant to therapy than is tuberculosis without silicosis.

4   References

Commission recommendation 2003/670/EC concerning the European schedule of occupational diseases

Council Directive 89/391/EEC on the introduction of measures to encourage improvements in the safety and health of workers at work

Council Directive 92/85/EEC on the introduction of measures to encourage improvements in the safety and health at work of pregnant workers and workers who have recently given birth or are breastfeeding

Council Directive 92/91/EEC concerning the minimum requirements for improving the safety and health protection of workers in the mineral-extracting industries through drilling

Council Directive 92/104/EEC on the minimum requirements for improving the safety and health protection of workers in surface and underground mineral-extracting industries

Council Directive 98/24/EC on the protection of the health and safety of workers from the risks related to chemical agents at work

European Network on Silica NEPSI (2007) Good Practice Guide on Workers Health Protection through the Good Handling and Use of Crystalline Silica and Products containing it. At: www.nepsi.eu/good-practice-guide.aspx

GESTIS-database on hazardous substances. BGIA
    at: www.dguv.de/bgia/gestis-database

GESTIS-international limit values for chemical agents. BGIA
    at: www.dguv.de/bgia/gestis-limit-values

International Labour Organisation. Guidelines for the Use of the ILO international Classification of radiographs of pneumoconioses. 2000 edition. Geneva: International Labour Office, 2002 (Occupational Safety and Health Series No. 22)

5   Forms

- Protocol sheet for anamnesis ("Mineral Dust", G 1.1, G 1.2, G 1.3)

Anamnesis "Mineral Dust" G 1.1, G 1.2, G 1.3

G 1.1

Surname	First name
Date of birth	Nationality
Address: street	
Postcode, town	
Employer	
Employer's address	
Job	
Exposures	

Examination according to the guideline   ☐ G 1.1   ☐ G 1.2   ☐ G 1.3   Date ___.___._____

Examination   ☐ initial   ☐ follow-up   ☐ when leaving the job

Work anamnesis	crystalline silica		asbestos		mineral fibres	
Have you been exposed to dust at work before you started work in the present firm?	☐ no	☐ yes	☐ no	☐ yes	☐ no	☐ yes
In which year were you first exposed to dust?	_____		_____		_____	
Kind of job						
For how long were you or have you been exposed to dust all together? (years, months)	___ years	___ months	___ years	___ months	___ years	___ months
Have you ever stopped working at a dusty workplace because of one or more of the following symptoms?						
a) respiratory symptoms	☐ no	☐ yes	☐ no	☐ yes	☐ no	☐ yes
b) heart problems	☐ no	☐ yes	☐ no	☐ yes	☐ no	☐ yes
c) problems with the circulatory system	☐ no	☐ yes	☐ no	☐ yes	☐ no	☐ yes

Symptom anamnesis

Have you or have you had any of the following diseases?

a) tuberculosis of the lungs	☐ no	☐ yes	☐ unsure	date of the illness ___.___._____
b) pneumonia	☐ no	☐ yes	☐ unsure	date of the illness ___.___._____
c) pleurisy	☐ no	☐ yes	☐ unsure	date of the illness ___.___._____
d) bronchitis several times a year	☐ no	☐ yes		date when it began ___.___._____
e) bronchial asthma	☐ no	☐ yes		date when it began ___.___._____
f) other chronic diseases?	☐ no	☐ yes		date when it began ___.___._____

Which?

Do you cough during at least three months of the year?   ☐ no   ☐ yes   date when it began month ___ and year _____

Do you expectorate during at least three months of the year?   ☐ no   ☐ yes   date when it began ___.___._____

a) haemoptysis (spitting blood)   ☐ no   ☐ yes   date when it began ___.___._____

Have you noticed recently persistent hoarseness, difficulty in swallowing, the feeling of having something stuck in your throat?   ☐ no   ☐ yes

Do you smoke?   ☐ no   ☐ not any longer   ☐ yes

If **yes** or **not any longer** please state how many pack years* _____

* a pack year is about 20 cigarettes daily per year

1–10 cigarettes/day from ___ till ___ (year)   11–20 cigarettes/day from ___ till ___ (year)

21–40 cigarettes/day from ___ till ___ (year)   >40 cigarettes/day from ___ till ___ (year)

☐ pipe   ☐ cigars

Have you lost weight during the last 6 months?   ☐ no   ☐ yes

Comments _____

Date, stamp, signature of the physician

G 1.2   Mineral Dust, Part 2: Dust containing asbestos fibre

Committee for occupational medicine, working group "Occupational risks for the lungs", Bergbau-Berufsgenossenschaft, Bochum

Preliminary remarks

The present guideline describes a scheme for occupational medical prophylaxis which aims to prevent or ensure early diagnosis of disorders which can be caused by inhalation of dust containing asbestos fibres.

Schedule

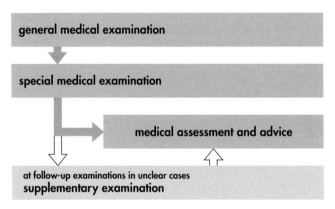

1 Medical examinations

Occupational medical examinations are to be carried out for persons at whose workplaces the asbestos fibre concentration of 15000 fibres/m^3 is exceeded during demolition, renovation and maintenance work.

Even when this exposure concentration is not exceeded or when tested procedures involving lower level exposures are used, persons exposed to asbestos fibres during demolition, renovation and maintenance work are to be offered occupational medical examinations.

1.1 Examinations, intervals between examinations

initial examination	before taking up the job
first follow-up examination	after 12–36 months
further follow-up examinations	after 12–36 months and when leaving the job
premature follow-up examination	• after an illness lasting for several weeks or when a physical handicap gives cause for concern about whether the work should be continued • in individual cases when the physician considers it necessary, e.g. when there is short-term concern about the person's health • when requested by an employee who suspects a causal association between his or her illness and work

1.2   Medical examination schedule

1.2.1   General medical examination

G 1.2

Initial examination	Follow-up examination

- general anamnesis, differentiated work anamnesis, detailed smoking anamnesis[1]
  - non-smokers, smokers, ex-smokers
  - cigarettes, cigars, pipes (number per day)
  - year of starting and, if applicable, ending tobacco consumption (number of cigarette pack years)
- because of the risk of larynx carcinoma, particular attention should be paid to persistent hoarseness (> 3 weeks), phonation disorders, malaise, alcohol consumption

1.2.2   Special medical examination

Initial examination	Follow-up examination

- examination of the respiratory and cardiocirculatory organs
- spirometry
- large format posterior-anterior thorax radiograph taken with high kilovolt technique unless results are available from such an x-ray examination which has been carried out within the previous year (or previous half-year for follow-up examinations)

1.2.3   Supplementary examination

Follow-up examination

Depending on the results seen on the posterior-anterior radiogram and any previous radiograms, a lateral radiogram may be required.

If the alterations detected radiographically do not permit an unambiguous statement as to their morphology, a computer tomogram of the thorax may be indicated. If the presence of a malignant disorder is suspected, further examinations should be arranged.

In cases where there is evidence of a larynx disorder, examination by an ENT specialist may be indicated.

---

[1] See protocol sheet for anamnesis ("Mineral Dust", G 1.1, G 1.2, G 1.3) and remarks concerning tobacco consumption in G 1.1.

1.3   Requirements for the medical examinations

- competent doctor or occupational health professional
- continual medical education in reading and classification of radiograms according to the international pneumoconiosis classification ILO 2000, specific x-ray diagnostic experience
- apparatus and other requirements for the examinations: x-ray examination, lung function tests, ILO standard x-ray images

2   Occupational medical assessment and advice

An assessment is only possible when the workplace situation and the exposure of the individual are known. For this purpose a risk assessment as defined in Article 4 Council directive 98/24/EC must have been carried out; it must specify which technical, organizational and individual protective measures have been applied.

2.1   Assessment criteria

2.1.1   Long-term concern about health

Initial examination	Follow-up examination

Persons with existing disorders and/or functional defects especially of the cardiopulmonary system for whom the exposure to dust containing asbestos fibres would be expected to result in a clinically relevant worsening of their state of health.
As examples are mentioned here especially:
- severe disorders of lung function and of the cardiocirculatory system
- chronic bronchitis, bronchial asthma, pulmonary emphysema
- pleuritis, chronic or recurrent
- radiographically detectable dust lung or other fibrotic or granulotamous lung alterations
- malformations, tumours, chronic inflammation, pleural fibrosis or other damage which significantly impairs the function of the airways or lungs or which favours the development of bronchopulmonary disorders
- deformities of the thorax or spine which have adverse effects on breathing
- condition following lung resection or injury with functional impairment of the thoracic organs
- chronic larynx disorders with functional deficits
- condition after tumour diagnosis with partial or total resection of the vocal cords or larynx or radiation therapy
- active, also latent tuberculosis, extensive inactive tuberculosis

G 1.2

- reduced nutritional status, weakness, body weight more than 30 % above the optimum weight determined by Broca's formula (height in cm minus 100 = optimum weight in kg), constitutional defects and weaknesses
- manifest or expected premature cardiac insufficiency, such as is found with cardiac valve defects, other organic cardiac damage or recent disorders which are known to result frequently in premature cardiac insufficiency
- high blood pressure especially when this does not respond to therapy
- other chronic disorders which reduce general resistance

2.1.2   Short-term concern about health

Initial examination   **Follow-up examination**

Persons like those described in Section 2.1.1 but who are expected to recover.

2.1.3   No concern about health under certain conditions

Initial examination

If the illnesses or physical deficits mentioned in Section 2.1.1 are less severe, the doctor should establish whether or not it is possible for the person to start work under certain conditions.

Follow-up examination

If the illnesses or physical deficits mentioned in Section 2.1.1 are less severe, the doctor should establish whether or not it is possible for the person to go on working under certain conditions, e.g. after transfer to a workplace with lower level exposure (<15000 fibres/m³).

2.1.4   No concern about health

Initial examination   **Follow-up examination**

All other persons, provided there are no restrictions on their employment.

2.2   Medical advice

The advice in an individual case should be commensurate with the workplace situation and the results of the medical examinations.
Cigarette smoking is the main cause of lung cancer. The combination of exposure to asbestos fibres and cigarette smoking has a synergistic effect. The physician is to inform the smoker of these facts and that treatment can be successful in helping him or her to stop smoking.

3   Supplementary notes

3.1   Exposure

3.1.1   Occurrence, sources of hazards

In the European Union asbestos is regulated by Council Directive 76/769/EEC. In addition several member countries have adopted specific and more stringent measures such as a ban on production and use of asbestos.

The main asbestos deposits which were most important for production lie in the old USSR, in Canada and South Africa. About 93 % of the asbestos used was chrysotile. During processing of asbestos minerals, transport and storage of crude asbestos (asbestos fibres) and during production and processing of products containing asbestos, asbestos fibres were released. Branches of industry with such exposures included: asbestos textile industry (threads, fabrics, ropes), asbestos cement industry (sheets, pipes), building industry (processing of asbestos cement products), chemical industry (fillers for paints and sealant materials, synthetic resin compression moulding materials, thermoplastics, rubber products), insulation industry (heat, sound and fire insulation), paper industry (asbestos paper and cardboard), brake and clutch lining manufacture, shipbuilding and wagon construction. In Germany the production and use of asbestos has been forbidden since 1.1.1993. Therefore in Germany exposure to asbestos fibres is possible only during demolition, renovation and maintenance work.

3.1.2   Physicochemical properties

Asbestos is a collective term for fibrous crystalline siliceous minerals which may be processed to yield technically useful fibres.

According to the WHO, these fibres are considered to be critical if they are <3 µm in diameter, >5 µm in length and have a length to diameter ratio $>5:1$.

The information system on hazardous substances (GESTIS) provides details of classification, evaluation and other substance-specific information (see Section 4).

	CAS number
asbestos	1332-21-4
actinolite	77536-66-4
amosite	12172-73-5
anthophyllite	77536-67-5
chrysotile	12001-29-5
crocidolite	12001-28-4
tremolite	77536-68-6

3.1.3   Uptake

The dust is taken up via the airways.

3.2   Functional disorders, symptoms

3.2.1   Mode of action

The effects of the dust depend on its content of asbestos (chrysotile, crocidolite, amosite, anthophyllite, actinolite, tremolite), the dose and the persistence of the dust which has entered the respiratory tract and on the individual disposition. Fibres up to 400 µm in length tend to find a way directly into the lower lung. The length, diameter and form of the asbestos fibres determines whether they are deposited in the alveoli, the peripheral or central airways including the larynx or whether they penetrate into the pleural region and whether phagocytosis and cell damage result. Cellular defence mechanisms result in the formation of asbestos bodies which can be detectable in sputum and in the lung tissues. The fibrogenic effects of inhaled asbestos fibres are put down to direct repeated cell damage and to discrete callous-forming inflammatory processes. The immediate result is peribronchial and perivascular diffuse connective tissue production. It leads to obliteration of the pulmonary alveoli, which are responsible for gas exchange, and therefore to restrictive ventilation disorders and impairment of alveolar gas exchange. These changes are referred to as asbestos-induced pulmonary fibrosis, asbestos pneumoconiosis or asbestosis. Pleural drift (pleurotropy of inhaled asbestos fibres) can lead to the development of diffuse pleural fibrosis and hyaline and calcifying pleural plaques. Pleural effusion (asbestos pleuritis) is observed and can be evidence of concomitant mesothelioma. In persons exposed to asbestos, the incidence of bronchial carcinoma and mesothelioma of the pleura, peritoneum and pericardium is increased. The effect seems to be greatest for mesothelioma in persons exposed to crocidolite. Even a short period of exposure can be sufficient to cause mesothelioma development. For larynx carcinoma caused by exposure to asbestos, exposure periods of less than 10 years are described only rarely. For persons who inhale cigarette smoke, the more than additive increase in the risk of developing lung cancer after exposure to asbestos fibres should be remembered.

3.2.2   Acute and subacute effects on health

not applicable

3.2.3   Chronic effects on health

The symptoms of asbestosis usually depend on the extent of the anatomical changes. Complications can make the symptoms much more severe.

The first symptoms are those of a restrictive functional disorder. In practice, chronic bronchitis with or without obstruction, and increased pressure in the pulmonary circulation with chronic cor pulmonale, bronchiectasis and bronchopneumonic processes are the most important sequelae of asbestosis. In addition, attention should be paid to pleural thickening, effusion and plaques. Pleural effusion occurs frequently together with mesotheliomas. It can, however, precede the manifestation of a mesothelioma by a long period.

In patients with asbestosis, the triad of symptoms – coughing, respiratory distress and expectoration – is determined essentially by the extent of the pulmonary fibrosis and the severity of the chronic bronchitis. The same is true for the ausculatory sounds, e.g. crepitations and dry respiratory sounds. Diagnosis of asbestosis is made on the basis of the radiogram, given the appropriate work history.

In addition, in the advanced stages of the disorder shrinkage may be seen in the most severely fibrotic lung sections.

Initially the radiogram reveals fine, irregular or linear opacities of size s, t or u in the ILO dust lung classification with a profusion of 1/0 to 1/1, mainly in the two middle and lower fields.

Of pathophysiological interest in asbestosis cases is especially the demonstration of a restrictive and/or obstructive ventilation disorder, disorders of respiratory gas exchange, disorders of ventilation distribution, pulmonary emphysema, and/or increased pressure in the pulmonary circulation. Asbestos-induced lung fibrosis generally progresses slowly.

In most cases of compensatable asbestosis, the persons were exposed to dust containing asbestos fibres for several years. However, it is possible to develop asbestosis after exposure periods of less than one year. The disorder can make its appearance after long latency periods, also long after the end of exposure.

Generally the latency period for bronchial carcinoma and mesothelioma caused by dust containing asbestos fibres is more than 10 years. Mesotheliomas can even be induced by relatively brief, low level exposure.

For the induction of bronchial carcinoma by asbestos fibres, a cumulative asbestos fibre dust dose caused by exposure at workplaces of at least 25 fibre years[2] is considered to be necessary. Specific non-malignant disorders of the pleura which are considered to be caused by asbestos fibres include:
• hyaline pleural connective tissue plaques
• calcified pleural plaques
• especially bilateral diffuse pleural fibrosis
• pleural effusion with/without fibrous thickening (hyalinosis complicata)

Larynx carcinoma caused by asbestos is not distinguishable clinically or diagnostically from larynx carcinomas of other aetiology. The disorder begins with hoarseness, difficulties in swallowing and the feeling of a foreign body in the throat. Later respiratory distress and swelling of the cervical lymph nodes develop as well.

---

[2] A "fibre year" represents the dose taken in during one year (240 days of whole-shift employment) of exposure at an average exposure concentration of 1×10^6 asbestos fibres per m^3 (equivalent to 1 fibre per cm^3) to fibres of the critical dimensions: length >5 μm, diameter <3 μm, ratio of length to diameter at least 3:1.

Diagnostic methods include laryngoscopy and biopsy for histological differentiation. Generally the tumours are keratinized squamous cell carcinomas, more rarely slightly differentiated or undifferentiated carcinomas.

G 1.2

4   References

Commission recommendation 2003/670/EC concerning the European schedule of occupational diseases

Council Directive 76/769/EEC on the approximation of the laws, regulations and administrative provisions of the Member States relating to restrictions on the marketing and use of certain dangerous substances and preparations

Council Directive 89/391/EEC on the introduction of measures to encourage improvements in the safety and health of workers at work

Council Directive 92/85/EEC on the introduction of measures to encourage improvements in the safety and health at work of pregnant workers and workers who have recently given birth or are breastfeeding

Council Directive 98/24/EC on the protection of the health and safety of workers from the risks related to chemical agents at work

GESTIS-database on hazardous substances. BGIA
   at: www.dguv.de/bgia/gestis-database

GESTIS-international limit values for chemical agents. BGIA
   at: www.dguv.de/bgia/gestis-limit-values

International Labour Organisation. Guidelines for the Use of the ILO international Classification of radiographs of pneumoconioses. 2000 edition. Geneva: International Labour Office, 2002 (Occupational Safety and Health Series No. 22)

G 1.3   Mineral Dust, Part 3: Man-made mineral fibres (aluminium silicate wool)

G 1.3

Committee for occupational medicine, working group "Occupational risks for the lungs", Bergbau-Berufsgenossenschaft, Bochum

Preliminary remarks

The present guideline describes a scheme for occupational medical prophylaxis which aims to prevent or ensure early diagnosis of disorders which can be caused by inhalation of dust containing aluminium silicate wool fibres.

Schedule

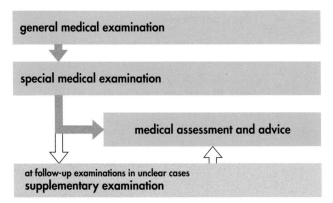

1   Medical examinations

Occupational medical examinations are to be offered to persons at workplaces where they can be exposed to fibres containing aluminium silicates.

1.1   Examinations, intervals between examinations

initial examination	before taking up the job
follow-up examinations	• up to 15 years after the start of exposure: 60 months • more than 15 years after the start of exposure: 36 months (depending on the cumulative exposure level, exposure to other fibres and results of the medical examination) Note: a follow-up examination planned because of (earlier) exposure to dust containing asbestos fibres should be combined with the follow-up examination according to G 1.3
premature follow-up examination	• after an illness lasting for several weeks or when a physical handicap gives cause for concern about whether the work should be continued • in individual cases when the physician considers it necessary, e.g. when there is short-term concern about the person's health • when requested by an employee who suspects a causal association between his or her illness and work

1.2   Medical examination schedule

1.2.1   General medical examination

| Initial examination | Follow-up examination |

- general anamnesis, differentiated work anamnesis taking special account of any inhalative exposure to fibrogenic dusts containing asbestos, quartz[1] or other fibres, detailed smoking anamnesis[2]
  - non-smokers, smokers, ex-smokers
  - cigarettes, cigars, pipes (number per day)
  - year of starting and, if applicable, ending tobacco consumption (number of cigarette pack years)

1.2.2   Special medical examination

| Initial examination | Follow-up examination |

- examination of the respiratory and cardiocirculatory organs
- spirometry
- large format posterior-anterior thorax radiograph taken with high kilovolt technique unless results are available from such an x-ray examination which has been carried out within the previous year

1.2.3   Supplementary examination

| Follow-up examination |

In individual cases it may be necessary to take lateral and/or oblique radiographs (RAO and LAO 35–40°). The decision must be based on the
- latency period (>15 years)
- duration and level of exposure
- inhalative smoking habits
- and previous radiograms

---

1 AES (alkaline earth silicate) fibres recrystallize at temperatures above 900°C to yield cristobalite.
2 See protocol sheet for anamnesis ("Mineral Dust", G 1.1, G 1.2, G 1.3) and remarks concerning tobacco consumption in G 1.1.

1.3   Requirements for the medical examinations
- competent doctor or occupational health professional
- continual medical education in reading and classification of radiograms according to the international pneumoconiosis classification ILO 2000, specific x-ray diagnostic experience
- apparatus and other requirements for the examinations: x-ray examination, lung function tests, ILO standard x-ray images

2   Occupational medical assessment and advice
An assessment is only possible when the workplace situation and the exposure of the individual are known. For this purpose a risk assessment as defined in Article 4 Council directive 98/24/EC must have been carried out; it must specify which technical, organizational and individual protective measures have been applied.

2.1   Assessment criteria

2.1.1   Long-term concern about health

| Initial examination | Follow-up examination |

Persons with existing disorders and/or functional defects especially of the cardiopulmonary system for whom the exposure to dust containing aluminium silicate fibres would be expected to result in a clinically relevant worsening of their state of health. As examples are mentioned here especially:
- severe disorders of lung function and of the cardiocirculatory system
- chronic, especially obstructive bronchitis with functional disorders, bronchial asthma, pulmonary emphysema
- radiographically detectable dust lung or other fibrotic or granulotamous lung alterations
- malformations, tumours, chronic inflammation, pleural fibrosis or other damage which significantly impairs the function of the airways or lungs or which favours the development of bronchopulmonary disorders
- deformities of the thorax or spine which have adverse effects on breathing
- condition following lung resection or injury with functional impairment of the thoracic organs
- active, also latent tuberculosis, extensive inactive tuberculosis and the condition following pleuritis which is perhaps not completely cured

- manifest or expected premature cardiac insufficiency, such as is found with cardiac valve defects, other organic cardiac damage or recent disorders which are known to result frequently in premature cardiac insufficiency
- high blood pressure especially when this does not respond to therapy
- other chronic disorders which reduce general resistance

G 1.3

2.1.2   Short-term concern about health

| **Initial examination** | **Follow-up examination** |

Persons like those described in Section 2.1.1 but who are expected to recover.

2.1.3   No concern about health under certain conditions

| **Initial examination** | **Follow-up examination** |

If the illnesses or alterations mentioned in Section 2.1.1 are less severe, the doctor should establish whether or not it is possible for the person to start work or go on working under certain conditions.
Such conditions could include:
- transfer to workplaces with exposure to lower concentrations of fibres containing aluminium silicates
- more frequent follow-up examinations
If necessary, details of exposure levels may be obtained by carrying out measurements at the individual workplace.

2.1.4   No concern about health

| **Initial examination** | **Follow-up examination** |

All other persons, provided there are no restrictions on their employment.

2.2   Medical advice

The advice in an individual case should be commensurate with the workplace situation and the results of the medical examinations.
Cigarette smoking is the main cause of lung cancer. The combination of exposure to dust containing aluminium silicate fibres and cigarette smoking has a synergistic effect. The physician is to inform the smoker of these facts and that treatment can be successful in helping him or her to stop smoking.

3   Supplementary notes

3.1   Exposure

3.1.1   Occurrence, sources of hazards

The group of high temperature wools includes
• AES wool (alkaline earth silicate wool)
Persons exposed to dust containing AES wool fibres should be examined according to the scheme described in G 1.4 Exposure to dust.
• aluminium silicate wool (RCF = refractory ceramic fibre)
Persons exposed to dust containing aluminium silicate wool fibres should be examined according to the scheme described in G 1.3.
• polycrystalline ceramic fibres (alumina wool)
Persons exposed to dust containing polycrystalline ceramic wool fibres should be examined according to the scheme described in G 1.4 Exposure to dust.
Scheme showing a classification of high-temperature wools with a classification temperature >1000°C (see also EN 1094):

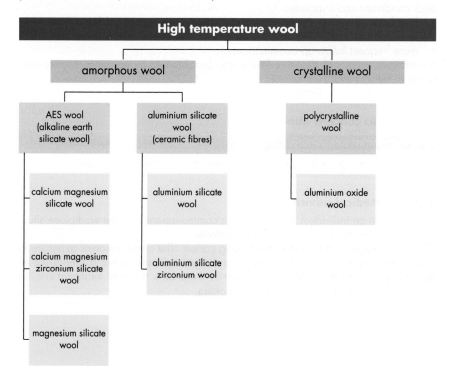

High temperature wool is generally used at temperatures above 900°C.
Aluminium silicate wool is still used today in the construction of furnaces and fire-
boxes, in heating systems in regions in direct contact with the flame, in exhaust systems in motorized vehicles, as mats for holding ceramic substrates or as heat insulation in hot end systems. The products are used in the form of felts and plates of
various densities and thicknesses, folded modules, vacuum-formed parts and many
other items.
During processing of these products the fibres may be broken and inhalable fibre
fragments produced; attention should be paid to the enrichment of short, thin
($\varnothing$ <1 µm) fibres in the workplace air.

3.1.2   Physicochemical properties

High temperature wools belong to the group of man-made mineral fibres (MMMF).
Aluminium silicate wool (combination of Al_2O_3 and SiO_2) and AES wool (combina-
tion von CaO, MgO, SiO_2 and ZrO_2) are produced by melting and blowing or cen-
trifuging processes.
The fibres produced in these processes have diameters between 0.5 and 5 µm and
are several centimetres long.
Polycrystalline wool is produced by the sol-gel process from an aqueous spin solution; the crystallization takes place in a subsequent heating step.
Products made of high temperature wool generally do not contain binder.
AES wool recrystallizes when used at temperatures above 900°C to yield cristobalite
(up to 45 % w/w), aluminium silicate wool recrystallizes too but only at higher temperatures (about 1150°C). During repair or demolition of products made with these
fibres, appropriate protective measures should be implemented.

3.1.3   Uptake

The dust is taken up via the airways.

3.2   Functional disorders, symptoms

3.2.1   Mode of action

Sufficient data for carcinogenicity of aluminium silicate fibres in man is not available
at present. However, the data which is available from (not very sensitive) experi-
ments with animals which inhaled such fibres suggests that they can cause both pulmonary fibrosis, lung tumours and pleural mesothelioma.
In an intrapleural test with animals a dose-dependent increase in proliferation of
pleural mesothelial cells was demonstrated.
In exposed persons especially benign pleural disorders (pleural plaques) have been
observed.

3.2.2   Acute and subacute effects on health

not applicable

3.2.3   Chronic effects on health

While taking into account exposure levels and latency periods, the physician should watch for signs of disorders like those which occur after exposure to asbestos or quartz.

4   References

Bunn WB, Bender JR, Hesterberg TW, Case GR, Konzen JL (1993) Recent studies on man-made vitreous fibers. Chronic animal inhalation studies. J Occup Med 35: 101–113

Council Directive 89/391/EEC on the introduction of measures to encourage improvements in the safety and health of workers at work

Council Directive 92/85/EEC on the introduction of measures to encourage improvements in the safety and health at work of pregnant workers and workers who have recently given birth or are breastfeeding

Council Directive 98/24/EC on the protection of the health and safety of workers from the risks related to chemical agents at work

EN 1094 "Insulating refractory products"

GESTIS-international limit values for chemical agents. BGIA
    at: www.dguv.de/bgia/gestis-limit-values

International Labour Organisation. Guidelines for the Use of the ILO international Classification of radiographs of pneumoconioses. 2000 edition. Geneva: International Labour Office, 2002, (Occupational Safety and Health Series No. 22)

G 1.4   Exposure to dust

Committee for occupational medicine, working group "Occupational risks for the lungs", Bergbau-Berufsgenossenschaft, Bochum

G 1.4

Preliminary remarks

The present guideline describes a scheme for occupational medical prophylaxis which aims to prevent if possible or to ensure early diagnosis of obstructive airway disorders, pulmonary emphysema and their sequelae which can be caused by exposure to high levels of dust at the workplace or to prevent further deterioration in persons with existing airway damage. If the exposures are to substances with germ cell mutagenic, carcinogenic, fibrogenic, allergenic, chemically irritating or other toxic effects, the relevant Guidelines for Occupational Medical Examinations should be consulted.

Schedule

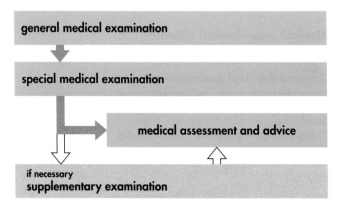

1   Medical examinations

Occupational medical examinations are to be carried out for persons at whose workplaces the occupational exposure limit values for respirable dust or inhalable dust are exceeded. At workplaces where the exposure limit values are observed, occupational medical examinations are to be offered to persons exposed to dust.

1.1   Examinations, intervals between examinations

initial examination	before taking up the job
follow-up examinations	after 36 months after 60 months for persons less than 40 years old and when leaving the job
premature follow-up examination	• after an illness lasting for several weeks or when a physical handicap gives cause for concern about whether the work should be continued • in individual cases when the physician considers it necessary, e.g. when there is short-term concern about the person's health • when requested by an employee who suspects a causal association between his or her illness and work

1.2   Medical examination schedule

1.2.1   General medical examination

Initial examination

Review of past history (general anamnesis, paying particular attention to disorders which could cause concern about the person's health, see Section 2.1)
- anamnesis of coughing/expectoration (since when, how often, how long)
- respiratory distress (during physical work, at rest, since when)
- work anamnesis
- previous jobs (periods and levels of exposure to dusts or other substances which damage the airways)
- current work
- kind and duration of work involving exposure to high levels of dust
- irritating and/or sensitizing substances encountered at the workplace
- symptoms associated with the workplace or particular jobs (e.g. coughing, expectoration, respiratory distress)

- detailed smoking anamnesis[1]
  - non-smokers, smokers, ex-smokers
  - cigarettes, cigars, pipes (number per day)
  - year of starting and, if applicable, ending tobacco consumption (number of cigarette pack years)
- any medications affecting the bronchi (dilating, constricting)
- other symptoms.

Medical examination, taking into account the work done by the person, and including extensive examination of the respiratory organs.

G 1.4

Follow-up examination

As for the initial examination. Interim anamnesis especially as to current work and dust exposure at the workplace, symptoms associated with the workplace, coughing, expectoration, respiratory distress, recently developed disorders of the respiratory system especially those spatially and temporally related to the workplace and perhaps whether the symptoms regress during work-free intervals.

1.2.2   Special medical examination

Initial examination

Spirometry and volume-flow curve as basic examination for documentation and later evaluation of changes[2].

Follow-up examination

As for the initial examination; determination of any changes in FEV_1 and in maximum vital capacity (VC_{max}) since the previous examination.

1.2.3   Supplementary examination

Initial examination

Supplementary examinations are necessary and indicated if an assessment is not possible without their results. Which supplementary examinations are necessary may be decided from the work anamnesis, respiratory symptoms, previous results and medical indications. Generally it is not necessary to carry out all the examinations listed below.

---

[1] See protocol sheet for anamnesis ("Mineral Dust", G 1.1, G 1.2, G 1.3) and remarks concerning tobacco consumption in G 1.1.

[2] Because of the great importance of slowly progressing impairment of lung function, appropriate measures should be taken to ensure that the test procedure and the evaluation of the results are subject to quality control.

Extended lung function tests
- where indicated, determination of the airway resistance, if possible by whole body plethysmography
- tests for reversibility of an obstructive ventilation disorder
- tests for unspecific bronchial hyperreactivity
- if clinically significant emphysema is suspected: whole body plethysmography, determination of diffusing capacity DL_{CO} or blood gas analysis at rest and during physical activity

Thorax radiogram
- large format posterior-anterior thorax radiograph taken with high kilovolt technique, only for specific diagnostic purposes, if indicated, in two planes. If a radiograph not more than one year old is available, this should be taken into consideration before deciding on the indicated procedure

Follow-up examination

As for the initial examination. Supplementary examinations are also necessary if the reduction in FEV_1 since the previous examination is reproducibly more than 50 ml per year. If clinically significant unspecific bronchial hyperreactivity is suspected, the lung function tests should be carried out before and after exposure at the workplace (spirometry, determination of peak flow).

1.3   Requirements for the medical examinations
- competent doctor or occupational health professional
- the physician should have specialist knowledge of the procedures and evaluation of lung function tests including the indications for whole body plethysmography, knowledge of indications for, procedures for and evaluation of unspecific bronchial inhalation tests (provocation tests).

2   Occupational medical assessment and advice

An assessment is only possible when the workplace situation and the individual exposure to dust are known. For this purpose a risk assessment as defined in Article 4 Council directive 98/24/EC must have been carried out; it must specify which technical, organizational and individual protective measures have been applied.

2.1   Assessment criteria

2.1.1   Long-term concern about health

| Initial examination | Follow-up examination |

Persons with
- manifest obstructive respiratory disease, especially bronchial asthma, chronic obstructive bronchitis and/or pulmonary emphysema with significant functional impairment
- symptomatic, irreversible bronchial hyperreactivity (for longer than 6 months)
- severe previous lung damage such as exogenous allergic alveolitis
- silicosis or asbestosis or other fibrotic or granulomatous lung alterations (e.g. sarcoidosis) which can be confirmed roentgenologically (conventional radiogram
  [silicosis 1/1 or more, asbestosis of the lung 1/1 and/or pleura] or HRCT), and
  thorax deformities, pleural thickening, etc. with functional effects
- manifest cardiac insufficiency
- cardiopulmonary disorders for which higher levels of dust exposure would mean
  an extra risk (e.g. in cases of congestive bronchitis)

G 1.4

2.1.2   Short-term concern about health

| Initial examination | Follow-up examination |

Persons with
- transient hypersensitivity of the upper and/or lower airways (e.g. as a result of
  bronchopneumonic infections) for which a worsening is to be expected on inhalation of even relatively low concentrations of noxious substances

2.1.3   No concern about health under certain conditions

| Initial examination | Follow-up examination |

If the illnesses or functional disorders mentioned in Section 2.1.1 are less severe, the
physician should establish whether or not it is possible for the person to start work or
go on working under certain conditions. Such conditions could include
- technical protective measures
- organizational protective measures, e.g., limitation of exposure periods
- transfer to workplaces known to involve lower levels of dust exposure in the sense
  of the general threshold limit value for dust (see Section 3.1.2)
- personal protective equipment which takes the individual's state of health into account
- more frequent follow-up examinations

2.1.4   No concern about health

| Initial examination | Follow-up examination |

All other persons.

2.2   Medical advice

The advice in an individual case should be commensurate with the workplace situation and the results of the medical examinations.

Cigarette smoking is the main reason for the development of chronic obstructive airway diseases. Giving up inhalative smoking of tobacco has been shown to result in an improvement in lung function and so to a more favourable course of the disease. The physician is to inform the smoker of these facts and that treatment can be successful in helping him or her to stop smoking.

If there are indications of chronic obstructive respiratory disease, the employee should be told that specific medical treatment is advisable and possible.

3   Supplementary notes

3.1   Exposure

3.1.1   Occurrence, sources of hazards

As stipulated in the definition of the general threshold limit value for dust (see Section 3.1.2), this threshold applies to all workplaces at which poorly soluble dust is released during handling of dusty or powdery products or is produced during handling, e.g. during mechanical processing. Such workplaces are to be found in practically all branches and sectors of industry. Although there are no precise data for the number of exposed persons, it has been estimated that several million workplaces are affected. The results of the exposure determinations in various work areas must be seen in this context; they can provide, on the one hand, only a limited survey of affected workplaces and, on the other, reveal a very large number of typical and especially critical areas of exposure to such dusts. Examples of areas/sectors in which the workplace exposure to dust is caused mainly by handling of dusty or powdery materials include the building industry, mining, natural rock, gravel, sand, lime, ceramic and glass industries, foundries, etc. Areas/sectors in which dust develops frequently or mainly during handling of materials include wood and plastics industries, trades, textile industry, paper industry and jobs involving grinding, mechanical processing, demolition work, etc. In most areas and sectors of industry, more or less of the jobs/workplaces involve both of these mechanisms of dust emission in parallel with exposure.

3.1.2 Physical properties and the general threshold limit value for dust

The general threshold limit value for dust applies to poorly soluble dusts for which no specific threshold limit value has been established for the dust constituents and to mixtures of dusts. It may not be applied to dusts from which germ cell mutagenic, carcinogenic, fibrogenic, toxic or allergenic effects are to be expected. For these dusts the general threshold limit value for dust applies as an additional general upper threshold. The general threshold limit value for dust does not apply to soluble dust, ultrafine or dispersed coarse particle fractions or to paint aerosols.

G 1.4

3.1.3 Uptake

Dusts are taken up only via the airways.

3.2 Functional disorders, symptoms

Chronic (obstructive) bronchitis[3] and/or emphysema, hyper-reactive bronchial system, bronchial asthma.

Inflammation of the deep airways is called bronchitis. In the terminology of the international classification of diseases (10th revision) "simple and mucopurulent chronic bronchitis" (J41) is distinguished from "other chronic obstructive pulmonary disease" (J44). This includes chronic obstructive bronchitis. The ICD-10 codes pulmonary emphysema as J43. The development of chronic bronchitis as a reaction to dust exposure takes years to decades. The initial changes in lung clearance are not noticed at all subjectively; the first signs which can be detected are coughing and expectoration. Even these symptoms are often not considered by the affected persons to be a sign of disease (e.g. as for the so-called smoker's cough). The first symptom which is always associated with a reduction in the performance of the affected person is respiratory distress (initially only during physical activity) or the diagnosis of an obstructive ventilation disorder.

Chronic bronchitis is a very wide-spread disease. Contributing factors are considered to include not only the exposure to dust at the workplace but also and especially the smoking habits of the population, repeated virus infections of the respiratory passages, general air pollution and certain predisposing factors. The incidence of the manifest, therapy-requiring obstructive lung disease in the working population without airway exposure is about 2 % at the age of 20 years and about 4 % at the age of 60 years.

---

[3] Definition WHO (1966): coughing and expectoration on most days during at least three months of two consecutive years.

3.2.1   Mode of action

Inhaled dust particles penetrate the airways to different extents depending on their aerodynamic diameters. Whereas the particles deposited in the bronchi are relatively rapidly (hours) transported back towards the mouth where they are eliminated by swallowing or being coughed up, the particles which penetrate to the alveoli, provided that they are insoluble, remain there for months or even years (biological half life up to 400 days). The main role in the elimination of particles deposited in the alveoli is played by the macrophages which ingest the particles and transport them away via the bronchial passages, lymph or blood vessels. The macrophages digesting the particles release so-called mediators which attract inflammatory cells. Such mediators are also released by bronchial epithelial cells exposed to foreign substances. If the exposure continues for years or decades and the bronchoalveolar clearance capacity is insufficient to cope, chronic inflammation can develop in the peripheral and central airways. This is characterized histologically by invasion of the mucous membrane by leukocytes, proliferation of the mucous-producing glands and fibrosis of the bronchial walls. The associated clinical signs are coughing and expectoration and later also respiratory distress. This kind of respiratory distress may be recognized objectively by determining lung function parameters diagnostic for obstructive ventilation disorders, distribution disorders and/or diffusion disorders.

Disturbance of the equilibrium between particle uptake and elimination (clearance) for longer periods towards excess uptake can result in the so-called overload phenomenon which has been clearly demonstrated in animal studies. This mechanism has been demonstrated in various small mammals (rat, hamster, etc.) and so it is likely that similar processes take place in man. The overload phenomenon is understood to involve reduction in the clearance of dust deposited in the alveoli from a certain level of particle load in the macrophages and total standstill when the system is overloaded (60 % of the macrophage volume filled with particles). Then the associated inflammatory processes become more intensive. Emphysema develops. In rodents even tumour-forming processes may be initiated in this way. This last has not yet been demonstrated with sufficient certainty for man.

3.3   Comments

For persons exposed mainly to welding fumes, Guideline G 39 is to be used for the occupational medical examinations.

In order to avoid repeat examinations, the necessity for examinations according to the guidelines G 1.1 and G 26 should be checked.

4   References

Barnes PJ (2000) Chronic obstructive pulmonary disease. New Engl J Med 343: 269–280

Council Directive 98/24/EC on the protection of the health and safety of workers from the risks related to chemical agents at work

Deutsche Forschungsgemeinschaft (German Research Foundation, DFG) (ed) List of MAK and BAT Values 2007. Maximum Concentrations and Biological Tolerance Values at the workplace. Wiley-VCH, Weinheim

Deutsche Forschungsgemeinschaft (German Research Foundation, DFG) (ed) The MAK-Collection for Occupational Health and Safety. Wiley-VCH at: www.mrw.interscience.wiley.com/makbat

GESTIS-international limit values for chemical agents. BGIA at: www.dguv.de/bgia/gestis-limit-values

Scanlon PD et al (2000) Smoking cessation and lung function in mild-to-moderate chronic obstructive pulmonary disease. Am J Resp Crit Care Med 161: 381–390

G 1.4

G 2   Lead and lead compounds (with the exception of alkyllead compounds)

Committee for occupational medicine, working group "Hazardous substances", Berufsgenossenschaft der chemischen Industrie, Heidelberg

Preliminary remarks

The present guideline describes a scheme for occupational medical prophylaxis which aims to prevent or ensure early diagnosis of disorders which can be caused by lead and lead compounds (with the exception of alkyllead compounds).

Schedule

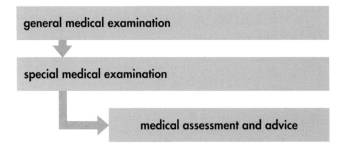

1 Medical examinations

Occupational medical examinations are to be carried out for persons at whose workplaces exposure to lead or lead compounds (with the exception of alkyllead compounds) could endanger health (e.g. the occupational exposure limit value is exceeded).

1.1 Examinations, intervals between examinations

initial examination	before taking up the job
first follow-up examination	after 12 months
further follow-up examinations	after 12 months and when leaving the job
premature follow-up examination	• after a serious or prolonged illness which could cause concern as to whether the activity should be continued • in individual cases when the physician considers it necessary, e.g. when there is short-term concern about the person's health • when requested by an employee who suspects a causal association between his or her illness and work

1.2 Medical examination schedule

1.2.1 General medical examination

Initial examination

• review of past history (general anamnesis, work anamnesis, symptoms)
  Particular attention should be paid to disorders of the haematopoietic system and gastrointestinal tract, the peripheral and central nervous systems and the kidneys. The physician carrying out the examination should be familiar with the conditions under which the person is exposed to lead at work.
• urinalysis (multiple test strips)

Follow-up examination

- interim anamnesis (including work anamnesis)
  Particular attention should be paid to symptoms typically caused by lead (see Section 3.2).
- urinalysis (multiple test strips)

1.2.2   Special medical examination

Initial examination

G 2

- full blood count
Not required, except in special cases when the physician considers lead-specific tests (see Section 3.1.4) to be necessary, e.g. if anamnesis suggests that the person has previously been exposed to lead.

Follow-up examination

- full blood count
- determination of the lead level in blood (see Section 3.1.4)
If the blood lead level (quality control!*) exceeds 300 µg/l in male employees and 100 µg/l in female employees, the examining physician is to explain the medical and toxicological situation and can advise individual persons as to the necessity for a premature follow-up examination.
If the blood lead level (quality control!*) exceeds 350 µg/l in male employees and 200 µg/l in female employees, levels of lead in biological material must be determined again at the latest within 3 months.

Important: the lead in blood is mainly bound to the erythrocyte membranes. Given the same levels of lead in blood, the erythrocytes of anaemic individuals are much more heavily loaded with lead than those of individuals who are not anaemic; this suggests that the risk associated with lead exposure is higher for anaemic persons.

1.3   Requirements for the medical examinations

- competent doctor or occupational health professional
- laboratory analyses carried out with appropriate quality control (Good Laboratory Practice)

---

* It has been shown in practice that certain quality control criteria are necessary for the analysis of lead in blood, e.g. that in the expected concentration range of 100–700 µg/l, the day to day standard deviation of the method used should not be above 6 %.

2   Occupational medical assessment and advice

An assessment is only possible when the workplace situation and the exposure of the individual are known. For this purpose a risk assessment as defined in Article 4 Council directive 98/24/EC must have been carried out; it must specify which technical, organizational and individual protective measures have been applied.

2.1   Assessment criteria

2.1.1   Long-term concern about health

Initial examination

Persons with severe disorders of
* the liver
* the kidneys
* the blood (anaemia, thalassaemia, etc)
* the peripheral and central nervous systems
* the endocrine system (especially diabetes and marked hyperactivity of the thyroid gland)
* the gastrointestinal tract
* the vessels (angioneuropathy, endangiitis, arteriosclerosis, etc.)

Also persons with
* marked hypertension
* tuberculosis
* general physical weakness

Follow-up examination

see initial examination
and in addition
* persons whose lead intake or lead-associated symptoms are repeatedly more pronounced than in persons working in similar jobs (e.g. because of diet, lack of personal hygiene or internal causes)
  Transfer of such persons to workplaces involving less lead exposure can often be a sufficient response; during this time blood lead levels are to be checked at shorter intervals.

2.1.2   Short-term concern about health

Initial examination

Persons with the disorders mentioned in Section 2.1.1, provided recovery is to be expected.

Follow-up examination

see initial examination.

In addition, male employees whose blood lead levels (quality control!*) exceed 400 µg/l and female employees whose blood lead levels (quality control!*) exceed 300 µg/l.

The findings are to be checked by repeating the assays in biological material at short intervals. Because of the half-life of lead in the biological system, short-term concern about health should apply for at least 3 months. During this period the person should not work or should work much less with substances containing lead.

G 2

2.1.3   No concern about health under certain conditions

Initial examination	Follow-up examination

If the illnesses or functional disorders mentioned in Section 2.1.1 are less severe, the doctor should establish whether or not it is possible for the person to start work or go on working under certain conditions. Such conditions could include

* technical protective measures
* organizational protective measures, e.g., limitation of exposure periods
* transfer to workplaces known to involve lower levels of exposure
* personal protective equipment which takes the individual's state of health into account
* more frequent follow-up examinations

2.1.4   No concern about health

Initial examination	Follow-up examination

All other persons, provided there are no restrictions on their employment.

2.2   Medical advice

The advice in an individual case should be commensurate with the workplace situation and the results of the medical examinations.

Employees are to be informed about the biomonitoring results and about the potential prenatal toxicity and the toxic effects of lead and its compounds on reproduction. The employees should be informed about general hygienic measures and personal protective equipment and especially about the risk of lead intake during eating, drinking and smoking at the workplace.

---

* see Section 1.2.2

If during the course of his work in the company the occupational physician finds indications that the risk assessment should be brought up to date to improve health and safety standards, he is to inform the employer. When this is necessary, the interests of the employee are to be protected (medical confidentiality).

3   Supplementary notes

3.1   External and internal exposure

3.1.1   Occurrence, sources of hazards

Listed below are the kinds of processes, workplaces or activities, including cleaning and repair work, for which exposure to lead or lead compounds (with the exception of alkyllead compounds) must be expected. This must be taken into account during the risk assessment:

- transport, storage and stacking of lead as bars, sheet metal, rods, and in other forms
- handling and loading of lead compounds in closed containers
- painting enamel, glass and ceramics with lead-containing paints in the form of pastes or solidified thermoplastics
- processing pastes with lead-containing pigments and paints containing lead as screen-printing pastes or thermoplastics
- soldering with solder containing lead
- smelting of lead ores and lead concentrates (primary lead smelting)
- recycling of waste and secondary raw materials containing lead (secondary lead smelting)
- loading containers with and removal of lead-containing ore fines (blue dust), ash or other dusty materials; emptying the containers
- refining of lead
- production and processing of leaded bronze, lead pigments, lead glazes, lead powder and dusty lead compounds
- lead coating
- preparation and charging of lead crystal mixtures
- spraying paints containing lead (restoration) or other lead-containing products
- use of powdery lead compounds in the production of paints (restoration), accumulators (storage batteries) and plastic objects
- production, transport and installation of charge carriers in the accumulator industry
- removal of coatings containing lead (e.g., by burning off, by abrasive processes such as brushing, sanding or sandblasting, or by chemical stripping)
- welding or oxygen cutting of metal parts containing lead or with coatings containing lead

- mechanical (sanding, polishing, machining) or thermal processing of lead, lead alloys or coatings containing lead
- repair, cleaning and servicing work in lead-producing and lead-processing areas
- roofing jobs with materials containing lead
- painting glass, lead glazing (especially during restoration of antique lead glazing)
- dismantling of old devices containing lead (e.g. electrical and electronic equipment)
- production and processing of free-machining steels containing lead
- use of explosives containing lead (munition and special explosives) and cleaning of places (e.g. shooting ranges) where these materials have been used

G 2

During work with substances containing lead it should be remembered that only a part of the lead dose taken up by the employee is inhaled in the form of lead dust and fumes. A very large part of the dose is taken up through the gastrointestinal tract (oral intake, e.g., by hand to mouth contact). Determination of the internal dose of lead is therefore also of decisive importance when the lead concentrations in the workplace air are low. It has been shown in practice that the blood lead levels depend to a very large extent on the cleanliness of the workplace and the person and on individual behaviour.

Occurrence and hazards for specific substances are documented in the information system on hazardous substances (GESTIS) (see Section 4).

3.1.2   Physicochemical properties and classification

The information system on hazardous substances (GESTIS) provides details of international threshold limit values, classification, evaluation and other substance-specific information (see Section 4).

Additional information is to be found in the recommendations of the DFG Commission for the Investigation of Health Hazards of Chemical Compounds in the Work Area (List of MAK and BAT Values).

Lead is a soft grey-blue metal which is obtained by smelting of lead ores – primarily of galena (PbS). In vapour form (begins to vaporize at temperatures as low as 550°C) it is oxidized in the air to lead oxide (PbO). "Lead fumes" consist of colloidal particles of lead oxide. Lead is found in divalent and tetravalent form, is readily soluble in nitric acid and is passivated by phosphoric, hydrochloric and sulfuric acids (formation of the insoluble salts). It is resistant to chlorine and hydrofluoric acid, but is attacked slowly by some organic acids.

Lead and lead compounds (with the exception of the alkyllead compounds)

Formula (lead)	Pb
CAS number (lead)	7439-92-1
OEL value[1]	0.15 mg/m^3 (inhalable aerosol)

---

[1] occupational exposure limit value of the European Community

3.1.3   Uptake

Lead is taken up mainly via the airways in the form of dust or fumes and through the gastrointestinal tract.

3.1.4   Biomonitoring

Information about biomonitoring may be found in Appendix 1 "Biomonitoring".

3.1.4.1 Blood sample and analysis

Sampling time
In spite of the long half-life of lead in biological systems, it is recommended that the blood sample not be taken immediately after a longer exposure-free interval.

Sampling
Meaningful results from analysis of the lead level in blood may only be obtained if the blood sample is taken under contamination-free conditions. For this purpose an appropriately fitted clean room is required. Personal hygienic measures – such as washing the arm – are necessary to ensure that the results are not falsified by lead from the skin or from other sources. Generally it is sufficient to carry out thorough cleansing of the skin and disinfection with alcohol before the sample is taken.
Whole venous blood (2–5 ml) samples are obtained with disposable blood collection devices such as Monovettes® or the Vacutainer® system. In both cases K-EDTA must be present as anticoagulant. Shaking is necessary to mix the venous blood sample thoroughly.
The tubes used must be certified as of suitable quality for blood sampling.

Storage and transport of blood samples
The samples for determination of blood lead levels may be stored at room temperature for several days. They should not be exposed to direct sunlight. If they are to be stored for longer periods (more than 5 days) they should be refrigerated.
The samples may be sent by post. The containers should be unbreakable and well closed so that they cannot leak. There are special regulations for dispatch of biological material. Details may be obtained from certified laboratories.

Choice of laboratory and analysis
When choosing a laboratory it should be established whether qualified support for sampling, storage and transport is offered. It must be clear that the laboratory is willing to provide assistance in the interpretation of the analytical results if this should be necessary. To check the quality of the analysis and if the results do not seem plausible, identical samples of whole blood should be sent to another certified laboratory for a repeat analysis.
Biomonitoring should be carried out with reliable methods and meet quality control requirements (see Appendix 1 "Biomonitoring").

3.2   Functional disorders, symptoms

3.2.1   Mode of action

Lead has effects especially on
- haemoglobin synthesis and erythropoiesis
- the smooth musculature
- the peripheral and central nervous systems
- the vascular system

For the second to fourth sites of action in this list, the mechanisms are still not fully understood. Lead inhibits certain of the enzymes of haemoglobin synthesis. This results in increased urinary excretion of δ-aminolaevulic acid and coproporphyrin III and inhibition of the incorporation of bivalent iron into protoporphyrin IX, a precursor of haemoglobin. Some of the lead taken up by the body is bound in the bones as the tertiary phosphate (lead depot).

G 2

3.2.2   Acute effects on health

Acute adverse effects of lead on health are rather rare.

3.2.3   Subacute/chronic effects on health

The disorders caused by lead are most usually subacute and chronic, and these are not always distinguishable; they have the following stages:

clinically silent precursor stage:
- increased lead level in the blood
- increased vegetative lability

critical initial stage:
- mild anaemia, basophilic punctate erythrocytes
- pale skin and mucous membranes
- general exhaustion
- anorexia
- headaches
- weakness, sometimes pain in limbs and joints
- gastrointestinal disorders
- constipation

marked lead poisoning:
- the symptoms listed above in more severe form
- lead colic (violent, often persistent colon spasms, sometimes with vomiting, stool like sheep's droppings)
- pale skin colouring

There is scientific evidence that lead has carcinogenic effects.

Decisive for the reduction of the biological threshold value to 400 µg/l were effects on the central nervous system (brain). It had been demonstrated that even at blood lead concentrations below 700 µg/l functional disorders developed including impairment of perceptiveness, learning, memory, concentration and attentiveness as well as other parameters of cognitive performance, motor functions and personality changes.

Parenteral or oral treatment of persons with occupational lead poisoning with chelating agents (EDTA) is generally contraindicated because of the risk of overloading the renal epithelium with unpredictably high levels of the toxic EDTA-lead complex.

4   References

Commission Recommendation 2003/670/EC concerning the European schedule of occupational diseases. Annex I

Council Directive 67/548/EEC on the approximation of the laws, regulations and administrative provisions relating to the classification, packaging and labelling of dangerous substances

Council Directive 98/24/EC on the protection of the health and safety of workers from the risks related to chemical agents at work

Deutsche Forschungsgemeinschaft (German Research Foundation, DFG) (ed) List of MAK and BAT Values 2007. Maximum Concentrations and Biological Tolerance Values at the workplace. Wiley-VCH, Weinheim

Deutsche Forschungsgemeinschaft (German Research Foundation, DFG) (ed) The MAK-Collection for Occupational Health and Safety. Wiley-VCH
at: www.mrw.interscience.wiley.com/makbat

GESTIS-database on hazardous substances. BGIA
at: www.dguv.de/bgia/gestis-database

GESTIS-international limit values for chemical agents. BGIA
at: www.dguv.de/bgia/gestis-limit-values

G 3   Alkyllead compounds

Committee for occupational medicine, working group "Hazardous substances", Berufsgenossenschaft der chemischen Industrie, Heidelberg

Preliminary remarks

The present guideline describes a scheme for occupational medical prophylaxis which aims to prevent or ensure early diagnosis of disorders which can be caused by alkyllead compounds.

G 3

Schedule

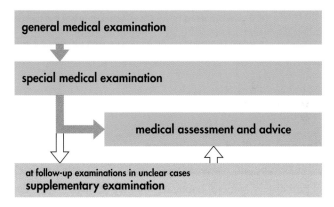

1 Medical examinations

Occupational medical examinations are to be carried out for persons exposed at work to levels of alkyllead compounds which could have adverse effects on health (e.g. when the occupational exposure limit value is exceeded) or for whom dermal absorption could endanger health.

1.1 Examinations, intervals between examinations

initial examination	before taking up the job
first follow-up examination	after 12–24 months
further follow-up examinations	after 12 months and when leaving the job
premature follow-up examination	• after a serious or prolonged illness which could cause concern as to whether the activity should be continued • in individual cases when the physician considers it necessary, e.g. when there is short-term concern about the person's health • when requested by an employee who suspects a causal association between his or her illness and work

1.2 Medical examination schedule

1.2.1 General medical examination

Initial examination

• review of past history (general anamnesis, work anamnesis, symptoms)
• urinalysis (multiple test strips, sediment)

Follow-up examination

• interim anamnesis (including work anamnesis)
  Particular attention should be paid to bad nightmares, sleeplessness, marked moodiness, weight loss, hand tremor, nausea, irritability, quarrelsomeness (no suggestive questions!)
• urinalysis (multiple test strips, sediment)

1.2.2   Special medical examination

Initial examination	Follow-up examination

• full blood count

1.2.3   Supplementary examination

Follow-up examination

In unclear cases:
If the symptoms listed in Section 1.2.1 or the results obtained according to Section 1.2.2 suggest that it is necessary, the urinary lead level should be determined quantitatively (see Section 3.1.4).

G 3

1.3   Requirements for the medical examinations

• competent doctor or occupational health professional
• laboratory analyses carried out with appropriate quality control (Good Laboratory Practice)

2   Occupational medical assessment and advice

An assessment is only possible when the workplace situation and the exposure of the individual are known. For this purpose a risk assessment as defined in Article 4 Council directive 98/24/EC must have been carried out; it must specify which technical, organizational and individual protective measures have been applied.

2.1   Assessment criteria

2.1.1   Long-term concern about health

Initial examination

Persons with severe disorders of
• the blood
• the heart and circulatory system
• the lungs (asthma, tuberculosis, etc.)
• the nasopharyngeal space
• the liver
• the kidneys

- the metabolism (diabetes, gout, etc.)
- the peripheral and central nervous systems
- the skin (allergic and degenerative eczema)

Also persons with

- mental disorders
- addiction to alcohol, medications, drugs
- untreated and incompletely cured syphilis

Follow-up examination

Persons with residual damage (see initial examination) if clear signs of intoxication persist (increased blood lead level – see G 2 "Lead and lead compounds", increased urinary lead level, depression, schizoid confusion, chronic disorders of the blood or nervous system).

2.1.2   Short-term concern about health

Initial examination

Persons with the disorders mentioned in Section 2.1.1, provided recovery is to be expected.
Persons who have worked for long periods in lead works and have taken up large amounts of lead or who have already suffered from lead poisoning.

Follow-up examination

See initial examination and

- persons with clear signs of lead poisoning or for whom it is strongly suspected
- and persons with a total urinary lead level of more than 50 µg/l until the symptoms have regressed

2.1.3   No concern about health under certain conditions

Initial examination   Follow-up examination

If the illnesses or functional disorders mentioned in Section 2.1.1 are less severe or if the laboratory results are close to the limits of the normal range (see Section 3.1.4), the doctor should establish whether or not it is possible for the person to start work or go on working under certain conditions.

Such conditions could include

- technical protective measures
- organizational protective measures, e.g., limitation of exposure periods
- transfer to workplaces known to involve lower levels of exposure
- personal protective equipment which takes the individual's state of health into account
- more frequent follow-up examinations

2.1.4   No concern about health

Initial examination	Follow-up examination

All other persons, provided there are no restrictions on their employment.

2.2   Medical advice

The advice in an individual case should be commensurate with the workplace situation and the results of the medical examinations.

Employees are to be informed about the biomonitoring results and about the potential prenatal toxicity and the toxic effects of the alkyllead compounds on reproduction.

Employees should be informed about general hygienic measures and personal protective equipment.

If during the course of his work in the company the occupational physician finds indications that the risk assessment should be brought up to date to improve health and safety standards, he is to inform the employer. When this is necessary, the interests of the employee are to be protected (medical confidentiality).

G 3

3   Supplementary notes

3.1   External and internal exposure

3.1.1   Occurrence, sources of hazards

Listed below are the kinds of processes, workplaces or activities, including cleaning and repair work, for which exposure to alkyllead compounds must be expected. This must be taken into account during the risk assessment:
- production
- adding to aviation fuel (for piston engines and propeller aircraft)
- filling and emptying of tankers and tank wagons with tetramethyllead or tetraethyllead, especially when attaching and detaching the hoses
- cleaning of tank wagons, tanks and pipes which have contained tetramethyllead or tetraethyllead or leaded fuels
- garages servicing veteran cars
- renovation of petrol stations where skin contact is conceivable.

Occurrence and hazards for specific substances are documented in the information system on hazardous substances (GESTIS) (see Section 4).

3.1.2 Physicochemical properties and classification

The information system on hazardous substances (GESTIS) provides details of international threshold limit values, classification, evaluation and other substance-specific information (see Section 4).

Additional information is to be found in the recommendations of the DFG Commission for the Investigation of Health Hazards of Chemical Compounds in the Work Area (List of MAK and BAT Values).

Alkyllead compounds are colourless, dense, oily fluids with a sweetish ether-like odour; they are miscible with organic solvents and practically insoluble in water. They react readily with most inorganic acids and many organic acids. Under rigorous reaction conditions Pb(II) salts are formed. In the light they are decomposed photolytically, at high temperatures (>100°C) thermolytically to yield lead and hydrocarbons or their oxidation products. The most important members of this group of compounds are tetramethyllead and tetraethyllead.

Tetramethyllead
Formula	$Pb(CH_3)_4$
CAS number	75-74-1
MAK value[1]	0.05 mg/m^3

Tetraethyllead
Formula	$Pb(C_2H_5)_4$
CAS number	78-00-2
MAK value[1]	0.05 mg/m^3

3.1.3 Uptake

The alkyllead compounds are taken up via the airways and the skin (high risk of absorption). Tetramethyllead is taken up through the skin much less readily than is tetraethyllead, but because of its higher volatility it is taken up more readily through the lungs.

3.1.4 Biomonitoring

Information about biomonitoring may be found in Appendix 1 "Biomonitoring".

---

[1] Maximale Arbeitsplatz-Konzentration (MAK) = maximum workplace concentration

Biological tolerance value for occupational exposures

Substance	Parameter	BAT[2]	Assay material	Sampling time
tetraethyllead	diethyllead	25 µg/l, calculated as Pb	urine	end of exposure or end of shift
	total lead (also applies for mixtures with tetramethyllead)	50 µg/l	urine	end of exposure or end of shift
tetramethyllead	see tetraethyllead			

Biomonitoring should be carried out with reliable methods and meet quality control requirements (see Appendix 1 "Biomonitoring").

3.2   Functional disorders, symptoms

3.2.1   Mode of action
Tetraalkyllead compounds are metabolized in the liver to yield trialkyllead compounds and lead. The trialkyllead compounds are responsible for the acute toxic effects. They are excreted only slowly in the urine and so can accumulate in the organism.

3.2.2   Acute and subacute effects on health
Alkyllead compounds are systemically highly toxic. They cause especially irritative and degenerative effects in the central nervous system. The following symptoms are often first noticed hours or even days after exposure:
• anorexia, nausea, vomiting
• sleeplessness, headaches, dizziness
• anxiety, confusion, irritability, excitability, tremor, hallucinations
• cardiovascular disorders (hypotension, bradycardia)
In severe cases: after a latency period acute psychosis, spasms, delirium, high temperature, coma.
After survival of the acute phase, recovery usually takes place within a few months.

---

[2] Biologischer Arbeitsstoff-Toleranzwert (BAT) = biological tolerance value for occupational exposures

3.2.3 Chronic effects on health

In chronic intoxications the nervous system is also the main target. Neurological disorders correlate with increased blood lead levels (see also G 2 "Lead and lead compounds"). The symptoms include:
- excitability, depression, hallucinations
- headaches
- low blood pressure
- tremor, ataxia, neurasthenia

The familiar signs of inorganic lead poisoning such as anaemia, increased number of basophilic punctate erythrocytes, motor nerve damage with radial paralysis and wristdrop and Burton sign (blue line along the gums) are not seen in cases of alkyl-lead poisoning. Also the symptoms listed in Sections 3.2.2 and 3.2.3 are not characteristic on their own and can be confused with the symptoms of alcoholism, drug addiction, schizophrenia and tertiary syphilis. Decisive for the differential diagnosis is only the relative lead level in blood (see G 2 "Lead and lead compounds") or in urine.

4 References

Commission Recommendation 2003/670/EC concerning the European schedule of occupational diseases. Annex I

Council Directive 98/24/EC on the protection of the health and safety of workers from the risks related to chemical agents at work

Deutsche Forschungsgemeinschaft (German Research Foundation, DFG) (ed) List of MAK and BAT Values 2007. Maximum Concentrations and Biological Tolerance Values at the workplace. Wiley-VCH, Weinheim

Deutsche Forschungsgemeinschaft (German Research Foundation, DFG) (ed) The MAK-Collection for Occupational Health and Safety. Wiley-VCH at: www.mrw.interscience.wiley.com/makbat

GESTIS-database on hazardous substances, BGIA at: www.dguv.de/bgia/gestis-database

GESTIS-international limit values for chemical agents, BGIA at: www.dguv.de/bgia/gestis-limit-values

G 4   Substances which cause skin cancer or skin alterations which tend to become cancerous

Committee for occupational medicine, working group "Hazardous substances", Berufsgenossenschaft der chemischen Industrie, Heidelberg

Preliminary remarks

The present guideline describes a scheme for occupational medical prophylaxis which aims to prevent or ensure early diagnosis of disorders which can be caused by substances which cause skin cancer or skin alterations which tend to become cancerous.

Schedule

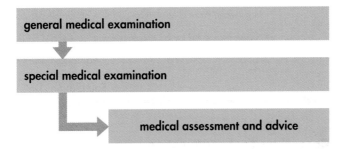

1   Medical examinations

Occupational medical examinations are to be carried out for persons exposed at work to levels of polycyclic aromatic hydrocarbons (PAH, pyrolysis products of organic materials, e.g. black coal tar, pitch, soot, etc) which could have adverse effects on health (e.g. when the occupational exposure limit value is exceeded) or for whom dermal absorption of such substances could endanger health.

1.1   Examinations, intervals between examinations

initial examination	before taking up the job
first follow-up examination	after 24–36 months
further follow-up examinations	after 24–36 months and when leaving the job
premature follow-up examination	• after a serious or prolonged illness which could cause concern as to whether the activity should be continued • in individual cases when the physician considers it necessary, e.g. when there is short-term concern about the person's health • when requested by an employee who suspects a causal association between his or her illness and work

1.2   Medical examination schedule

1.2.1   General medical examination

Initial examination

review of past history (general anamnesis, work anamnesis)

Follow-up examination

interim anamnesis (including detailed work anamnesis)

1.2.2   Special medical examination

Initial examination

- urinalysis (multiple test strips)
- examination of the skin

Follow-up examination

- urinalysis (multiple test strips)
- biomonitoring (1-hydroxypyrene in urine)
- specific anamnesis: skin changes and sensitivity to sunlight
- inspection of the whole body (including scrotal region); particular attention to be paid to suspicious skin changes such as comedos, folliculitis, cysts, circumscribed melanosis, keratosis, hyperkeratosis, eczema, pseudoscleroderma, leukomelanoderma, flat papillomas, leukoplakia, tar keratosis, farmers' or sailors' skin, basaloma, squamous epithelial carcinoma
- if warts are found, examination by a skin specialist, perhaps excision and histology
- if appropriate, photographic documentation of the skin for comparison with later findings

G 4

1.3   Requirements for the medical examinations

- competent doctor or occupational health professional
- the physician should have experience in the assessment of occupational dermatosis
- laboratory analyses carried out with appropriate quality control (Good Laboratory Practice)

2   Occupational medical assessment and advice

2.1   Assessment criteria

An assessment is only possible when the workplace situation and the exposure of the individual are known. For this purpose a risk assessment as defined in Article 4 Council directive 98/24/EC must have been carried out; it must specify which technical, organizational and individual protective measures have been applied.

2.1.1   Long-term concern about health

| Initial examination | Follow-up examination |

Persons with severe disorders:
- sensitivity of the skin to UV light reported in anamnesis, marked seborrhoea
- extensive vitiligo
- marked skin changes of the kind seen in farmers' or sailors' skin
- skin cancer and/or its precursors, also after successful treatment
- marked ichthyosis
- porphyria cutanea tarda

2.1.2   Short-term concern about health

not applicable

2.1.3   No concern about health under certain conditions

| Initial examination | Follow-up examination |

If the illnesses or functional disorders mentioned in Section 2.1.1 are less severe, the doctor should establish whether or not it is possible for the person to start work or go on working under certain conditions. Such conditions could include
- technical protective measures
- organizational protective measures, e.g., limitation of exposure periods
- transfer to workplaces known to involve lower levels of exposure
- personal protective equipment which takes the individual's state of health into account
- more frequent follow-up examinations.

At 12-month intervals persons with, e.g., the following symptoms should be examined
- particularly light-sensitive skin (check sensitivity to UV light)
- acne (apart from acne juvenilis)
- moderate seborrhoea
- a tendency to eczema

2.1.4   No concern about health

| Initial examination | Follow-up examination |

All other persons, provided there are no restrictions on their employment.

2.2   Medical advice

The advice in an individual case should be commensurate with the workplace situation and the results of the medical examinations.

Employees are to be informed about the biomonitoring results.

Employees should be informed about general hygienic measures and personal protective equipment.

Because these substances may be readily absorbed through the skin, skin protection is particularly important.

Employees should be advised that PAH and pyrolysis products of organic materials may have carcinogenic effects in other organs (e.g. airways) and have germ cell mutagenic and prenatal toxic effects and toxic effects on reproduction.

Instruction of the employees in inspection of their own skin; motivation of the employees to do this regularly and, if appropriate, to protect their skin from sunlight.

If during the course of his work in the company the occupational physician finds indications that the risk assessment should be brought up to date to improve health and safety standards, he is to inform the employer. When this is necessary, the interests of the employee are to be protected (medical confidentiality).

G 4

3   Supplementary notes

3.1   External and internal exposure

3.1.1   Occurrence, sources of hazards

Listed below are the kinds of processes, workplaces or activities, including cleaning and repair work, for which exposure to PAH/pyrolysis products of organic material must be expected. This must be taken into account during the risk assessment:

- work on or close to the ovens of a coking plant including tar separation
- in the production of carbon (high-fired carbon) and electrographite in open processes without direct exhaust systems, where tar and pitch can be encountered (e.g., pitch store, mixer, press, impregnation, oven)
- aluminium production in the following areas: production of anodes, Söderberg electrolysis works, prebaked anode production in open ovens, cathode production from hot/cold carbon ramming paste, anode forge if products containing pitch are used.
- tar impregnation systems
- in foundries during running off and emptying of moulds if coal dust or coal-tar pitch preparations or other such organic materials are used as sources of carbon
- processing of lenses in the optical industry when coal-tar pitch is used
- cleaning chimneys
- loading tar

- servicing, maintenance and inspection of plants for gas treatment and recovery of carbonaceous materials in coking plants
- in blast furnace plants in the area of the casting house especially if there is no house or trough exhaust system, when cleaning the clay gun machine, in the production of clays containing pitch, when filling the clay gun machine and preparing the trough with ramming pastes containing pitch
- in steel works in the production and processing of ramming pastes containing tar or pitch and in the preparation and use of these pastes and of carbon bricks bonded with tar or pitch for repair and relining of converters, melting pots and pans
- when heating converters and pans which are lined with pastes or blocks containing tar or pitch and when smelting steel after relining the smelter
- in metal smelters and foundries when heating ovens and pans newly relined with pastes containing pitch
- briquetting with coal-tar pitch
- production of silicon carbide crucibles
- impregnation of wood with coal-tar oil
- application of insulating coatings of coal-tar pitch, coal-tar oil and of preparations containing coal-tar pitch (e.g. for ships)
- pitch-processing units in tar refineries
- roofing jobs where coal-tar pitch and preparations containing coal-tar pitch are handled
- insulation with coal-tar pitch
- road construction where coal-tar pitch is used
- application of spray-coatings containing coal-tar oil and coal-tar pitch
- smoking of fish and meat
- use of oil quenching baths in hardening plants

Occurrence and hazards for specific substances are documented in the information system on hazardous substances (GESTIS) (see Section 4).

3.1.2   Physicochemical properties and classification

At present it makes sense to select benzo[a]pyrene as reference substance for pyrolysis products containing carcinogenic polycyclic aromatic hydrocarbons.

Benzo[a]pyrene
Formula $C_{20}H_{12}$
CAS number   50-32-8

The information system on hazardous substances (GESTIS) provides details of international threshold limit values, classification, evaluation and other substance-specific information (see Section 4).

Additional information is to be found in the recommendations of the DFG Commission for the Investigation of Health Hazards of Chemical Compounds in the Work Area (List of MAK and BAT Values).

3.1.3   Uptake

Uptake is via the skin and by inhalation. It is currently not known whether the incidence of skin tumours is also increased in persons exposed only via the airways.

3.1.4   Biomonitoring

Biomonitoring should be carried out with reliable methods and meet quality control requirements. Information about biomonitoring may be found in Appendix 1 "Biomonitoring".

3.2   Functional disorders, symptoms

Exposure at the workplaces listed in Section 3.1.1 can result inflammatory reddening of the skin and dermatitis (eczema) with itching and increased sensitivity to sunlight. After longer exposures diffuse hyperpigmentation develops and can progress to diffuse or circumscribed melanosis, folliculitis and acne. On skin in this state, but also without these preliminary signs, tar keratosis can develop: single or multiple variously sized warty lesions, in appearance not distinguishable from verruca vulgaris. These warts tend to become cancerous. Tar keratosis can develop after relatively short exposures but more often after several years and even after the end of exposure, especially on the face, ears, back of the hands, sometimes also on the forearms, lower abdomen and scrotum.

The substances mentioned in Section 3.1.1 are liquid or solid mixtures of high molecular weight hydrocarbons (from aliphatic to polycyclic aromatics). At some workplaces and depending on the processing temperatures, inhalation of the substances may be expected and in individual cases systemic carcinomas such as larynx or lung cancer can develop. It is at present unclear whether the development of bladder cancer can also be associated with such exposures. This should be taken into account during the medical examinations.

3.2.1   Mode of action

Chemical carcinogens can damage the skin after direct exposure but also after contact with dust, vapour or clothing contaminated with the substances. Heat and mechanical skin damage can promote such effects.

Physical carcinogens, e.g. UV light, especially in the UV-B spectral region, can damage exposed skin. The duration of exposure to the substances mentioned above which is necessary for the development of skin cancer or skin changes which tend to become cancerous is generally several years to several decades; it can, however, be much less. Even after the end of exposure, such developments are possible.

G 4

4   References

Commission Recommendation 2003/670/EC concerning the European schedule of occupational diseases. Annex I

Council Directive 67/548/EEC on the approximation of the laws, regulations and administrative provisions relating to the classification, packaging and labelling of dangerous substances

Council Directive 98/24/EC on the protection of the health and safety of workers from the risks related to chemical agents at work

Deutsche Forschungsgemeinschaft (German Research Foundation, DFG) (ed) List of MAK and BAT Values 2007. Maximum Concentrations and Biological Tolerance Values at the workplace. Wiley-VCH, Weinheim

Deutsche Forschungsgemeinschaft (German Research Foundation, DFG) (ed) The MAK-Collection for Occupational Health and Safety. Wiley-VCH
at: www.mrw.interscience.wiley.com/makbat

GESTIS-database on hazardous substances. BGIA
at: www.dguv.de/bgia/gestis-database

GESTIS-international limit values for chemical agents. BGIA
at: www.dguv.de/bgia/gestis-limit-values

Letzel S, Drexler H (1998) Occupational-Related Tumors in Tar Refinery Workers. Journal of the American Academy of Dermatology 39: 712–720

G 5   Ethylene glycol dinitrate and glycerol trinitrate (glycol dinitrate and nitroglycerin)

Committee for occupational medicine, working group "Hazardous substances", Berufsgenossenschaft der chemischen Industrie, Heidelberg

Preliminary remarks

The present guideline describes a scheme for occupational medical prophylaxis which aims to prevent or ensure early diagnosis of disorders which can be caused by ethylene glycol dinitrate (glycol dinitrate) or glycerol trinitrate (nitroglycerin).

G 5

Schedule

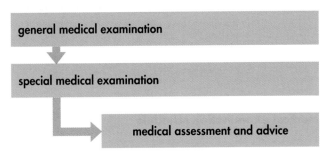

1 Medical examinations

Occupational medical examinations are to be carried out for persons exposed at work to levels of ethylene glycol dinitrate (glycol dinitrate) or glycerol trinitrate (nitroglycerin) which could have adverse effects on health (e.g. when the occupational exposure limit value is exceeded) or for whom dermal absorption could endanger health.

1.1 Examinations, intervals between examinations

initial examination	before taking up the job
first follow-up examination	after 6–12 months
further follow-up examinations	after 12–24 months and when leaving the job
premature follow-up examination	• after a serious or prolonged illness which could cause concern as to whether the activity should be continued • in individual cases when the physician considers it necessary, e.g. when there is short-term concern about the person's health • when requested by an employee who suspects a causal association between his or her illness and work

1.2 Medical examination schedule

1.2.1 General medical examination

Initial examination

• review of past history (general anamnesis, work anamnesis, symptoms)
• urinalysis (multiple test strips, sediment)

Follow-up examination

• interim anamnesis (including work anamnesis)
• urinalysis (multiple test strips, sediment)

1.2.2   Special medical examination

Initial examination	Follow-up examination

- full blood count
- ergometry
- if other additives (e.g. TNT) are used, their specific toxic effects are also to be taken into account

Also helpful:
- cardiocirculatory function test (e.g. Schellong test)
- long-term blood pressure monitoring

1.3.1   Requirements for the medical examinations

- competent doctor or occupational health professional
- laboratory analyses carried out with appropriate quality control (Good Laboratory Practice)

G 5

2   Occupational medical assessment and advice

An assessment is only possible when the workplace situation and the exposure of the individual are known. For this purpose a risk assessment as defined in Article 4 Council directive 98/24/EC must have been carried out; it must specify which technical, organizational and individual protective measures have been applied.

2.1   Assessment criteria

2.1.1   Long-term concern about health

Initial examination	Follow-up examination

Persons with
- cardiac disorders
- relevant ECG changes
- blood pressure values (long-term blood pressure monitoring!) of
  a) systolic   more than 20 kPa (150 mm Hg) or
                  less than 13 kPa (100 mm Hg)
  b) diastolic   more than 12 kPa (90 mm Hg) or
                  less than   8 kPa (60 mm Hg)
  c) pulse pressure less than   4 kPa (30 mm Hg)
- strain for the cardiovascular system because of other organ damage

2.1.2   Short-term concern about health

| Initial examination | Follow-up examination |

Persons with the disorders mentioned in Section 2.1.1, provided recovery is to be expected.

2.1.3   No concern about health under certain conditions

| Initial examination | Follow-up examination |

If the illnesses or functional disorders mentioned in Section 2.1.1 are less severe, the doctor should establish whether or not it is possible for the person to start work or go on working under certain conditions. Such conditions could include
- technical protective measures
- organizational protective measures, e.g., limitation of exposure periods
- transfer to workplaces known to involve lower levels of exposure
- personal protective equipment which takes the individual's state of health into account
- more frequent follow-up examinations

2.1.4   No concern about health

| Initial examination | Follow-up examination |

All other persons, provided there are no restrictions on their employment.

2.2   Medical advice

The advice in an individual case should be commensurate with the workplace situation and the results of the medical examinations. Employees should be advised to have their blood pressure checked regularly and informed about general hygienic measures and personal protective equipment.

If during the course of his work in the company the occupational physician finds indications that the risk assessment should be brought up to date to improve health and safety standards, he is to inform the employer. When this is necessary, the interests of the employee are to be protected (medical confidentiality).

3   Supplementary notes

3.1   External and internal exposure

3.1.1   Occurrence, sources of hazards

Listed below are the kinds of processes, workplaces or activities, including cleaning and repair work, for which exposure to ethylene glycol dinitrate (glycol dinitrate) or glycerol trinitrate (nitroglycerin) must be expected. This must be taken into account during the risk assessment:
- nitration of glycerol or ethylene glycol
- transport of blasting oils and explosives within the plant
- gelatinization of the nitrate ester
- production of powder cake (powder paste)
- mixing of explosives and filling cartridges
- processing
- destruction of reject material

Occurrence and hazards for specific substances are documented in the information system on hazardous substances (GESTIS) (see Section 4).

3.1.2   Physicochemical properties and classification

Ethylene glycol dinitrate (glycol dinitrate) and glycerol trinitrate (nitroglycerin) are nitric acid esters of polyhydric alcohols (glycerol, glycol).
They are colourless oily liquids. They are sensitive to shock, impact, friction, and concussion and to sudden heating or other ignition sources and react with rapid decomposition forming large amounts of gas (steam, carbon monoxide, carbon dioxide, nitrogen oxides). With ethylene glycol dinitrate there is also a risk of build-up of electrostatic charge (risk of explosion!). The substances are readily soluble in most organic solvents and poorly soluble in water.
At normal temperatures they are stable, that is, they can be stored for unlimited periods of time. Ethylene glycol dinitrate has a higher vapour pressure than glycerol trinitrate (about 30-fold), that is, it is much more volatile.
The substances are often combined in the production of explosives. This increases the stability of the explosive to frost (because of the lower melting point of ethylene glycol dinitrate).

G 5

Glycerol trinitrate
Formula

$$CH_2-O-NO_2$$
$$|$$
$$CH-O-NO_2$$
$$|$$
$$CH_2-O-NO_2$$

CAS number   55-63-0

Ethylene glycol dinitrate (glycol dinitrate)
Formula

$$CH_2-O-NO_2$$
$$|$$
$$CH_2-O-NO_2$$

CAS number   628-96-6
MAK value[1]   0.32 mg/m^3 (0.05 ppm)

The information system on hazardous substances (GESTIS) provides details of international threshold limit values, classification, evaluation and other substance-specific information (see Section 4).

3.1.3   Uptake

The substances are taken up via the airways and the skin.

3.2   Functional disorders, symptoms

3.2.1   Mode of action

The substances are readily and rapidly absorbed via the skin and the mucous membranes of the airways and digestive tract and cause dilation of the blood vessels and consequent reductions in blood pressure, first systolic and then diastolic.

In addition to the peripheral effects on the circulatory system and their consequences, these substances can also have central effects.

Chronic exposure to low doses of the substances causes a slow increase in the diastolic blood pressure, also an expression of counter-regulation. The result is a reduction in pulse pressure.

3.2.2   Acute and subacute effects on health

Symptoms of acute poisoning include:
* headaches
* dizziness

---

[1] Maximale Arbeitsplatz-Konzentration (MAK) = maximum workplace concentration

- nausea
- flushing
- peripheral paraesthesia
- anxiety
- pains in the heart region
- low blood pressure
- bradycardia or tachycardia
- unconsciousness
- circulatory collapse

3.2.3   Chronic effects on health

The symptoms described after chronic exposures include:
- headaches
- feeling hot
- inebriation
- anorexia
- alcohol intolerance
- chest pains (as in angina pectoris)
- arteriosclerotic changes

G 5

After many years of high level exposure, e.g. as a mix-house worker or cartridge filler, sudden death from acute heart failure can occur.

4   References

Commission Recommendation 2003/670/EC concerning the European schedule of occupational diseases. Annex I

Council Directive 67/548/EEC on the approximation of the laws, regulations and administrative provisions relating to the classification, packaging and labelling of dangerous substances

Council Directive 98/24/EC on the protection of the health and safety of workers from the risks related to chemical agents at work

Deutsche Forschungsgemeinschaft (German Research Foundation, DFG) (ed) List of MAK and BAT Values 2007. Maximum Concentrations and Biological Tolerance Values at the workplace. Wiley-VCH, Weinheim

Deutsche Forschungsgemeinschaft (German Research Foundation, DFG) (ed) The MAK-Collection for Occupational Health and Safety. Wiley-VCH
    at: www.mrw.interscience.wiley.com/makbat

GESTIS-database on hazardous substances. BGIA
    at: www.dguv.de/bgia/gestis-database

GESTIS-international limit values for chemical agents. BGIA
    at: www.dguv.de/bgia/gestis-limit-values

G 6   Carbon disulfide

Committee for occupational medicine, working group "Hazardous substances", Berufsgenossenschaft der chemischen Industrie, Heidelberg

Preliminary remarks

The present guideline describes a scheme for occupational medical prophylaxis which aims to prevent or ensure early diagnosis of disorders which can be caused by carbon disulfide.

Schedule

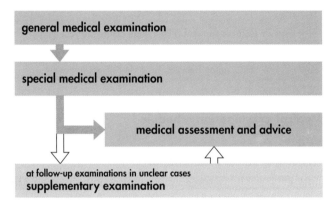

1   Medical examinations

Occupational medical examinations are to be carried out for persons exposed at work to levels of carbon disulfide which could have adverse effects on health (e.g. when the occupational exposure limit value is exceeded) or for whom dermal absorption could endanger health.

1.1   Examinations, intervals between examinations

initial examination	before taking up the job
first follow-up examination	after 6–12 months
further follow-up examinations	after 6–12 months and when leaving the job
premature follow-up examination	• after an illness lasting for several weeks or when a physical handicap gives cause for concern about whether the work should be continued • in individual cases when the physician considers it necessary, e.g. when there is short-term concern about the person's health • when requested by an employee who suspects a causal association between his or her illness and work

1.2   Medical examination schedule

1.2.1   General medical examination

Initial examination

• review of past history (general anamnesis, work anamnesis)
  Particular attention should be paid to extensive skin changes (e.g. as in psoriasis vulgaris).
• urinalysis (multiple test strips, sediment)

Follow-up examination

- interim anamnesis (including detailed work anamnesis)
  Particular attention should be paid to:
  - levels of exposure to carbon disulfide (any dermal exposure, any brief exposure peaks above the threshold value for air)
  - symptoms such as lack of appetite, alcohol intolerance, sleep disorders, memory problems, confusion, dulling of intellect, occasional euphoria, irritability, quarrelsomeness
  - extensive skin changes (e.g. as in psoriasis vulgaris)

- *Job-related examinations*
  Particular attention should be paid to:
  - sensitivity disorders (distal paresthesia, hypoaesthesia, hypoalgesia, dysaesthesia)
  - disorders of reflexes (weakening of the Achilles tendon reflex relative to the reflexes of the upper extremities)
  - tremor of the extremities, parkinsonian symptoms
  - disorders of colour vision
  - psychic symptoms (irritability, depression)
  - weight loss
  - palpation of the arteria dorsalis pedis and the arteria tibialis posterior
- urinalysis (multiple test strips, sediment)

G 6

1.2.2   Special medical examination

Initial examination

- ergometry
- determination of the vibratory sensibility by means of a 128 Hz tuning fork

Also helpful:
- cholesterol and triglycerides
- γ-GT, SGPT(ALT)
- blood count

Follow-up examination

Like the initial examination but, in addition,
- biomonitoring (see Section 3.1.4)

1.2.3   Supplementary examination

Follow-up examination

In cases which are still unclear after the general medical examination described in Section 1.2, specialist neurological and/or psychiatric examinations may be carried out, perhaps with EEG and electroneuromyography and electromyography.

1.3   Requirements for the medical examinations

- competent doctor or occupational health professional
- laboratory analyses carried out with appropriate quality control (Good Laboratory Practice)

2   Occupational medical assessment and advice

An assessment is only possible when the workplace situation and the exposure of the individual are known. For this purpose a risk assessment as defined in Article 4 Council directive 98/24/EC must have been carried out; it must specify which technical, organizational and individual protective measures have been applied.

2.1   Assessment criteria

2.1.1   Long-term concern about health

| Initial examination | Follow-up examination |

Persons with
- disorders of the peripheral and/or central nervous systems, especially with anamnestic or clinical indications of polyneuropathy and/or psychic disorders
- cardiac disorders affecting the circulatory system
- arteriosclerosis
- marked vegetative lability
- high blood pressure with systolic blood pressure values above 21 kPa (160 mm Hg), diastolic above 13 kPa (100 mm Hg)
- primary or secondary anaemia
- gastrointestinal ulcers
- renal disorders
- damaged liver parenchyma
- extensive skin changes (e.g. as in psoriasis vulgaris)
- alcohol or drug addiction

2.1.2   Short-term concern about health

Initial examination

Persons with the disorders mentioned in Section 2.1.1 provided recovery is to be expected.

Follow-up examination

Like the initial examination but, in addition,
- persons with signs of carbon disulfide poisoning as a result of an unusually high-level exposure during a break-down or accident for the period until the clinical findings return to normal

Note: persons returning to work may be hypersensitive to carbon disulfide.

2.1.3   No concern about health under certain conditions

Initial examination   **Follow-up examination**

If the illnesses or functional disorders mentioned in Section 2.1.1 are less severe, the doctor should establish whether or not it is possible for the person to return to work or go on working under certain conditions. Such conditions could include

G 6

- technical protective measures
- organizational protective measures, e.g., limitation of exposure periods
- transfer to workplaces known to involve lower levels of exposure
- personal protective equipment which takes the individual's state of health into account
- more frequent follow-up examinations

2.1.4   No concern about health

Initial examination   **Follow-up examination**

All other persons, provided there are no restrictions on their employment.

2.2   Medical advice

The advice in an individual case should be commensurate with the workplace situation and the results of the medical examinations.

Employees are to be informed about the biomonitoring results.

They should be informed about general hygienic measures and personal protective equipment. Because carbon disulfide readily penetrates the skin, the wearing of protective clothing is of particular significance.

Substance-specific protective measures are documented in the information system on hazardous substances (GESTIS) in the section "Handling and usage" (see Section 4).

Employees should be advised as to the potential reproductive and prenatal toxicity of carbon disulfide.

If during the course of his work in the company the occupational physician finds indications that the risk assessment should be brought up to date to improve health and safety standards, he is to inform the employer. When this is necessary, the interests of the employee are to be protected (medical confidentiality).

3   Supplementary notes

3.1   External and internal exposure

3.1.1   Occurrence, sources of hazards

Occurrence and hazards are documented in the information system on hazardous substances (GESTIS) (see Section 4).
Health surveillance is necessary for persons working with carbon disulfide especially for the following kinds of processes, workplaces or activities, including cleaning and repair work:
• production of carbon disulfide
• production of carbon tetrachloride from carbon disulfide
• production and processing of viscose
• extraction of fats from oily seeds, bones, wool, skins
• extraction of sulfur from rock
• purification of crude paraffin

3.1.2   Physicochemical properties and classification

Carbon disulfide is – depending on its purity – a colourless to yellowish, highly refractive, poorly water-soluble liquid which smells like rotten radishes. It is very readily absorbed on activated charcoal. Because of its high vapour pressure, carbon disulfide evaporates very readily at normal room temperature. The vapour is heavier than air and can accumulate at floor level.

Carbon disulfide
Formula CS_2
CAS number   75-15-0
MAK value[1]   16 mg/m^3 (5 ppm)

---

[1] Maximale Arbeitsplatz-Konzentration (MAK) = maximum workplace concentration

The information system on hazardous substances (GESTIS) provides details of international threshold limit values, classification, evaluation and other substance-specific information (see Section 4).

3.1.3   Uptake
Carbon disulfide is taken up via the airways and the skin.

3.1.4   Biomonitoring
Information about biomonitoring may be found in Appendix 1 "Biomonitoring".

Biological tolerance value for occupational exposures

Substance	Parameter	BAT[2]	Assay material	Sampling time
carbon disulfide	2-thio-thiazoli-dine-4-carboxylic acid (TTCA)	8 mg/l	urine	end of exposure or end of shift

The level of TTCA in the urine can be increased after consumption of raw cabbage. This has, however, probably no significance for occupational medical practice. Biomonitoring should be carried out with reliable methods and meet quality control requirements (see Appendix 1 "Biomonitoring").

3.2   Functional disorders, symptoms

3.2.1   Mode of action
Carbon disulfide (CS_2) taken up by the body is transported in erythrocytes and plasma in bound and free form and distributed rapidly in the tissues. The high lipid-solubility of the substance and its ability to form covalent bonds with amino groups explains the high affinity of CS_2 to all organs. CS_2 is metabolized to carbonyl sulfide and atomic sulfur mostly by the enzyme system cytochrome P450 in the endoplasmic reticulum of the liver cells. The reactive sulfur binds to sulfhydryl groups of proteins and so probably disrupts enzyme function. Direct reaction of CS_2 with amino and sulfhydryl groups of amino acids yields compounds such as dithiocarbamic acids, trithiocarbamic acids and xanthogenic acids. The condensation product of the reaction of CS_2 with the amino acid cysteine, 2-thio-thiazolidine-4-carboxylic acid (TTCA), is excreted in the urine in concentrations directly related to the level of CS_2 exposure and so is a suitable parameter of internal exposure.

---

[2] Biologischer Arbeitsstoff-Toleranzwert (BAT) = biological tolerance value for occupational exposures

The biochemical pathomechanism of the neurotoxic effects of CS_2 has still not been clarified definitively in spite of intensive research. CS_2 can damage the peripheral and central nervous systems. It causes swelling and disintegration of the axons of peripheral nerves in the sense of a wallerian degeneration, primary axon degeneration. In the central nervous system after exposure to CS_2, primary neuron degeneration with swelling or shrinkage of the cytoplasm is found. The affected central nervous system structures appear to differ in different species. Central nervous system lesions can also result from CS_2-induced vascular changes which induce circulatory disorders.

Of clinical relevance are also the effects of CS_2 on the cardiovascular system because these could be detected in persons exposed long term, especially under the exposure conditions which prevailed in the viscose industry before the exposure threshold was introduced. An association of increased mortality from coronary heart disorders with chronic CS_2-exposure has been found independently in several study collectives. At present, the adverse effects of CS_2 on the cardiocirculatory and peripheral nervous systems must be considered to be the critical toxic effects.

3.2.2 Acute and subacute effects on health

After high doses the substance has marked narcotic effects, causing agitation, sleeplessness, logorrhoea, psychic disorders, rapid deep unconsciousness and even death.

3.2.3 Chronic effects on health

- signs of damage in the central, peripheral or autonomic nervous system (especially polyneuropathy with distal sensitivity disorders, weakened distal muscle reflexes)
- vessel damage in the sense of vessel sclerosis affecting the blood supply to the brain, heart, kidneys and extremities
- psychic changes mainly of the excitatory or depressive kind
- psychoses, performance insufficiency, loss of the ability to concentrate, rapid fatigue, emotional lability, encephalopathy
- tendency to gastrointestinal disorders, constant weight loss, lack of appetite

4   References

Commission Recommendation 2003/670/EC concerning the European schedule of occupational diseases. Annex I

Council Directive 98/24/EC on the protection of the health and safety of workers from the risks related to chemical agents at work

Deutsche Forschungsgemeinschaft (German Research Foundation, DFG) (ed) List of MAK and BAT Values 2007. Maximum Concentrations and Biological Tolerance Values at the workplace. Wiley-VCH, Weinheim

Deutsche Forschungsgemeinschaft (German Research Foundation, DFG) (ed) The MAK-Collection for Occupational Health and Safety. Wiley-VCH
at: www.mrw.interscience.wiley.com/makbat

GESTIS-database on hazardous substances. BGIA
at: www.dguv.de/bgia/gestis-database

GESTIS-international limit values for chemical agents. BGIA
at: www.dguv.de/bgia/gestis-limit-values

G 6

G 7   Carbon monoxide

Committee for occupational medicine, working group "Hazardous substances", Berufsgenossenschaft der chemischen Industrie, Heidelberg

Preliminary remarks

The present guideline describes a scheme for occupational medical prophylaxis which aims to prevent or ensure early diagnosis of disorders which can be caused by carbon monoxide.

Schedule

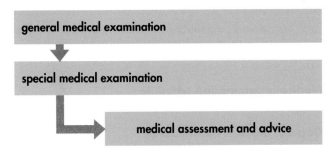

1   Medical examinations

Occupational medical examinations are to be carried out for persons at whose workplaces exposure to carbon monoxide could endanger health (e.g. the occupational exposure limit value is exceeded).

1.1   Examinations, intervals between examinations

initial examination	before taking up the job
first follow-up examination	after 24 months
further follow-up examinations	after 24 months and when leaving the job
premature follow-up examination	• after a serious or prolonged illness which could cause concern as to whether the activity should be continued • in individual cases when the physician considers it necessary, e.g. when there is short-term concern about the person's health • when requested by an employee who suspects a causal association between his or her illness and work

1.2   Medical examination schedule

1.2.1   General medical examination

Initial examination

• review of past history (general anamnesis, work anamnesis, smoking habits, symptoms)
Particular attention should be paid to cardiac findings and to neurological and psychic symptoms.

Follow-up examination

• interim anamnesis (including work anamnesis)
Attention is to be paid to headaches, dizziness, general lassitude, fatigability, irritability, sleeplessness and similar neurasthenic symptoms, memory problems (avoid suggestive questions!); perhaps also neurovegetative and ataxic disorders (equivocal!)

1.2.2   Special medical examination

Initial examination

- haemoglobin, erythrocytes
- spirometry
- ergometry

Follow-up examination

If "chronic carbon monoxide poisoning" is suspected, CO-Hb in blood should be determined repeatedly (see Section 3.1.4); the blood sample should be taken at the workplace towards the end of the shift and CO-Hb determined or the sample sent to an appropriate laboratory for this purpose.
When sending a sample it must be kept cool (not frozen) and have a gas-tight seal. The assay must be carried out within 24 h of sampling.

1.3   Requirements for the medical examinations

- competent doctor or occupational health professional
- laboratory analyses carried out with appropriate quality control (Good Laboratory Practice)
- necessary equipment:
  - ECG/ergometer
  - spirometer which displays flow-volume and volume-time curves simultaneously

G 7

2   Occupational medical assessment and advice

An assessment is only possible when the workplace situation and the exposure of the individual are known. For this purpose a risk assessment as defined in Article 4 Council directive 98/24/EC must have been carried out; it must specify which technical, organizational and individual protective measures have been applied.

2.1   Assessment criteria

2.1.1   Long-term concern about health

Initial examination   **Follow-up examination**

Persons with severe disorders of
- the heart
- the vascular system (severe arteriosclerosis)
- the lungs
- the thyroid gland (hyperthyroidism)

- the blood (anaemia)
- the central nervous system

2.1.2   Short-term concern about health

| Initial examination | Follow-up examination |

Persons with the disorders mentioned in Section 2.1.1, provided recovery is to be expected.

2.1.3   No concern about health under certain conditions

| Initial examination | Follow-up examination |

If the illnesses or functional disorders mentioned in Section 2.1.1 are less severe, the doctor should establish whether or not it is possible for the person to start work or go on working under certain conditions. Such conditions could include
- technical protective measures
- organizational protective measures, e.g., limitation of exposure periods
- transfer to workplaces known to involve lower levels of exposure
- personal protective equipment which takes the individual's state of health into account
- more frequent follow-up examinations

2.1.4   No concern about health

| Initial examination | Follow-up examination |

All other persons, provided there are no restrictions on their employment.

2.2   Medical advice

The advice in an individual case should be commensurate with the workplace situation and the results of the medical examinations. Employees are to be informed about the biomonitoring results.

Employees should be informed about general hygienic measures and personal protective equipment.

Women should be informed of the prenatal toxic effects of carbon monoxide.

Smokers should be advised that carbon monoxide is also taken up when smoking.

If during the course of his work in the company the occupational physician finds indications that the risk assessment should be brought up to date to improve health and safety standards, he is to inform the employer. When this is necessary, the interests of the employee are to be protected (medical confidentiality).

3   Supplementary notes

3.1   External and internal exposure

3.1.1   Occurrence, sources of hazards

Listed below are the kinds of processes, workplaces or activities, including cleaning and repair work, for which exposure to carbon monoxide must be expected. This must be taken into account during the risk assessment:

- workplaces at which carbon monoxide, a product of incomplete oxidation, is produced during burning of materials containing carbon
- workplaces at which carbon monoxide occurs in producer gas, coke-oven gas, blast-furnace gas, flue gas, clouds of smoke from an explosion, etc.
- workplaces near blast-furnaces and heat-treatment furnaces (annealing ovens)
- work at blast furnaces above tuyère level (hot-metal furnaces)
- work on cupola furnaces
- in foundries during draining off moulds and in the cooling zone
- near coke-ovens, also at times in metallurgical laboratories
- work at the hardening furnace
- work in furnace and chimney construction when the work must be done in or close to operating plant
- work in largely closed rooms in which carbon monoxide emissions in exhaust gases – especially from petrol motors, less from diesel motors – must be expected, e.g. near calender machines or generators, in garages servicing motor cars, enclosed garages for parking cars, car decks and road tunnels
- work for the fire brigade
- work in construction of furnaces and chimneys, in installation of heating, firing and gas-fired systems
- work in containers and enclosed spaces in which carbon monoxide can be produced, e.g., soldering with a white flame
- how far the employer must go in his considerations is shown by the fact that exposure to carbon monoxide must even be expected on ferries: for the employees who work on the car decks, sometimes for hours at a time, during loading and unloading of vehicles.

Occurrence and hazards are documented in the information system on hazardous substances (GESTIS) (see Section 4).

G 7

3.1.2   Physicochemical properties and classification

Carbon monoxide is a colourless, tasteless, odourless, inflammable, toxic gas. It has a very high diffusivity (penetrates ceilings and walls).

Carbon monoxide
Formula   CO
CAS number   630-08-0
MAK value[1]   35 mg/m^3 (30 ppm)

The information system on hazardous substances (GESTIS) provides details of international threshold limit values, classification, evaluation and other substance-specific information (see Section 4).
Additional information is to be found in the recommendations of the DFG Commission for the Investigation of Health Hazards of Chemical Compounds in the Work Area (List of MAK and BAT Values).

3.1.3   Uptake
Carbon monoxide is taken up mainly via the airways.

3.1.4   Biomonitoring
Information about biomonitoring may be found in Appendix 1 "Biomonitoring".

Biological tolerance value for occupational exposures

Substance	Parameter	BAT[2]	Assay material	Sampling time
carbon monoxide	CO-Hb	5 %	whole blood	end of exposure or end of shift

Biomonitoring should be carried out with reliable methods and meet quality control requirements (see Appendix 1 "Biomonitoring").
It must be taken into account that the CO-Hb level in smokers can be as high as 25 % (average level 10 %); the normal CO-Hb level in man is about 1 %.
Preliminary information as to whether or not and to what extent a person is suffering from acute carbon monoxide poisoning is obtained by determining the CO concentration in exhaled air, either with
• gas collection bag, Draeger tube and the appropriate suction pump, or with
• an assay apparatus with an electrochemical reaction cell and digital display

---

[1] Maximale Arbeitsplatz-Konzentration (MAK) = maximum workplace concentration
[2] Biologischer Arbeitsstoff-Toleranzwert (BAT) = biological tolerance value for occupational exposures

3.2   Functional disorders, symptoms

3.2.1   Mode of action

Carbon monoxide is a respiratory poison. Its toxicity is a result of its high affinity for haemoglobin and of the hypoxaemia caused by the formation of carboxyhaemoglobin. The binding of carbon monoxide to haemoglobin is, however, reversible. The affinity of carbon monoxide for haemoglobin is about three hundred times that of oxygen for haemoglobin. The toxicity is primarily a function of the formation of CO-Hb. This depends on the concentration of carbon monoxide in the inhaled air, the respiratory minute volume, the exposure time and the haemoglobin level. Carbon monoxide is not metabolized and is eliminated by exhalation.

3.2.2   Acute and subacute effects on health

Symptoms seen from CO-Hb levels of about 20 % and increasing
- headaches
- dizziness
- nausea
- tachycardia and increased blood pressure
- occasionally angina pectoris-like symptoms
- buzzing in the ears
- flickering in front of the eyes
- generalized weakness (weak knees)
- apathy
- occasional cramps
- sometimes confusion
- unconsciousness (at about 50 % CO-Hb)
- death (at 60 % to 70 % CO-Hb)

Sequelae affect mainly the central nervous system and the heart.

For acute carbon monoxide poisoning:
- immediate determination of carbon monoxide in the exhaled air and/or determination of CO-Hb in the blood (see Section 3.1.5)
- immediate ECG
- check ECG again at the latest before the person returns to work
- in some cases EEG

3.2.3   Chronic effects on health

Chronic carbon monoxide poisoning in the real sense has been considered to date to be rather unlikely. As a result of chronic poisoning caused by exposure to low levels of carbon monoxide (CO-Hb >5 %) symptoms such as headaches, tiredness, dizziness, nausea and reduced mental performance have been described. In this context, however, it must be pointed out that the CO-Hb levels in smokers can be as

G 7

high as 25 %. It has been suggested that psychovegetative disorders could be a result of frequently repeated abortive or subacute intoxications.

4   References

Commission Recommendation 2003/670/EC concerning the European schedule of occupational diseases. Annex I

Council Directive 67/548/EEC on the approximation of the laws, regulations and administrative provisions relating to the classification, packaging and labelling of dangerous substances

Council Directive 98/24/EC on the protection of the health and safety of workers from the risks related to chemical agents at work

Deutsche Forschungsgemeinschaft (German Research Foundation, DFG) (ed) List of MAK and BAT Values 2007. Maximum Concentrations and Biological Tolerance Values at the workplace. Wiley-VCH, Weinheim

Deutsche Forschungsgemeinschaft (German Research Foundation, DFG) (ed) The MAK-Collection for Occupational Health and Safety. Wiley-VCH
at: www.mrw.interscience.wiley.com/makbat

GESTIS-database on hazardous substances. BGIA
at: www.dguv.de/bgia/gestis-database

GESTIS-international limit values for chemical agents. BGIA
at: www.dguv.de/bgia/gestis-limit-values

G 8   Benzene

Committee for occupational medicine, working group "Hazardous substances",
Berufsgenossenschaft der chemischen Industrie, Heidelberg

Preliminary remarks

The present guideline describes a scheme for occupational medical prophylaxis
which aims to prevent or ensure early diagnosis of disorders which can be caused
by benzene.

Schedule

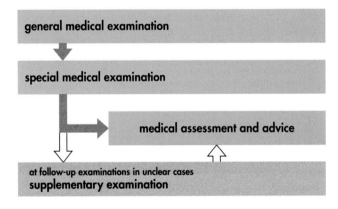

G 8

1   Medical examinations

Occupational medical examinations are to be carried out for persons exposed at work to levels of benzene which could have adverse effects on health (e.g. when the occupational exposure limit value is exceeded) or for whom dermal absorption could endanger health.

1.1   Examinations, intervals between examinations

initial examination	before taking up the job
first follow-up examination	after 6–12 months
further follow-up examinations	after 6–12 months and when leaving the job
premature follow-up examination	• after a serious or prolonged illness which could cause concern as to whether the activity should be continued • in individual cases when the physician considers it necessary, e.g. when there is short-term concern about the person's health • when requested by an employee who suspects a causal association between his or her illness and work

1.2   Medical examination schedule

1.2.1   General medical examination

Initial examination

• review of past history (general anamnesis, work anamnesis)
• urinalysis (multiple test strips)

Follow-up examination

• interim anamnesis (including work anamnesis); particular attention should be paid to an increased tendency to bleed (e.g. bleeding of the gums, bruising even after slight trauma, menorrhagia)
• urinalysis (multiple test strips)

1.2.2   Special medical examination

Initial examination

• full blood count

Follow-up examination

• full blood count
Also helpful:
• biomonitoring (see Section 3.1.4)

1.2.3   Supplementary examination

Follow-up examination

In unclear cases, haematology

1.3   Requirements for the medical examinations

• competent doctor or occupational health professional
• laboratory analyses carried out with appropriate quality control (Good Laboratory Practice)

G 8

2   Occupational medical assessment and advice

An assessment is only possible when the workplace situation and the exposure of the individual are known. For this purpose a risk assessment as defined in Article 4 Council directive 98/24/EC must have been carried out; it must specify which technical, organizational and individual protective measures have been applied.

2.1   Assessment criteria

2.1.1   Long-term concern about health

Initial examination   **Follow-up examination**

Persons with
• blood disorders
• disorders of the haematopoietic organs
• chronic bacterial infections
• alcohol addiction

2.1.2   Short-term concern about health

| Initial examination | Follow-up examination |

Persons with the disorders mentioned in Section 2.1.1, provided recovery is to be expected.

2.1.3   No concern about health under certain conditions

| Initial examination | Follow-up examination |

If the illnesses or functional disorders mentioned in Section 2.1.1 are less severe, the doctor should establish whether or not it is possible for the person to start work or go on working under certain conditions. Such conditions could include
- technical protective measures
- organizational protective measures, e.g., limitation of exposure periods
- transfer to workplaces known to involve lower levels of exposure
- personal protective equipment which takes the individual's state of health into account
- more frequent follow-up examinations

2.1.4   No concern about health

| Initial examination | Follow-up examination |

All other persons, provided there are no restrictions on their employment.

2.2   Medical advice

The advice in an individual case should be commensurate with the workplace situation and the results of the medical examinations.

Employees are to be informed about the biomonitoring results.

They should be informed about general hygienic measures and personal protective equipment. Because benzene readily penetrates the skin, the wearing of protective clothing is of particular significance. Substance-specific protective measures are documented in the information system on hazardous substances (GESTIS) in the section "Handling and usage" (see Section 4).

The effect of alcohol consumption, which can amplify the haematotoxicity of benzene, should also be discussed.

Employees should be advised as to the carcinogenic and germ cell mutagenic effects of benzene.

If during the course of his work in the company the occupational physician finds indications that the risk assessment should be brought up to date to improve health and safety standards, he is to inform the employer. When this is necessary, the interests of the employee are to be protected (medical confidentiality).

3   Supplementary notes

3.1   External and internal exposure

3.1.1   Occurrence, sources of hazards

Occurrence and hazards are documented in the information system on hazardous substances (GESTIS) (see Section 4).
Health surveillance is necessary for persons working with benzene, especially for the following kinds of processes, workplaces or activities, including cleaning and repair work:

- filling and emptying of containers involving disconnection of hoses and pipes or lifting of dipping pipes, and drawing liquid from containers during production, recovery, processing and transport of benzene or products containing benzene
- changing filters and catalysts, and taking samples during production, recovery, processing and transport of benzene and products containing benzene
- demolition and repair work on production systems for benzene
- automobile production (filling tanks of goods vehicles with internal combustion engines in the production factory without a fume extractor)
- petrol motor test stands (attaching and detaching the petrol hoses)
- servicing and cleaning of petrol pumps and tanks
- mechanical work on car petrol delivery systems involving frequent exposure
- work near the upper part of the coking-oven in coking plants

G 8

3.1.2   Physicochemical properties and classification

Benzene is a colourless, highly refractive, sparingly water-soluble, inflammable liquid with a characteristic odour. It is stable to heat (up to about 650°C) and oxidation; however, it evaporates very readily. The vapour is heavier than air and can accumulate at floor level.

Benzene
Formula $\qquad$ C_6H_6
CAS number $\qquad$ 71-43-2
OEL value[1] $\qquad$ 3.25 mg/m^3 (1 ppm)

The information system on hazardous substances (GESTIS) provides details of international threshold limit values, classification, evaluation and other substance-specific information (see Section 4).

---

[1] occupational exposure limit value of the European Community

3.1.3   Uptake

Benzene is taken up mainly via the airways. Moistening of large areas of skin with benzene may be expected to result in percutaneous uptake.

3.1.4   Biomonitoring

Information about biomonitoring may be found in Appendix 1 "Biomonitoring". Various internal and external factors (e.g. alcohol consumption) can influence the biomonitoring results and must be taken into account when interpreting these.

Exposure equivalents for carcinogenic materials (EKA[2]) from the List of MAK and BAT Values

		Sampling time: end of exposure or end of shift		
air		whole blood	urine	
benzene (ml/m^3)	benzene (mg/m^3)	benzene $(\mu g/l)$	S-phenyl-mercapturic acid (mg/g creatinine)	trans, trans-muconic acid (mg/l)
0.3	1	0.9	0.010	–
0.6	2	2.4	0.025	1.6
0.9	3	4.4	0.040	–
1.0	3.3	5	0.045	2
2	6.5	14	0.090	3
4	13	38	0.180	5
6	19.5	–	0.270	7

Biomonitoring should be carried out with reliable methods and meet quality control requirements (see Appendix 1 "Biomonitoring").

3.2   Functional disorders, symptoms

3.2.1   Mode of action

Benzene irritates the skin and mucous membranes. The amount absorbed through the skin depends on the exposure conditions.

About 50 % of inhaled benzene is exhaled and about 50 % metabolized. The benzoquinones which are formed in metabolism via epoxybenzene are probably the reaction products which can react with DNA and so must be seen as the ultimately carcinogenic metabolites.

---

[2] Expositionsäquivalente für Krebserzeugende Arbeitsstoffe = exposure equivalents for carcinogenic materials

The urinary metabolites include phenol, S-phenylmercapturic acid and *trans,trans*-muconic acid; the choice of sampling times and sampling intervals has a marked effect on the findings.

In acute intoxications resulting from inhalation of high concentrations of benzene, the narcotic effects predominate.

Long-term exposure to benzene can cause damage especially in the haematopoietic system and can have adverse effects on all or any of the functions of the bone marrow. Thus after long-term or discontinuous exposure to benzene in concentrations markedly higher than the OEL value, both reversible effects on the haematopoietic system such as aplastic anaemia and pancytopenia and also the development of leukaemia have been described; the latency period can be up to 20 years.

3.2.2   Acute and subacute effects on health

Narcotic effects.

3.2.3   Chronic effects on health

Disorders of or damage to the haematopoietic system.

G 8

4   References

Commission Recommendation 2003/670/EC concerning the European schedule of occupational diseases. Annex I

Council Directive 98/24/EC on the protection of the health and safety of workers from the risks related to chemical agents at work

Deutsche Forschungsgemeinschaft (German Research Foundation, DFG) (ed) List of MAK and BAT Values 2007. Maximum Concentrations and Biological Tolerance Values at the workplace. Wiley-VCH, Weinheim

Deutsche Forschungsgemeinschaft (German Research Foundation, DFG) (ed) The MAK-Collection for Occupational Health and Safety. Wiley-VCH
    at: www.mrw.interscience.wiley.com/makbat

GESTIS-database on hazardous substances. BGIA
    at: www.dguv.de/bgia/gestis-database

GESTIS-international limit values for chemical agents. BGIA
    at: www.dguv.de/bgia/gestis-limit-values

G 9   Mercury and mercury compounds

Committee for occupational medicine, working group "Hazardous substances", Berufsgenossenschaft der chemischen Industrie, Heidelberg

Preliminary remarks

The present guideline describes a scheme for occupational medical prophylaxis which aims to prevent or ensure early diagnosis of disorders which can be caused by mercury or mercury compounds.

Schedule

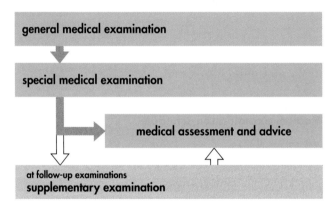

general medical examination

special medical examination

medical assessment and advice

at follow-up examinations
supplementary examination

G 9

1　Medical examinations

Occupational medical examinations are to be carried out for persons exposed at work to levels of mercury or mercury compounds which could have adverse effects on health (e.g. when the occupational exposure limit value is exceeded) or for whom dermal absorption could endanger health.

1.1　Examinations, intervals between examinations

initial examination	before taking up the job
first follow-up examination	for persons exposed to alkylmercury compounds, metallic mercury, inorganic and organic non-alkyl mercury compounds after 6–12 months
further follow-up examinations	after 6–12 months and when leaving the job
premature follow-up examination	• after a serious or prolonged illness which could cause concern as to whether the activity should be continued • in individual cases when the physician considers it necessary, e.g. when there is short-term concern about the person's health • when requested by an employee who suspects a causal association between his or her illness and work

1.2　Medical examination schedule

1.2.1　General medical examination

Initial examination

- review of past history (general anamnesis, work anamnesis, symptoms) Particular attention is to be given to:
  - the state of the teeth, amalgam fillings
  - renal damage
  - neurological and mental abnormalities
  - psycho-vegetative disorders
  - evidence of addiction to alcohol, drugs, medications
  - hyperactivity of the thyroid gland
- urinalysis (multiple test strips, sediment)

Follow-up examination

- interim anamnesis (including work anamnesis)
  Attention is to be paid to:
  - complaints of listlessness, headaches, pains in the limbs
  - inspection of the oral cavity (stomatitis, gingivitis)
  - look for mercurial line at the gingival margin (rare)
  - neurological and mental state (tremor, psellism, emotional lability, erethism, vegetative disorders, handwriting test, see also Section 3.2.3).
- urinalysis (multiple test strips, sediment)

1.2.2   Special medical examination

| **Initial examination** | **Follow-up examination** |

- biomonitoring (see Section 3.1.4); at the initial examination only if the person has previously been exposed to mercury
Also helpful:
- quantitative determination of urinary protein
If a renal disorder is suspected:
- α_1-microglobulin or N-acetyl-β-D-glucosaminidase in urine

1.2.3   Supplementary examination

Follow-up examination

- supervised handwriting test (see also Section 3.2.2)

1.3   Requirements for the medical examinations

- competent doctor or occupational health professional
- laboratory analyses carried out with appropriate quality control (Good Laboratory Practice)

2   Occupational medical assessment and advice

An assessment is only possible when the workplace situation and the exposure of the individual are known. For this purpose a risk assessment as defined in Article 4 Council directive 98/24/EC must have been carried out; it must specify which technical, organizational and individual protective measures have been applied.

G 9

2.1   Assessment criteria

2.1.1   Long-term concern about health

Initial examination	Follow-up examination

Persons with severe disorders such as
*   previous severe mercury poisoning
*   renal disorders (tubular damage)
*   neurological disorders
*   marked psycho-vegetative disorders
*   manifest thyroid hyperactivity
*   addiction to alcohol, drugs or medication

2.1.2   Short-term concern about health

Initial examination	Follow-up examination

Persons with the disorders mentioned in Section 2.1.1, provided recovery is to be expected (apart from previous severe mercury poisoning).

2.1.3   No concern about health under certain conditions

Initial examination	Follow-up examination

If the illnesses or functional disorders mentioned in Section 2.1.1 are less severe, the doctor should establish whether or not it is possible for the person to start work or go on working under certain conditions. Such conditions could include
*   technical protective measures
*   organizational protective measures, e.g., limitation of exposure periods
*   transfer to workplaces known to involve lower levels of exposure
*   personal protective equipment which takes the individual's state of health into account
*   more frequent follow-up examinations

2.1.4   No concern about health

Initial examination	Follow-up examination

All other persons, provided there are no restrictions on their employment.

2.2   Medical advice

The advice in an individual case should be commensurate with the workplace situation and the results of the medical examinations. Employees are to be informed about the biomonitoring results.

Employees should be informed about general hygienic measures and personal protective equipment.

If during the course of his work in the company the occupational physician finds indications that the risk assessment should be brought up to date to improve health and safety standards, he is to inform the employer. When it is necessary to inform the employer, the interests of the employee are to be protected (medical confidentiality).

3   Supplementary notes

3.1   External and internal exposure

3.1.1 Occurrence, sources of hazards

Listed below are the kinds of processes, workplaces or activities, including cleaning and repair work, for which exposure to mercury or mercury compounds must be expected. This must be taken into account during the risk assessment:

- production and processing of mercury and mercury compounds (filtering, purification, oxidation, distillation)
- production of measuring instruments (barometer, thermometer) and control devices containing mercury, and especially their maintenance and repair (glassblowers)
- use of mercury in electrical engineering (rectifiers, circuit-breakers, mercury arc lamps, fluorescent lamps, pelleting mercuric oxide for button cells)
- high vacuum techniques (mercury pumps)
- production of mercury-containing fluorescent tubes for neon signs
- production and recycling of mercury switches
- use of sealing liquid in gas laboratories
- recycling of fluorescent lamps
- electrolysis with mercury cathodes (electrolysis of alkali-metal chlorides)
- use as a catalyst (aldehyde production)
- amalgamation (e.g. battery production)
- production and processing of mercury compounds to produce pyrotechnical devices and explosives (fulminates, thiocyanates)
- production of alkoxides (reaction of sodium amalgam with alcohols)
- renovation of surfaces coated with antifouling paints containing mercury
- dismantling and renovation work in areas contaminated with mercury or mercury compounds

G 9

Occurrence and hazards for specific substances are documented in the information system on hazardous substances (GESTIS) (see Section 4).

3.1.2   Physicochemical properties and classification

Mercury is a silvery liquid metal. It is volatile even at room temperature. The vapour pressure of mercury at 30°C is 6 times that at 10°C. The vapour is odourless and tasteless and very poisonous. Mercury can dissolve many metals (amalgam formation). It exists in monovalent and divalent forms. The mercury(II) compounds are most stable.

Mercury and mercury compounds
Formula   Hg
CAS number   7439-97-6
MAK value[1]   0.1 mg/m^3

The information system on hazardous substances (GESTIS) provides details of international threshold limit values, classification, evaluation and other substance-specific information (see Section 4).
Additional information is to be found in the recommendations of the DFG Commission for the Investigation of Health Hazards of Chemical Compounds in the Work Area (List of MAK and BAT Values).

3.1.3   Uptake

Mercury is taken up via the airways in the form of vapour of metallic mercury or organic mercury compounds (especially alkylmercury compounds) or in the form of dust containing mercury compounds and also through the skin (only organic mercury compounds).

---

[1] Maximale Arbeitsplatz-Konzentration (MAK) = maximum workplace concentration

3.1.4   Biomonitoring

Information about biomonitoring may be found in Appendix 1 "Biomonitoring".

Biological tolerance values for occupational exposures

Substance	Parameter	BAT[2]	Assay material	Sampling time
mercury, metallic and inorganic mercury compounds	mercury	25 µg/l	whole blood	not fixed
	mercury	100 µg/l	urine	not fixed
mercury, organic mercury compounds	mercury	100 µg/l	whole blood	not fixed

Biomonitoring should be carried out with reliable methods and meet quality control requirements (see Appendix 1 "Biomonitoring").

3.2   Functional disorders, symptoms

G 9

3.2.1   Mode of action

Mercury and mercury compounds have specific effects on certain parts of the central nervous system and on some enzymes in the renal tubules. They function as enzyme inhibitors by blocking sulfhydryl (SH) groups; they also interact with phosphate, carboxy, amino and other groups.

Inorganic mercury compounds
Divalent mercury compounds are more poisonous than the monovalent compounds when ingested. The toxicity of the compounds increases with increasing solubility in water or dilute hydrochloric acid. Divalent mercury compounds are generally more soluble in water than the monovalent compounds.
Inorganic mercury compounds accumulate especially in the renal cortex and to a slightly less extent also in the liver. The corrosive inorganic mercury compounds precipitate protein (denaturation).

---

[2] Biologischer Arbeitsstoff-Toleranzwert (BAT) = biological tolerance value for occupational exposures

Organic mercury compounds
The organic mercury compounds are readily lipoid-soluble. They have a high affinity for the central nervous system and adipose tissue and some have a long half-life in the organism. Therefore they tend to accumulate. From the toxicological point of view, two groups of organic mercury compounds must be distinguished:

a) The unstable (rapidly metabolized) organic non-alkyl mercury compounds. To this group belong the arylmercury and alkoxyalkylmercury compounds and their derivatives. The toxicological behaviour of these compounds is largely the same as that of the inorganic mercury compounds.

b) The alkylmercury compounds are highly volatile (high saturation concentrations which increase from propylmercury to methylmercury compounds) They are relatively stable and can readily cross the blood-brain barrier. Here dimethylmercury is dominant. Inorganic mercury compounds in aqueous solution can be converted to methylmercury compounds by bacteria.

The reported symptoms are like those produced by mercury or inorganic mercury salts. The main effects of stable alkylmercury compounds are central nervous system disorders.

3.2.2   Acute and subacute effects on health

- disorders of renal function (increased diuresis, albuminuria, erythrocyturia) and even anuria
- after inhalation of the substances, irritation of the airways (tracheobronchitis, bronchopneumonia)
- inflammation of the oral mucosa (stomatitis, gingivitis, coated ulcers mainly close to carious teeth, loosening of the teeth)

3.2.3   Chronic effects on health

Disorders of the central nervous system such as:
- hyperexcitability
- anxious self-consciousness and emotional lability (erethismus mercurialis)
- tremor of the fingers, shaking of the arms, legs and head (tremor mercurialis) stuttering unclear speech (psellismus mercurialis)
- marked vegetative stigmata
- irreversible brown discoloration of the anterior capsule of the crystalline lens (mercurialentis) only after exposure to very high levels
- peripheral polyneuropathy
- allergic contact eczema

4   References

Commission Recommendation 2003/670/EC concerning the European schedule of occupational diseases. Annex I

Council Directive 67/548/EEC on the approximation of the laws, regulations and administrative provisions relating to the classification, packaging and labelling of dangerous substances

Council Directive 98/24/EC on the protection of the health and safety of workers from the risks related to chemical agents at work

Deutsche Forschungsgemeinschaft (German Research Foundation, DFG) (ed) List of MAK and BAT Values 2007. Maximum Concentrations and Biological Tolerance Values at the workplace. Wiley-VCH, Weinheim

Deutsche Forschungsgemeinschaft (German Research Foundation, DFG) (ed) The MAK-Collection for Occupational Health and Safety. Wiley-VCH
at: www.mrw.interscience.wiley.com/makbat

GESTIS-database on hazardous substances. BGIA
at: www.dguv.de/bgia/gestis-database

GESTIS-international limit values for chemical agents. BGIA
at: www.dguv.de/bgia/gestis-limit-values

G 9

References

Commission Recommendation 2003/670/EC concerning the European schedule of occupational diseases, Annex I

Council Directive 67/548/EEC on the approximation of the laws, regulations and administrative provisions relating to the classification, packaging and labelling of dangerous substances

Council Directive 98/24/EC on the protection of the health and safety of workers from the risks related to chemical agents at work

Deutsche Forschungsgemeinschaft (German Research Foundation) DFG, List of MAK and BAT Values 2002, Maximum Concentrations and Biological Tolerance Values at the workplace, Wiley-VCH, Weinheim

BGIA – Berufsgenossenschaftliches Institut für Arbeitsschutz, International Limit Values for Occupational Health and Safety, Wiley-VCH or www.hvbg.de/e/bia/fac/limit/index.html

GESTIS database on hazardous substances, BGIA or www.hvbg.de/e/bia/fac/limit

GESTIS International limit values for chemical agents, BGIA or www.dguv.de/bia/gestis/limit_values

G 10   Methanol

Committee for occupational medicine, working group "Hazardous substances", Berufsgenossenschaft der chemischen Industrie, Heidelberg

Preliminary remarks

The present guideline describes a scheme for occupational medical prophylaxis which aims to prevent or ensure early diagnosis of disorders which can be caused by methanol.

Schedule

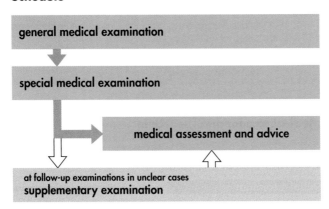

general medical examination

special medical examination

medical assessment and advice

at follow-up examinations in unclear cases
supplementary examination

G 10

1   Medical examinations

Occupational medical examinations are to be carried out for persons exposed at work to levels of methanol which could have adverse effects on health (e.g. when the occupational exposure limit value is exceeded) or for whom dermal absorption could endanger health.

1.1   Examinations, intervals between examinations

initial examination	before taking up the job
first follow-up examination	after 12–24 months
further follow-up examinations	after 24 months and when leaving the job
premature follow-up examination	• after an illness lasting for several weeks or when a physical handicap gives cause for concern about whether the work should be continued • in individual cases when the physician considers it necessary, e.g. when there is short-term concern about the person's health • when requested by an employee who suspects a causal association between his or her illness and work

1.2   Medical examination schedule

1.2.1   General medical examination

Initial examination	Follow-up examination

- review of past history (general anamnesis, work anamnesis)
- urinalysis (multiple test strips, sediment)

1.2.2   Special medical examination

Initial examination

- eyesight test including colour vision (if colour vision is abnormal, visual field to be examined by an ophthalmologist)
- SGPT (ALT)

Also helpful:

- ophthalmoscopy of the ocular fundus

Follow-up examination

- eyesight test including colour vision (if colour vision is abnormal, visual field to be examined by an ophthalmologist)
- SGPT (ALT)
- biomonitoring (see Section 3.1.4)

1.2.3   Supplementary examination

Follow-up examination

In unclear cases:

- examination by an ophthalmologist
- perhaps examination of liver-specific parameters
- examination by a neurologist

1.3   Requirements for the medical examinations

- competent doctor or occupational health professional
- laboratory analyses carried out with appropriate quality control (Good Laboratory Practice)

G 10

2   Occupational medical assessment and advice

An assessment is only possible when the workplace situation and the exposure of the individual are known. For this purpose a risk assessment as defined in Article 4 Council directive 98/24/EC must have been carried out; it must specify which technical, organizational and individual protective measures have been applied.

2.1   Assessment criteria

2.1.1   Long-term concern about health

| Initial examination | Follow-up examination |

Persons with
- disorders of the peripheral or central nervous system
- changes in the optic nerve
- chronic liver and kidney disorders
- diabetes mellitus
- alcoholism

2.1.2   Short-term concern about health

| Initial examination | Follow-up examination |

Persons with the disorders mentioned in Section 2.1.1, provided recovery is to be expected.

2.1.3   No concern about health under certain conditions

| Initial examination | Follow-up examination |

If the illnesses or functional disorders mentioned in Section 2.1.1 are less severe, the doctor should establish whether or not it is possible for the person to return to work or go on working under certain conditions. Such conditions could include
- technical protective measures
- organizational protective measures, e.g., limitation of exposure periods
- transfer to workplaces known to involve lower levels of exposure
- personal protective equipment which takes the individual's state of health into account
- more frequent follow-up examinations

2.1.4   No concern about health

| Initial examination | Follow-up examination |

All other persons, provided there are no restrictions on their employment.

2.2   Medical advice

The advice in an individual case should be commensurate with the workplace situation and the results of the medical examinations.

Employees are to be informed about the biomonitoring results.

They should be informed about general hygienic measures and personal protective equipment. Because methanol readily penetrates the skin, the wearing of protective clothing is of particular significance. Substance-specific protective measures are documented in the information system on hazardous substances (GESTIS) in the section "Handling and usage" (see Section 4).

The employees are to be advised that alcohol consumption potentiates the effects of the substance.

If during the course of his work in the company the occupational physician finds indications that the risk assessment should be brought up to date to improve health and safety standards, he is to inform the employer. When this is necessary, the interests of the employee are to be protected (medical confidentiality).

3   Supplementary notes

3.1   External and internal exposure

3.1.1   Occurrence, sources of hazards

Occurrence and hazards are documented in the information system on hazardous substances (GESTIS) (see Section 4).

Health surveillance is necessary for persons working with methanol, especially for the following kinds of processes, workplaces or activities, including cleaning and repair work:

- production and filling of containers
- use of methanol in the synthesis of formaldehyde, methyl acrylate, dimethyl sulfide, formic acid, acetic acid, methylamines, dimethyl sulfate, etc.
- use as antifreeze and refrigerant, solvent, aircraft fuel and carburetting additive, as inhibitor (reaction inhibitor), plasticizing agent, diluent and cleaning fluid
- use of methanol-containing undercoats and glues for floor-coverings
- use as a component of cold cleaning agents for defatting of metals in open systems
- filling of motor vehicle tanks with methanol-containing fuel as a petrol pump attendant or in a similar function

G 10

3.1.2   Physicochemical properties and classification

Methanol (methyl alcohol) is a colourless, inflammable, poisonous, readily volatile liquid which is miscible with water in all proportions.
It is, however, not very effective as a fat solvent.

Methanol (methyl alcohol)
Formula CH_3OH
CAS number   67-56-1
OEL value[1]   260 mg/m^3 (200 ppm)

The information system on hazardous substances (GESTIS) provides details of international threshold limit values, classification, evaluation and other substance-specific information (see Section 4).

3.1.3   Uptake

Methanol is taken up via the airways and the skin.

3.1.4   Biomonitoring

Information about biomonitoring may be found in Appendix 1 "Biomonitoring".
The oxidation of methanol is inhibited competitively by ethanol. In persons exposed simultaneously to both substances, methanol excretion can be increased.

Biological tolerance value for occupational exposures

Substance	Parameter	BAT[2]	Assay material	Sampling time
methanol	methanol	30 mg/l	urine	end of exposure or end of shift; for long-term exposures after several shifts

Biomonitoring should be carried out with reliable methods and meet quality control requirements (see Appendix 1 "Biomonitoring").

---

[1] occupational exposure limit value of the European Community
[2] Biologischer Arbeitsstoff-Toleranzwert (BAT) = biological tolerance value for occupational exposures

3.2   Functional disorders, symptoms

3.2.1   Mode of action

Methanol vapour is irritating for the eyes and the airway mucosa.

Skin moistened with methanol is defatted, dries out and becomes cracked; this can result in eczema or an increased susceptibility to infections.

Inhalation or oral intake of methanol leads to narcotic symptoms (similar to those caused by ethanol); oral intake by mistake can be lethal after consumption of as little as 30 ml methanol. Whereas a part of the methanol taken up is exhaled via the lungs (30 % to 60 %), the rest is oxidized in the body to formaldehyde which is rapidly converted to formic acid. Formic acid accumulates in the organism and is considered to be the main toxic metabolite of methanol because its detoxification in C1 metabolism is limited in man by low levels of folic acid. This results in severe acidosis with a marked reduction of alkali levels which can cause the typical symptoms of methanol poisoning: neurotoxic damage and especially damage to the optic nerve with consequent visus disorders and even blindness. Therefore an early symptom is considered to be the development of defective colour vision. However, the sensitivity to methanol differs greatly from person to person because of differences in detoxification capacity.

3.2.2   Acute and subacute effects on health

Almost only after uptake through the mouth, rarely through the airways or skin

* symptoms of a hangover: dizziness, weakness, headaches, early visus disorders (cloudy vision), nausea, vomiting, colic-like gastrointestinal pains, convulsions, respiratory distress or even paralysis of the respiratory centre, circulatory failure
* irritation of the eyes and airway mucosa caused by methanol vapour

G 10

3.2.3   Chronic effects on health

Central nervous disorders, signs of peripheral polyneuritis, acoustic neuritis, optic neuritis, parkinsonian symptoms, damage to the liver parenchyma (liver cirrhosis).

4   References

Commission Recommendation 2003/670/EC concerning the European schedule of occupational diseases. Annex I

Council Directive 98/24/EC on the protection of the health and safety of workers from the risks related to chemical agents at work

Deutsche Forschungsgemeinschaft (German Research Foundation, DFG) (ed) List of MAK and BAT Values 2007. Maximum Concentrations and Biological Tolerance Values at the workplace. Wiley-VCH, Weinheim

Deutsche Forschungsgemeinschaft (German Research Foundation, DFG) (ed) The
MAK-Collection for Occupational Health and Safety. Wiley-VCH
at: www.mrw.interscience.wiley.com/makbat
GESTIS-database on hazardous substances. BGIA
at: www.dguv.de/bgia/gestis-database
GESTIS-international limit values for chemical agents. BGIA
at: www.dguv.de/bgia/gestis-limit-values

G 11   Hydrogen sulfide

Committee for occupational medicine, working group "Hazardous substances", Berufsgenossenschaft der chemischen Industrie, Heidelberg

Preliminary remarks

The present guideline describes a scheme for occupational medical prophylaxis which aims to prevent or ensure early diagnosis of disorders which can be caused by hydrogen sulfide.

Schedule

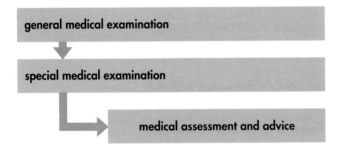

general medical examination

special medical examination

medical assessment and advice

G 11

1   Medical examinations

Occupational medical examinations are to be carried out for persons at whose workplaces exposure to hydrogen sulfide could endanger health (e.g. the occupational
exposure limit value is exceeded).

1.1   Examinations, intervals between examinations

initial examination	before taking up the job
first follow-up examination	after 12–24 months
further follow-up examinations	after 12–24 months or when leaving the job
premature follow-up examination	• after a serious or prolonged illness which could cause concern as to whether the activity should be continued • in individual cases when the physician considers it necessary, e.g. when there is short-term concern about the person's health • when requested by an employee who suspects a causal association between his or her illness and work

1.2   Medical examination schedule

1.2.1   General medical examination

Initial examination

• review of past history (general anamnesis, work anamnesis, symptoms)
Particular attention is to be given to:
• disorders of the upper and lower respiratory tract
• cardiocirculatory damage
• neurological and mental abnormalities

Follow-up examination

- interim anamnesis (including work anamnesis)

Particular attention is to be given to:

- mucous membranes: conjunctivitis, tracheopharyngitis, bronchitis, shortness of breath
- nervous system: headaches, balance disorders, tiredness, irritability, dizziness, mental abnormalities (especially confusion), extrapyramidal disorders
- circulatory system: low blood pressure (systolic value < 13 kPa, < 100 mm Hg), cardiac muscle damage, extrasystoles, stenocardia
- gastrointestinal tract: metallic taste, vomiting, diarrhoea, loss of appetite, weight loss
- skin: acute and chronic inflammation

1.2.2   Special medical examination

Initial examination	Follow-up examination

- ergometry

Also helpful:

- haemoglobin, erythrocytes (oxidative metabolism, release of O_2)

1.3   Requirements for the medical examinations

- competent doctor or occupational health professional
- laboratory analyses carried out with appropriate quality control (Good Laboratory Practice)
- necessary equipment: ECG/ergometer

G 11

2   Occupational medical assessment and advice

An assessment is only possible when the workplace situation and the exposure of the individual are known. For this purpose a risk assessment as defined in Article 4 Council directive 98/24/EC must have been carried out; it must specify which technical, organizational and individual protective measures have been applied.

2.1   Assessment criteria

2.1.1   Long-term concern about health

Initial examination   Follow-up examination

Persons with severe disorders such as
- haemodynamic cardiocirculatory disorders
- pulmonary emphysema or other lung changes associated with marked functional disorder
- disorders and irritation of the conjunctiva and the mucous membranes of the upper and lower respiratory tract
- olfactory dysfunction
- anaemia
- marked psychovegetative disorders
- marked neurological and mental disorders

2.1.2   Short-term concern about health

Initial examination   Follow-up examination

Persons with the disorders mentioned in Section 2.1.1, provided recovery is to be expected.

2.1.3   No concern about health under certain conditions

Initial examination   Follow-up examination

If the illnesses or functional disorders mentioned in Section 2.1.1 are less severe, the doctor should establish whether or not it is possible for the person to start work or go on working under certain conditions. Such conditions could include
- technical protective measures
- organizational protective measures, e.g., limitation of exposure periods
- transfer to workplaces known to involve lower levels of exposure
- personal protective equipment which takes the individual's state of health into account
- more frequent follow-up examinations

2.1.4   No concern about health

Initial examination   Follow-up examination

All other persons, provided there are no restrictions on their employment.

2.2   Medical advice

The advice in an individual case should be commensurate with the workplace situation and the results of the medical examinations.

Employees should be informed about general hygienic measures and personal protective equipment and also about the warning effect of the typical smell of hydrogen sulfide (like rotten eggs) which, however, soon disappears because of numbing of the sense of smell.

If during the course of his work in the company the occupational physician finds indications that the risk assessment should be brought up to date to improve health and safety standards, he is to inform the employer. When it is necessary to inform the employer, the interests of the employee are to be protected (medical confidentiality).

3   Supplementary notes

3.1   External and internal exposure

3.1.1   Occurrence, sources of hazards

Listed below are the kinds of processes, workplaces or activities, including cleaning and repair work, for which exposure to hydrogen sulfide must be expected. This must be taken into account during the risk assessment.

- emptying pits or tanks of liquid manure
- in water treatment works where water containing sulfides is processed
- in the rubber, plastics, viscose and sugar industries
- in gasworks, refineries, oil fields
- precipitating of metals as sulfides
- filling and discharging coke-oven batteries
- natural gas treatment works
- work on pipes for natural gas (crude gas)
- biogas works
- work in sewers

Occurrence and hazards for specific substances are documented in the information system on hazardous substances (GESTIS) (see Section 4).

G 11

3.1.2   Physicochemical properties and classification

Hydrogen sulfide is a colourless poisonous gas which smells intensely of rotten eggs even at very low concentrations. Hydrogen sulfide is flammable and may form explosive mixtures with air.

Hydrogen sulfide is readily soluble in water (2.6 l H_2S/l water at 20°C) and very readily soluble in alcohol (11.8 l H_2S/l alcohol at 10°C). In aqueous solution hydrogen sulfide is a weak acid; it is also a good reducing agent and so is readily oxidized to yield water, sulfur, sulfur dioxide and sulfate. Above 1000°C it is decomposed into its elements; it is decomposed by UV-irradiation and is known to be a catalytic poison. It reacts readily with metals and metal oxides to yield the sulfides.

Hydrogen sulfide
Formula H_2S
CAS number   7783-06-4

The information system on hazardous substances (GESTIS) provides details of international threshold limit values, classification, evaluation and other substance-specific information (see Section 4).

3.1.3   Uptake

The substance is taken up via the airways and through the skin and mucous membranes.

3.2   Functional disorders, symptoms

3.2.1   Mode of action

At high concentrations (300 ppm), hydrogen sulfide causes paralysis of the olfactory nerves so that the typical smell of rotten eggs can no longer be detected.

The substance irritates mucous membranes because of the formation of disulfides.

Depending on the exposure concentration, hydrogen sulfide is absorbed partly as the alkali metal sulfide and partly as free hydrogen sulfide. The alkali metal sulfides are hydrolysed in blood so that here too the hydrogen sulfide is present in free form. Because hydrogen sulfide is readily oxidized, it is converted to sulfate which may be detected in the urine.

In vitro H_2S blocks the activity of metalloenzymes either by formation of sulfides with the central metal atoms or by SH-blockage. The symptoms of H_2S poisoning, however, do not yield any evidence of whether and, if so, which enzymes are affected *in vivo*.

The effects of uptake of H_2S must, however, be a result of metabolic disturbances which finally result in oxygen deficiency.

The effect depends on the exposure concentration, shown below in cm^3 H_2S per m^3 of air:

1800	respiratory paralysis, instantaneous death
1000–1500	loss of consciousness, spasms, death after a few minutes exposure
700– 900	severe poisoning, death after 30–60 minutes exposure
300– 700	subacute poisoning after 15–30 minutes exposure
200– 300	severe local irritation of the mucous membranes with general symptoms of H_2S poisoning after 30 minutes exposure
100– 150	irritation of the eyes and airways
under 10	no signs of H_2S poisoning

3.2.2   Acute and subacute effects on health

The symptoms are dependent on the exposure concentration (see Section 3.2.1):

- unconsciousness, spasms and at high concentrations so-called instantaneous death due to respiratory paralysis (the heart goes on beating for 4–8 minutes);
- a mixture of symptoms resulting from irritation of the mucosa in contact with the gas, damage to the nervous system and hypoxia
  - mucosa:
    mainly irritation of the conjunctiva, also irritation of the throat, trachea, bronchi and via bronchitis leading to pulmonary oedema (given sufficient exposure concentration and duration), asphyxia; viscose-spinner keratoconjunctivitis develops almost exclusively under the specific conditions found in the viscose industry
  - nervous system:
    headaches, listlessness, nausea, vomiting, restlessness, anxiety, fits of agitation, confusion, tonic convulsions, areflexia, balance disorders, unconsciousness, also disorders of the olfactory and auditory nerves, speech disorders and other polyneuritic symptoms
  - circulatory system:
    low blood pressure, ECG changes (the T-wave becomes flatter or negative), atrial fibrillation, dysrhythmia with ventricular extrasystoles

The potential sequelae which have been described include cerebral damage and damage to the central nervous system, mental disorders, psychovegetative syndrome, low blood pressure and disorders of sugar metabolism.

G 11

3.2.3   Chronic effects on health

There is still no agreement as to whether H_2S can have chronic effects on health.

4 References

Commission Recommendation 2003/670/EC concerning the European schedule of occupational diseases. Annex I

Council Directive 67/548/EEC on the approximation of the laws, regulations and administrative provisions relating to the classification, packaging and labelling of dangerous substances

Council Directive 98/24/EC on the protection of the health and safety of workers from the risks related to chemical agents at work

Deutsche Forschungsgemeinschaft (German Research Foundation, DFG) (ed) List of MAK and BAT Values 2007. Maximum Concentrations and Biological Tolerance Values at the workplace. Wiley-VCH, Weinheim

Deutsche Forschungsgemeinschaft (German Research Foundation, DFG) (ed) The MAK-Collection for Occupational Health and Safety. Wiley-VCH
    at: www.mrw.interscience.wiley.com/makbat

GESTIS-database on hazardous substances. BGIA
    at: www.dguv.de/bgia/gestis-database

GESTIS-international limit values for chemical agents. BGIA
    at: www.dguv.de/bgia/gestis-limit-values

G 12   Phosphorus (white, yellow)

Committee for occupational medicine, working group "Hazardous substances",
Berufsgenossenschaft der chemischen Industrie, Heidelberg

Preliminary remarks

The present guideline describes a scheme for occupational medical prophylaxis
which aims to prevent or ensure early diagnosis of disorders which can be caused
by white phosphorus.

Schedule

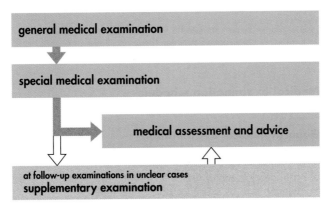

1　　Medical examinations

Occupational medical examinations are to be carried out for persons at whose workplaces exposure to white phosphorus could endanger health (e.g. the occupational exposure limit value is exceeded).

1.1　　Examinations, intervals between examinations

initial examination	before taking up the job
first follow-up examination	after 12–24 months
further follow-up examinations	after 12–24 months and when leaving the job
premature follow-up examination	• after a serious or prolonged illness which could cause concern as to whether the activity should be continued • in individual cases when the physician considers it necessary, e.g. when there is short-term concern about the person's health • when requested by an employee who suspects a causal association between his or her illness and work

1.2　　Medical examination schedule

1.2.1　　General medical examination

Initial examination

- review of past history (general anamnesis, work anamnesis, symptoms)
  Particular attention is to be given to: state of the teeth
- urinalysis (multiple test strips)

Follow-up examination

- interim anamnesis (including work anamnesis)
  Particular attention is to be given to:
  - anorexia, weight loss, pallor
  - mucosal bleeding
  - dental caries
  - albuminuria
- urinalysis (multiple test strips)

1.2.2   Special medical examination

Initial examination

- haemoglobin
- ALT
- γ-GT

Also helpful:

if previous liver damage is suspected

- other liver-specific tests (electrophoresis)

Follow-up examination

- erythrocyte sedimentation rate, haemoglobin
- ALT
- γ-GT

1.2.3   Supplementary examination

Follow-up examination

In unclear cases:

- other liver-specific tests (electrophoresis, perhaps biopsy)
- x-ray diagnosis (bones, especially jaw bone)

1.3   Requirements for the medical examinations

- competent doctor or occupational health professional
- laboratory analyses carried out with appropriate quality control (Good Laboratory Practice)

G 12

2   Occupational medical assessment and advice

An assessment is only possible when the workplace situation and the exposure of the individual are known. For this purpose a risk assessment as defined in Article 4 Council directive 98/24/EC must have been carried out; it must specify which technical, organizational and individual protective measures have been applied.

2.1   Assessment criteria

2.1.1   Long-term concern about health

Initial examination	Follow-up examination

Persons with
- severe liver or kidney disorders
- chronic disorders of the skeletal system

2.1.2   Short-term concern about health

Initial examination	Follow-up examination

Persons with the disorders mentioned in Section 2.1.1, provided recovery is to be expected.

2.1.3   No concern about health under certain conditions

Initial examination	Follow-up examination

If the illnesses or functional disorders mentioned in Section 2.1.1 are less severe, the doctor should establish whether or not it is possible for the person to start work or go on working under certain conditions. Such conditions could include
- technical protective measures
- organizational protective measures, e.g., limitation of exposure periods
- transfer to workplaces known to involve lower levels of exposure
- personal protective equipment which takes the individual's state of health into account
- more frequent follow-up examinations

2.1.4   No concern about health

Initial examination	Follow-up examination

All other persons, provided there are no restrictions on their employment.

2.2.   Medical advice

The advice in an individual case should be commensurate with the workplace situation and the results of the medical examinations.

Employees should be informed about general hygienic measures and personal protective equipment.

If during the course of his work in the company the occupational physician finds indications that the risk assessment should be brought up to date to improve health and safety standards, he is to inform the employer. When it is necessary to inform the employer, the interests of the employee are to be protected (medical confidentiality).

3   Supplementary notes

3.1   External and internal exposure

3.1.1   Occurrence, sources of hazards

Listed below are the kinds of processes, workplaces or activities, including cleaning and repair work, for which exposure to phosphorus must be expected; this must be taken into account during the risk assessment:

- production (furnace room)
- filling and emptying (cleaning) operations
- processing with sulfur to yield sulfides or with halogens to yield halogenides
- burning elemental phosphorus to produce thermal phosphoric acid
- repair and cleaning of apparatus and piping in which phosphorus is processed or transported
- demolition and restoration jobs in areas contaminated with white phosphorus

Occurrence and hazards for specific substances are documented in the information system on hazardous substances (GESTIS) (see Section 4).

G 12

3.1.2   Physicochemical properties and classification

Phosphorus exists as several allotropic modifications which have very different properties. The present document concerns the white (yellow) allotrope of phosphorus. The other phosphorus modifications are much less reactive and very much less poisonous than white phosphorus.

White phosphorus is a soft waxy translucent mass which is oxidized in the air even at room temperature to form a white vapour (phosphorus pentoxide). The heat produced in this reaction causes the substance to self-ignite at about 50°C. Because of these properties, white phosphorus is stored under water in which it is insoluble. In organic solvents, on the other hand, it is very readily to moderately soluble (solubility in 100 g solvent at 20°C: about 900 g in carbon disulfide, about 3 g in benzene, about 1.3 g in ether). Phosphorus is noticeably volatile even at room temperature. It is an effective reducing agent (e.g. sulfuric acid is reduced by phosphorus to sulfur dioxide, nitric acid to nitrogen oxides) and reacts directly also with many metals. Its valencies range from −3 to +5.

Phosphorus (white)
Formula   P
CAS number   7723-14-0

The information system on hazardous substances (GESTIS) provides details of international threshold limit values, classification, evaluation and other substance-specific information (see Section 4).

3.1.3   Uptake

White phosphorus is taken up via the airways.

3.2   Functional disorders, symptoms

3.2.1   Mode of action

Burning phosphorus causes very painful skin injuries which are slow to heal. White phosphorus is very poisonous; the lethal dose for an adult is probably less than 50 mg. Because phosphorus is a reducing agent, it inhibits intracellular oxidation. It can disturb the metabolic functions of the liver and kidney. Because of metabolic interaction between phosphorus and calcium, especially the bones are also affected.

3.2.2   Acute and subacute effects on health

It causes caustic burns of skin and mucous membranes. The burning substance on the skin causes very severe injuries (burns). The vapour and fumes of burning phosphorus irritate the respiratory tract.
Nausea, repeated diarrhoea, vomiting blood (the vomit can be luminescent), swelling of the liver and perhaps the spleen, jaundice, acute yellow liver atrophy, renal parenchymal damage, bleeding in other organs.
Sequelae of acute phosphorus poisoning can include the fibrotic alteration of liver tissue and even cirrhosis.
After exposure to large amounts of the substance, sudden death with the symptoms of circulatory failure can occur within a few hours.

3.2.3   Chronic effects on health

Anorexia, tiredness, digestive disorders, weight loss, tendency to bleeding of the skin, mucous membranes and fundus of the eye, osteoporosis of the bones, especially the jaw bone; attention should be paid to the susceptibility of the altered bone to infection (osteomyelitis).

A route of entry to the jaw bone for elemental phosphorus may be provided by dental granuloma as the final stage of dental caries.

The damage can first appear after months or years.

4   References

Commission Recommendation 2003/670/EC concerning the European schedule of occupational diseases. Annex I

Council Directive 67/548/EEC on the approximation of the laws, regulations and administrative provisions relating to the classification, packaging and labelling of dangerous substances

Council Directive 98/24/EC on the protection of the health and safety of workers from the risks related to chemical agents at work

Deutsche Forschungsgemeinschaft (German Research Foundation, DFG) (ed) List of MAK and BAT Values 2007. Maximum Concentrations and Biological Tolerance Values at the workplace. Wiley-VCH, Weinheim

Deutsche Forschungsgemeinschaft (German Research Foundation, DFG) (ed) The MAK-Collection for Occupational Health and Safety. Wiley-VCH
     at: www.mrw.interscience.wiley.com/makbat

GESTIS-database on hazardous substances. BGIA
     at: www.dguv.de/bgia/gestis-database

GESTIS-international limit values for chemical agents. BGIA
     at: www.dguv.de/bgia/gestis-limit-values

G 12

G 14   Trichloroethene (trichloroethylene) and other chlorinated hydrocarbon solvents

Committee for occupational medicine, working group "Hazardous substances", Berufsgenossenschaft der chemischen Industrie, Heidelberg

Preliminary remarks

The present guideline describes a scheme for occupational medical prophylaxis which aims to prevent or ensure early diagnosis of disorders which can be caused by trichloroethene and other chlorinated hydrocarbon solvents.

Schedule

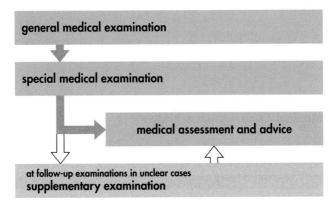

G 14

1   Medical examinations

Occupational medical examinations are to be carried out for persons exposed at work to levels of trichloroethene or other chlorinated hydrocarbon solvents which could have adverse effects on health (e.g. when the occupational exposure limit value is exceeded) or for whom dermal absorption could endanger health.

1.1   Examinations, intervals between examinations

initial examination	before taking up the job
first follow-up examination	after 12–24 months
further follow-up examinations	after 12–24 months and when leaving the job
premature follow-up examination	• after an illness lasting for several weeks or when a physical handicap gives cause for concern about whether the work should be continued • in individual cases when the physician considers it necessary, e.g. when there is short-term concern about the person's health • when requested by an employee who suspects a causal association between his or her illness and work

1.2   Medical examination schedule

1.2.1   General medical examination

Initial examination

• review of past history (general anamnesis, work anamnesis)
• urinalysis (multiple test strips, sediment)

Follow-up examination

• interim anamnesis (including work anamnesis)
Particular attention should be paid to
• headaches, dizziness, inebriation, concentration disorders, forgetfulness, disorders of sensitivity, of gait, of the sense of taste and smell, of sight and hearing, irritation of the eyes, upper airways, skin, reported lack of appetite, weight loss, nausea, vomiting, palpitations
• neurological screening
• urinalysis (multiple test strips, sediment)

1.2.2   Special medical examination

Initial examination

- SGPT (ALT)
- γ-GT

and in addition, only for persons exposed to trichloroethene
- α_1-microglobulin in the urine

Also helpful:
- SGOT (AST)
- serum creatinine
- blood count

Follow-up examination

Like the initial examination but, in addition,
- biomonitoring, when valid biomarkers are available (see Section 3.1.4)

1.2.3   Supplementary examination

Follow-up examination

In cases which could not be clarified with the methods listed above
- further kidney and liver diagnostics, e.g. ultrasonography of the kidneys when the latency period (exposure to trichloroethene) is at least 10 years and/or when microscopic haematuria or increased excretion of α_1-microglobulin has been detected
- ECG
- neurological-psychiatric examination, perhaps with psychological test methods

1.3   Requirements for the medical examinations

- competent doctor or occupational health professional
- laboratory analyses carried out with appropriate quality control (Good Laboratory Practice)

G 14

2   Occupational medical assessment and advice

An assessment is only possible when the workplace situation and the exposure of the individual are known. For this purpose a risk assessment as defined in Article 4 Council directive 98/24/EC must have been carried out; it must specify which technical, organizational and individual protective measures have been applied.

2.1   Assessment criteria

2.1.1   Long-term concern about health

Initial examination	Follow-up examination

Persons with
- disorders of the central and/or peripheral nervous system
- cardiocirculatory disorders (especially clinically relevant dysrhythmia, coronary heart disease, peripheral arterial circulatory disorders, inadequately treated high blood pressure)
- liver and kidney diseases with functional effects
- florid or chronically recurrent ulceration of the stomach or duodenum
- addiction to alcohol, drugs or medication

2.1.2   Short-term concern about health

Initial examination	Follow-up examination

Persons with the disorders mentioned in Section 2.1.1, provided recovery is to be expected.

2.1.3   No concern about health under certain conditions

Initial examination	Follow-up examination

If the illnesses or functional disorders mentioned in Section 2.1.1 are less severe, the doctor should establish whether or not it is possible for the person to start work or go on working under certain conditions. Such conditions could include
- technical protective measures
- organizational protective measures, e.g., limitation of exposure periods
- transfer to workplaces known to involve lower levels of exposure
- personal protective equipment which takes the individual's state of health into account
- more frequent follow-up examinations

2.1.4   No concern about health

Initial examination	Follow-up examination

All other persons, provided there are no restrictions on their employment.

2.2   Medical advice

The advice in an individual case should be commensurate with the workplace situation and the results of the medical examinations.

Employees are to be informed about the biomonitoring results.

They should be informed about general hygienic measures and personal protective equipment. For persons exposed to chlorinated hydrocarbons which can be absorbed through the skin, protection of the skin and wearing of protective clothing are particularly important. Substance-specific protective measures are documented in the information system on hazardous substances (GESTIS) in the section "Handling and usage" (see Section 4).

The employees are to be advised that alcohol consumption and smoking can potentiate the effects of these substances and that smoking is forbidden at the workplace (also because of the danger of formation of pyrolysis products); in addition it must be pointed out that various chlorinated hydrocarbons have been classified as carcinogenic, mutagenic or toxic for reproduction or are suspected of having such effects.

If during the course of his work in the company the occupational physician finds indications that the risk assessment should be brought up to date to improve health and safety standards, he is to inform the employer. When it is necessary to inform the employer, the interests of the employee are to be protected (medical confidentiality).

3   Supplementary notes

3.1   External and internal exposure

3.1.1   Occurrence, sources of hazards

Occurrence and hazards for specific substances are documented in the information system on hazardous substances (GESTIS) (see Section 4).

Chlorinated hydrocarbons occur especially in the following processes, products, workplaces or activities, including cleaning and repair work:

G 14

Trichloroethene
- production and filling of containers
- processing
- use as solvent for oils, fats, waxes, resins, rubber and during processing of these preparations
- use as an extractant in road construction laboratories
- use in paint removers and rust inhibitors
- vulcanization (rubber solution)

Tetrachloroethene
- production and filling of containers
- processing
- production of fluorochlorohydrocarbons from tetrachloroethene
- use as a solvent for oils, fats, waxes, resins, rubber, asphalt, paints and lacquers
- use in paint removers and rust inhibitors
- dry cleaning of textiles

Dichloromethane
- aerosols (spray paints, hair spray)
- paint remover, varnish remover
- defatting (of metal and plastic moulds)
- sponging agent (for foam plastics)
- extractant (e.g. in the pharmaceutical industry, for isolation of lipids, for preparation of hop and spice extracts, to decaffeinate coffee, in the deparaffinization of petroleum fractions)
- heat-exchanging medium
- coating tablets in the pharmaceutical industry
- production of glues (e.g. for acrylic glass)
- cleaning agents in the graphics industry
- components of fire-extinguishing agents
- insecticidal fumigants for cereals
- refrigerants

1,1,1-Trichloroethane
- plastics industry: cleaning plastic surfaces and films
- textile industry: defatting of production machines and yarns, removal of tacking threads
- glue industry: component of glues
- paint, lacquer and ink industry: solvent for air-drying paints and for flexographic and gravure printing inks
- electronic industry: development of dry film photoresist polymers in the production of printed circuit boards; removal of solder flux; *in situ* production of plasma etching agents in semi-conductor production
- paper industry: carrier solution for silicon coatings and other protective films
- cutting oils
- in aerosols for reducing vapour pressure: especially for body care products but also paints, insecticides and car cleaning agents

3.1.2   Physicochemical properties and classification

The information system on hazardous substances (GESTIS) provides details of classification, evaluation and other substance-specific information (see Section 4).

Trichloroethene – often called simply "tri" – is a non-flammable mobile liquid which is sparingly soluble in water and has a sweetish aromatic odour. It is decomposed by light, air and moderately high temperatures (>120°C). The pyrolysis products are carbon, carbon monoxide, carbon dioxide, chlorine, hydrochloric acid and phosgene. Trichloroethene is stabilized by additives such as phenols, amines and terpenes. It is highly volatile; the vapour is much heavier than air and accumulates at floor level.

Trichloroethene (trichloroethylene)
Formula $CHCl=CCl_2$
CAS number   79-01-6

Tetrachloroethene – also called perchloroethylene or "per" – is a colourless, non-flammable liquid which is very sparingly soluble in water and has a chloroform-like odour. It is the most stable chlorinated ethylene and may be stored for long periods without a stabilizer.
It is oxidized by oxygen to dichloroacetyl chloride. Pyrolysis (thermal decomposition) begins at 150°C; the products include hexachloroethane and dichloroacetylene. Tetrachloroethene is volatile; the vapour is much heavier than air and accumulates at floor level.

Tetrachloroethene (perchloroethylene)
Formula $CCl_2=CCl_2$
CAS number   127-18-4

Dichloromethane – also called methylene chloride – is a colourless non-flammable liquid with a sweetish chloroform-like odour. It is slightly soluble in water. Dichloromethane is highly volatile and the vapour is heavier than air.

Dichloromethane
Formula CH_2Cl_2
CAS number   75-09-2

G 14

1,1,1-Trichloroethane is a colourless non-combustible liquid with a sweetish ethereal odour. It is sparingly soluble in water. 1,1,1-Trichloroethane is highly volatile and the vapour is much heavier than air.

1,1,1-Trichloroethane
Formula CH_3CCl_3
CAS number   71-55-6
MAK[1] value   200 ml/m^3, 1100 mg/m^3

3.1.3   Uptake

At the workplace, the substances can be taken up via the airways and/or through the skin. The possibility of dermal uptake must be taken into account especially for those substances classified as toxic after percutaneous absorption.

3.1.4   Biomonitoring

Biomonitoring should be carried out with reliable methods and meet quality control requirements. Additional information about biomonitoring may be found in Appendix 1 "Biomonitoring". There data may also be found for other chlorinated hydrocarbons which are not included in the table below.

Trichloroethene: in persons exposed simultaneously to toluene the rate of metabolism of trichloroethene can be reduced. Ethanol has a marked inhibitory effect. These and other concomitant factors are to be taken into account when evaluating the biomonitoring results.

Dichloromethane: in smokers, CO-Hb levels above 5 % can be detected even without exposure to dichloromethane or carbon monoxide.

---

[1] Maximale Arbeitsplatz-Konzentration = maximum workplace concentration

Exposure equivalents for carcinogenic materials (EKA)[2] from the List of MAK and BAT Values

Trichloroethene			
	air trichloroethene		Sampling time: end of shift
(ml/m^3)		(mg/m^3)	urine trichloroacetic acid (mg/l)
10		55	20
20		109	40
30		164	60
50		273	100

Tetrachloroethene			
	air tetrachloroethene		Sampling time: 16 hours after the end of a shift
(ml/m^3)		(mg/m^3)	whole blood tetrachloroethene (mg/l)
10		69	0.2
20		138	0.4
30		206	0.6
50		344	1.0

Dichloromethane			
	air dichloromethane		Sampling time: during exposure, at least 2 hours after beginning of exposure
(ml/m^3)		(mg/m^3)	whole blood dichloromethane (mg/l)
10		35	0.1
20		70	0.2
50		175	0.5
100		350	1

G 14

---

[2] Expositionsäquivalente für Krebserzeugende Arbeitsstoffe = exposure equivalents for carcinogenic materials

Biological tolerance value for occupational exposures – see Appendix 1 "Biomonitoring"

Substance	Parameter	BAT[3]	Assay material	Sampling time
1,1,1-trichloro-ethane	1,1,1-trichloro-ethane	550 µg/l	whole blood	for long-term exposures: after several shifts; at the beginning of the next shift

3.2   Functional disorders, symptoms

3.2.1   Mode of action

Trichloroethene: because of its high solubility in lipids and the resulting slow satura-tion of and delayed release from adipose tissue, trichloroethene is a highly cumula-tive narcotic. Inhalation of high concentrations causes paralysis of the medullary res-piratory and/or cardiac centres. The sensitization of the conduction system of the heart caused by trichloroethene is more pronounced than that caused by other nar-cotic chlorinated hydrocarbons, the toxic effects on liver and kidney parenchyma, on the other hand, relatively slight and more often observed after long-term exposure. Deep narcosis develops at a concentration of about 5000 ml/m^3; sedative (subnar-cotic) effects begin at about 200 ml/m^3.

After short-term inhalation, trichloroethene is mostly exhaled; only a small part of the dose is metabolized and excreted via the kidneys.

Under the conditions normally found at the workplace, i.e. during continuous in-halation of low levels of the substance, it may be assumed that 50 % to 60 % of the inhaled trichloroethene is retained. Metabolism takes place mainly in the liver. The products (formed via trichloroethene epoxide and chloral) include trichloroacetic acid (TCA) and trichloroethanol (TCE). 5 % to 8 % of the TCA is excreted in the urine. The TCE binds to glucuronic acid and is excreted as urochloralic acid (trichloroethyl glucosiduronic acid). The excretion patterns of TCA and TCE are not constant and depend on individual factors, on the exposure profile and duration, on the concen-tration, etc. Only for the total amount of excreted TCA and TCE is there a fixed lin-ear relationship with the amount of trichloroethene taken up.

Recent studies with rats have revealed a glutathione-dependent metabolic pathway which is responsible for the induction of renal cell tumours. The genotoxic and cyto-toxic metabolites formed via this pathway have also been detected in man. Epi-demiological studies have reported an increased incidence of renal cell tumours in persons exposed for many years to high levels of trichloroethene. Thus, together with

---

[3] Biologischer Arbeitsstoff-Toleranzwert (BAT) = biological tolerance value for occupational exposures

the data for the mechanism of action, these results demonstrate a causal relationship between occupational exposure to high trichloroethene concentrations and the development of renal cell tumours in man.

Alcohol potentiates the toxic effects.

Liquid trichloroethene defats the skin and causes marked irritation, especially after repeated contact; in high concentrations trichloroethene vapour irritates the eyes and the mucous membranes of the upper airways.

The polyneuropathy observed in persons working with trichloroethene, especially cranial nerve damage and psycho-organic syndrome, is most probably caused by the dichloroacetylene formed from trichloroethene by splitting off HCl in the presence of alkali; even very small amounts of dichloroacetylene appear to have toxic effects.

Tetrachloroethene is soluble in lipids and is a narcotic with peripheral and central nervous effects; its narcotic effects are like those of trichloroethene. It also causes liver and kidney damage. Tetrachloroethene is eliminated mainly via the lungs. There is a fixed relationship between the concentration of tetrachloroethene in the exhaled air and the preceding exposure levels. Tetrachloroethene can still be detected in the exhaled air after several days. A small proportion of the dose appears in the urine in the form of the metabolites trichloroacetic acid and the glucuronic acid conjugate of trichloroethanol. It accumulates in the organism and so there is no clear association between levels of exposure to tetrachloroethene and the concentration of trichloroacetic acid in single urine samples. The half life of tetrachloroethene in the organism is about 4 days. Because it is readily soluble in lipids it defats the skin and can cause skin damage.

Dichloromethane in high concentrations has depressant effects on the central nervous system and can increase the sensitivity of the heart muscle to catecholamines. The hepatotoxic and nephrotoxic potential is considered to be slight.

Dichloromethane is metabolized via two pathways. Oxidative metabolism leads to the formation of carbon monoxide and carbon dioxide. Via a second glutathione-dependent metabolic pathway, dichloromethane can be converted to formaldehyde/formate and enter C1 metabolism. For this metabolic pathway, marked species differences have been demonstrated which correlate with differences in carcinogenic effects of dichloromethane. Tumour development in the liver and lungs of the mouse were explained in terms of the high level of metabolism of dichloromethane via the glutathione-dependent pathway in these organs of this species. The actual genotoxic metabolite is thought to be the intermediate S-(chloromethyl)glutathione. To date, a clear association between exposure to dichloromethane and the development of tumours in man could not be demonstrated.

The critical toxic effect of the substance is the formation of carbon monoxide. The CO-haemoglobin level should be kept under 5 %, to protect in particular employees with coronary heart disease or peripheral arterial circulatory disorders.

G 14

1,1,1-Trichloroethane has prenarcotic sedative effects and irritates both the airway and eye mucosa and the skin. In individual cases after high level exposures, damage in the central or peripheral nervous system has been described.

In the organism only a small part of the 1,1,1-trichloroethane is metabolized; mostly the substance is exhaled unchanged.

3.2.2   Acute and subacute effects on health

Trichloroethene
- narcotic effects including all stages of intoxication and even fatal deep narcosis
- anorexia, abdominal symptoms
- nausea, vomiting, abdominal pain/spasms
- headaches, dizziness
- lassitude
- motility, sensibility and trophic disorders of the extremities
- rare: acute irritation of the skin and mucous membranes (coughing, dyspnoea)
- occasional sudden deaths caused by ventricular fibrillation after physical effort and alcohol consumption

Survivors of an acute intoxication have generally no residual organ damage.

Tetrachloroethene
- narcotic effects including all stages of intoxication and even fatal deep narcosis
- in rare cases direct exposure to tetrachloroethene vapour results in pulmonary oedema
- gastrointestinal disorders and even haemorrhagic enteritis
- anorexia, abdominal symptoms
- nausea, vomiting, abdominal pain/spasms
- headaches, dizziness
- lassitude
- motility, sensibility and trophic disorders of the extremities
- rare: acute irritation of the skin and mucous membranes (coughing, dyspnoea)
- occasional sudden deaths caused by ventricular fibrillation after physical effort and alcohol consumption

Survivors of an acute intoxication have generally no residual organ damage.

Dichloromethane
- narcotic effects including all stages of intoxication and even fatal deep narcosis
- anorexia, nausea
- headaches, dizziness
- signs of irritation of the eyes, airways and skin
- cardiac arrhythmia
- angina pectoris-like symptoms

Survivors of an acute intoxication have generally no residual organ damage.

1,1,1-Trichloroethane
- narcotic effects including all stages of intoxication and even fatal deep narcosis
- signs of irritation of the eyes, airways and skin
- cardiac arrhythmia

Survivors of an acute intoxication have generally no residual organ damage.

3.2.3   Chronic effects on health

Trichloroethene
neurasthenic symptoms (see also subacute effects), damage to the CNS, the myocardium, the liver and kidneys; epidemiological studies indicate an increased risk of developing renal cell tumours after high level exposures; changes in the blood and haematopoietic organs are rare and doubtful; mucosal irritation in the upper airways; eczema

Tetrachloroethene
dermatitis of very variable kinds, mucosal irritation in the upper airways, encephalopathy, increased psycho-vegetative hyperexcitability, gastrointestinal disorders
Effects on parenchymatous organs are possible but liver damage is mostly slight. There are rare severe cases of liver cell necrosis, sometimes with involvement of the kidneys in a hepatorenal syndrome.

Dichloromethane
The critical toxic effect is the formation of carbon monoxide or CO-haemoglobin. In persons exposed to high levels of the substance at work, central nervous effects have been described.

1,1,1-Trichloroethane
The critical effect of the substance is its prenarcotic effect. In occasional individuals exposed long-term to 1,1,1-trichloroethane, peripheral neuropathy has been described without proof of a causal relationship. Skin contact can cause defatting and drying out of the skin.

G 14

5   References

Brüning T, Pesch B, Wiesenhütter B et al. (2003) Renal cell cancer risk and occupational exposure to trichloroethylene: results of a consecutive case-control study in Arnsberg, Germany. Am J Ind Med 43: 274-285
Commission Recommendation 2003/670/EC concerning the European schedule of occupational diseases. Annex I
Council Directive 98/24/EC on the protection of the health and safety of workers from the risks related to chemical agents at work

Deutsche Forschungsgemeinschaft (German Research Foundation, DFG) (ed) List of
    MAK and BAT Values 2007. Maximum Concentrations and Biological Tolerance
    Values at the workplace. Wiley-VCH, Weinheim
Deutsche Forschungsgemeinschaft (German Research Foundation, DFG) (ed) The
    MAK-Collection for Occupational Health and Safety. Wiley-VCH
    at: www.mrw.interscience.wiley.com/makbat
GESTIS-database on hazardous substances. BGIA
    at: www.dguv.de/bgia/gestis-database
GESTIS-international limit values for chemical agents. BGIA
    at: www.dguv.de/bgia/gestis-limit-values
Henschler D, Vamvakas S, Lammert M, Dekan W, Kraus B, Thomas B, Ulm K (1995)
    Increased incidence of renal well tumors in a cohort of cardboard workers ex-
    posed to trichloroethene. Arch Toxicol 69: 291–299
Kaneko T, Wang P-Y, Sato A (1997) Assessment of the health effects of trichloro-
    ethylene. Industrial Health 35: 301–324

G 15   Chromium(VI) compounds

Committee for occupational medicine, working group "Hazardous substances",
Berufsgenossenschaft der chemischen Industrie, Heidelberg

Preliminary remarks

The present guideline describes a scheme for occupational medical prophylaxis
which aims to prevent or ensure early diagnosis of disorders which can be caused
by chromium(VI) compounds.
Not covered by this guideline is the induction of allergies by exposure to traces of
chromium(VI) compounds which can take place during the processing of metals or on
contact with, e.g., chromium(III) compounds, cement, used aqueous metal-working
fluids.

Schedule

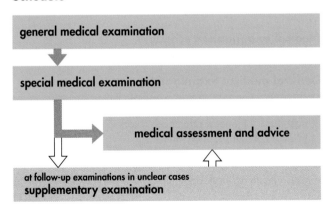

1   Medical examinations

Occupational medical examinations are to be carried out for persons at whose work-places exposure to chromium(VI) compounds could endanger health (e.g. the occupational exposure limit value is exceeded).

1.1   Examinations, intervals between examinations

initial examination	before taking up the job
first follow-up examination	after 6–12 months
further follow-up examinations	after 12–24 months and when leaving the job
premature follow-up examination	• after a serious or prolonged illness which could cause concern as to whether the activity should be continued • in individual cases when the physician considers it necessary, e.g. when there is short-term concern about the person's health • when requested by an employee who suspects a causal association between his or her illness and work

1.2   Medical examination schedule

1.2.1   General medical examination

Initial examination

- review of past history (general anamnesis, work anamnesis, symptoms)
- urinalysis (multiple test strips, sediment)

Follow-up examination

Interim anamnesis (including work anamnesis) with particular attention to:
- secretions
- encrustations and bleeding in the nose
- coughing
- expectoration
- respiratory difficulties
- shortness of breath
- skin disorders
- urinalysis (multiple test strips, sediment)

1.2.2   Special medical examination

Initial examination

- examination of the nose with the speculum
- spirometry
- large or medium sized x-ray picture of the thorax (not smaller than 10×10 cm) or use of an x-ray diagnosis which is less than 1 year old
- full blood count
- erythrocyte sedimentation reaction
- examination of the skin; attention to be paid to:
  eczema, fissures, allergic manifestations, venous circulatory disorders resulting from surface varicose veins

Also helpful:

- immunoglobulin E
- determination of chromium in urine and erythrocytes (basis level)

Follow-up examination

- as for the initial examination: the x-ray examination of the thorax should be carried out for persons aged 40 years or more or who have been exposed for more than 10 years and should be repeated at 12-month intervals unless results are available from such an x-ray examination which has been carried out within the previous year
- every 6–12 months: determination of chromium levels in biological material (see Section 3.2.3)

1.2.3   Supplementary examination

Follow-up examination

In unclear cases: examination by an ENT specialist

1.3   Requirements for the medical examinations

- competent doctor or occupational health professional
- laboratory analyses and x-ray examination carried out with appropriate quality control (Good Laboratory Practice)
- necessary equipment:
  - spirometer
  - nasal speculum

G 15

2   Occupational medical assessment and advice

An assessment is only possible when the workplace situation and the exposure of the individual are known. For this purpose a risk assessment as defined in Article 4 Council directive 98/24/EC must have been carried out; it must describe the levels of exposure to chromium(VI) compounds and specify which technical, organizational and individual protective measures have been applied.

2.1   Assessment criteria

2.1.1   Long-term concern about health

Initial examination	Follow-up examination

Persons with severe disorders:
- chronic disorders, inflammation and growths in the nasal sinuses or throat
- pleural fibrosis or other damage which significantly impairs the function of the airways or lungs or which favours the development of bronchopulmonary disorders
- venous circulatory disorders resulting from surface varicose veins
- severe skin fissures
- recurrent allergic manifestations
- chronic eczema

2.1.2   Short-term concern about health

Initial examination	Follow-up examination

Persons with the disorders mentioned in Section 2.1.1, provided recovery is to be expected.

2.1.3   No concern about health under certain conditions

Initial examination	Follow-up examination

If the illnesses or functional disorders mentioned in Section 2.1.1 are less severe, the doctor should establish whether or not it is possible for the person to start work or go on working under certain conditions. Such conditions could include
- technical protective measures
- organizational protective measures, e.g., limitation of exposure periods
- transfer to workplaces known to involve lower levels of exposure
- personal protective equipment which takes the individual's state of health into account
- more frequent follow-up examinations

- persons without clinical symptoms for whom the laboratory findings or the impairment of lung function is borderline

2.1.4   No concern about health

Initial examination	Follow-up examination

All other persons, provided there are no restrictions on their employment.

2.2   Medical advice

The advice in an individual case should be commensurate with the workplace situation and the results of the medical examinations.

Employees are to be informed about the biomonitoring results.

The persons should be told of the possibility of skin sensitization.

Employees whose work involves potential skin contact should be informed about the necessary measures for skin protection (protection, cleaning and care of the skin) and of the correct use of appropriate gloves.

The risk associated with smoking cigarettes especially if the airways are also exposed to chromium(VI) compounds should be made clear.

Attention to general hygienic measures is to be recommended.

If during the course of his work in the company the occupational physician finds indications that the risk assessment should be brought up to date to improve health and safety standards, he is to inform the employer. When this is necessary, the interests of the employee are to be protected (medical confidentiality).

3   Supplementary notes

3.1   External and internal exposure

3.1.1   Occurrence, sources of hazards

Listed below are the kinds of processes, workplaces or activities, including cleaning and repair work, for which exposure to chromium(VI) compounds must be expected. This must be taken into account during the risk assessment.

- production of the carcinogenic chromium(VI) compounds and of preparations containing these substances
- spraying of coatings containing more than 0.1 % w/w of carcinogenic chromium(VI) compounds
- thermal cutting and welding and removal of coatings on objects containing chromium(VI) compounds

G 15

- manual arc welding with high alloy coated electrodes (containing 5 % w/w or more chromium)
- work at chromic acid galvanic baths which are agitated and heated (≥70°C)
- metal active gas welding with high alloy filler wire (with ≥5 % w/w chromium in the alloy or slag formers)
- flame, arc and plasma arc spraying with high alloy spray materials (with ≥5 % w/w chromium)
- plasma arc and laser cutting of nickel-chromium objects ((with ≥5 % w/w chromium)
- demolition work on production plants for chromium(VI) compounds

Occurrence and hazards for specific substances are documented in the information system on hazardous substances (GESTIS) (see Section 4).

3.1.2   Physicochemical properties and classification

Chromium can exist in its compounds in valencies between +1 and +6; technically and toxicologically the chromium(VI) compounds are most important.

Potassium, sodium and magnesium chromates are readily soluble in water, calcium chromate is moderately soluble (at 20°C between 2 % and 10 % depending on the content of water of crystallization).

Barium, lead, strontium and zinc chromates are practically insoluble in water but barium, strontium and zinc chromates are readily soluble in acids.

The information system on hazardous substances (GESTIS) provides details of international threshold limit values, classification, evaluation and other substance-specific information (see Section 4).

Additional information is to be found in the recommendations of the DFG Commission for the Investigation of Health Hazards of Chemical Compounds in the Work Area (List of MAK and BAT Values).

3.1.3   Uptake

The substances are taken up mainly via the airways and through the gastrointestinal tract.

3.1.4   Biomonitoring

Information about biomonitoring may be found in Appendix 1 "Biomonitoring".

Exposure equivalents for carcinogenic substances (EKA: see the current List of MAK and BAT Values) give the relationships between the concentration of a substance in the workplace air and that of the substance or its metabolites in biological material. From these relationships, the body burden which results from uptake of the substance exclusively by inhalation may be determined. They are intended to provide the physician with a tool to help in the assessment of the analytical results. The EKA are not threshold values but data from occupational medical examinations.

Exposure equivalents for carcinogenic materials (EKA)[1] from the List of MAK and BAT Values

alkali metal chromates (Cr(VI))		
Concentration in the air calculated as CrO_3	Sampling time: for long-term exposures after several shifts	Sampling time: end of exposure or end of shift
(mg/m^3)	erythrocytes[2] chromium (µg/l whole blood)	urine[3] chromium (µg/l)
0.03	9	12
0.05	17	20
0.08	25	30
0.10	35	40

Biomonitoring should be carried out with reliable methods and meet quality control requirements (see Appendix 1 "Biomonitoring").

3.2   Functional disorders, symptoms

3.2.1   Mode of action

Chromic acid (H_2CrO_4), its anhydride (CrO_3, often wrongly called chromic acid) and their salts, the chromates (chromium(VI) compounds) are powerful oxidizing agents and so cause cell damage.

Chromium(VI) compounds can cause sensitization of the skin and induce bronchial carcinomas.

It has been suggested that the carcinogenicity of the chromium(VI) compounds results from redox processes in which the solubility of the various compounds plays a role. In smokers syncarcinogenicity is possible.

Neither acute nor chronic poisoning has been reported for chromium(III) compounds at the workplace.

G 15

---

[1] Expositionsäquivalente für Krebserzeugende Arbeitsstoffe = exposure equivalents for carcinogenic materials
[2] not applicable for exposure to welding fumes
[3] also applicable for exposure to welding fumes

3.2.2   Acute and subacute effects on health

Eye
Acute local exposure to dust and vapour of chromium trioxide, chromates or dichromates causes conjunctivitis with lacrimation and corneal damage.

Skin
Penetration of chromium trioxide, chromates or dichromates into skin wounds, especially grazes or fissures, produces the characteristic "chrome ulcers" which heal very poorly.
Chromium(VI) compounds can cause sensitization, especially of the skin.

Gastrointestinal tract
Oral uptake of large amounts of these substances causes immediate yellow discoloration of the mucous membranes and the oral cavity, difficulty in swallowing, corrosion of the glottis, burning pains in the stomach area, vomiting of yellow and green material (perhaps aspiratory pneumonia), diarrhoea with blood in the stool, circulatory failure, spasms, unconsciousness, renal failure, death in coma.

Airways
Inhalation of dust or vapour of chromium trioxide, chromates or dichromates in higher concentrations causes damage to the nasal mucosa (hyperaemia, catarrh, epithelial necrosis) and also irritation of the upper airways and lungs.

3.2.3   Chronic effects on health

Skin
The development of ulcers, sometimes deep ulcers (painless, red wall-like edges, necrotic ground, sometimes scabbing); these deep ulcers develop only where the skin is cracked, fissured or has small wounds, not on intact skin. Epicutaneous allergy induction can result in dermatitis or eczema especially on the hands. Note the marked tendency to recurrence.

Nose
Typical septum changes with the following stages:
A: reddening, swelling, increased secretion
B: ulceration, bleeding, scabs and encrustations
C: septum perforation
C I: pin-head sized perforation
C II: lentil sized perforation
C III: large to subtotal septum defect
Septum changes can develop after just weeks or months of such exposures; they are usually painless. Occasional rhinitis atrophicans, occasional loss of the sense of smell and taste.

Throat and larynx
chronic catarrh

Bronchi
chronic bronchitis, sometimes with spastic components, concomitant emphysema, in rare cases bronchial asthma; bronchial carcinoma possible but not distinguishable from bronchial carcinoma of other genesis

Gastrointestinal tract
So-called "chrome enteropathy" – gastrointestinal disorders resulting from swallowing small amounts of chromium with the saliva – is disputed. Nausea, stomach pain, diarrhoea (sometimes with blood) and involvement of the liver have been described.

4   References

Commission Recommendation 2003/670/EC concerning the European schedule of occupational diseases. Annex I

Council Directive 67/548/EEC on the approximation of the laws, regulations and administrative provisions relating to the classification, packaging and labelling of dangerous substances

Council Directive 98/24/EC on the protection of the health and safety of workers from the risks related to chemical agents at work

Deutsche Forschungsgemeinschaft (German Research Foundation, DFG) (ed) List of MAK and BAT Values 2007. Maximum Concentrations and Biological Tolerance Values at the workplace. Wiley-VCH, Weinheim

Deutsche Forschungsgemeinschaft (German Research Foundation, DFG) (ed) The MAK-Collection for Occupational Health and Safety. Wiley-VCH
    at: www.mrw.interscience.wiley.com/makbat

GESTIS-database on hazardous substances. BGIA
    at: www.dguv.de/bgia/gestis-database

GESTIS-international limit values for chemical agents. BGIA
    at: www.dguv.de/bgia/gestis-limit-values

G 15

G 16   Arsenic and arsenic compounds (with the exception of arsine)

Committee for occupational medicine, working group "Hazardous substances", Berufsgenossenschaft der chemischen Industrie, Heidelberg

Preliminary remarks

The present guideline describes a scheme for occupational medical prophylaxis which aims to prevent or ensure early diagnosis of disorders which can be caused by arsenic and arsenic compounds (with the exception of arsine).

Schedule

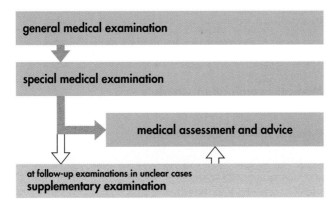

1   Medical examinations

Occupational medical examinations are to be carried out for persons at whose work-places exposure to arsenic or arsenic compounds could endanger health (e.g. the occupational exposure limit value is exceeded).

1.1   Examinations, intervals between examinations

initial examination	before taking up the job
first follow-up examination	after 6–12 months
further follow-up examinations	after 6–12 months or when leaving the job
premature follow-up examination	• after a serious or prolonged illness which could cause concern as to whether the activity should be continued • in individual cases when the physician considers it necessary, e.g. when there is short-term concern about the person's health • when requested by an employee who suspects a causal association between his or her illness and work

1.2   Medical examination schedule

1.2.1   General medical examination

Initial examination

Review of past history (general anamnesis, smoking anamnesis, work anamnesis – also with respect to previous exposures to carcinogenic substances, symptoms)
• urinalysis (multiple test strips, sediment)

Follow-up examination

• interim anamnesis (including work anamnesis)
• urinalysis (multiple test strips, sediment)

1.2.2   Special medical examination

Initial examination

- erythrocyte sedimentation reaction
- γ-GT
- examination of the skin; attention to: hyperkeratosis, pigmentation changes, eczema

Follow-up examination

Like the initial examination but, in addition,
- chest x-ray for persons aged 40 years or more and for persons who have been exposed for more than 10 years

Also helpful:
- determination of arsenic in the urine, immediately after the last shift after exposure on at least 3 consecutive days (see Section 3.1.4)

1.2.3   Supplementary examination

Follow-up examination

In unclear cases:
determination of arsenic in biological material (see Section 3.1.4)

1.3   Requirements for the medical examinations

- competent doctor or occupational health professional
- laboratory analyses and x-ray examination carried out with appropriate quality control (Good Laboratory Practice)

2   Occupational medical assessment and advice

An assessment is only possible when the workplace situation and the exposure of the individual are known. For this purpose a risk assessment as defined in Article 4 Council directive 98/24/EC must have been carried out; it must describe the levels of exposure to arsenic or arsenic compounds and specify which technical, organizational and individual protective measures have been applied.

2.1 Assessment criteria

2.1.1 Long-term concern about health

Initial examination	Follow-up examination

Persons with severe disorders of
* the liver
* the kidneys
* the gastrointestinal tract
* the skin (e.g. chronic eczema, chronic dermatosis in the form of, e.g., psoriasis, ichthyosis, hypersensitivity to light, farmer's skin, multiple hyperkeratosis, known hypersensitivity to arsenic)
* the vessels
* the blood
* the peripheral and central nervous systems
* the bronchi

Also persons with
* alcohol addiction

2.1.2 Short-term concern about health

Initial examination	Follow-up examination

Persons with the disorders mentioned in Section 2.1.1, provided recovery is to be expected.

2.1.3 No concern about health under certain conditions

Initial examination	Follow-up examination

If the illnesses or functional disorders mentioned in Section 2.1.1 are less severe, the doctor should establish whether or not it is possible for the person to start work or go on working under certain conditions. Such conditions could include
* technical protective measures
* organizational protective measures, e.g., limitation of exposure periods
* transfer to workplaces known to involve lower levels of exposure
* personal protective equipment which takes the individual's state of health into account
* more frequent follow-up examinations

2.1.4   No concern about health

Initial examination	**Follow-up examination**

All other persons, provided there are no restrictions on their employment.

2.2   Medical advice

The advice in an individual case should be commensurate with the workplace situation and the results of the medical examinations.

Employees are to be informed about the biomonitoring results.

Employees should be informed about general hygienic measures and personal protective equipment. The germ cell mutagenicity of arsenic and arsenic compounds should be mentioned.

The risk associated with smoking cigarettes especially if the airways are also exposed to arsenic or arsenic compounds should be made clear.

If during the course of his work in the company the occupational physician finds indications that the risk assessment should be brought up to date to improve health and safety standards, he is to inform the employer. When it is necessary to inform the employer, the interests of the employee are to be protected (medical confidentiality).

3   Supplementary notes

3.1   External and internal exposure

3.1.1   Occurrence, sources of hazards

Listed below are the kinds of processes, workplaces or activities, including cleaning and repair work, for which exposure to arsenic or arsenic compounds must be expected. This must be taken into account during the risk assessment.

- production and processing of arsenic compounds when dust is produced
- extraction of non-ferrous metals from ores and other starting materials containing arsenic
- roasting of iron pyrites
- repair or cleaning of flue dust systems, filters, etc
- processing of lead chamber residues in the production of sulfuric acid
- dismantling and renovation work in areas contaminated with arsenic or arsenic compounds

Occurrence and hazards for specific substances are documented in the information system on hazardous substances (GESTIS) (see Section 4).

3.1.2   Physicochemical properties and classification

Arsenic exists in several modifications of which the grey metallic form is most stable. In its compounds arsenic can have the valencies +3, +5 and −3. The arsenic(III) halogenides are poisonous liquids which hydrolyse readily. In water the alkali metal arsenites are readily soluble, the alkaline earth arsenites poorly soluble, and the heavy metal arsenites insoluble. White arsenic (arsenic(III) oxide) is readily soluble in hydrochloric acid and also in alkalis. Arsenic(III) compounds are more poisonous than arsenic(V) compounds.

The information system on hazardous substances (GESTIS) provides details of international threshold limit values, classification, evaluation and other substance-specific information (see Section 4).

Additional information is to be found in the recommendations of the DFG Commission for the Investigation of Health Hazards of Chemical Compounds in the Work Area (List of MAK and BAT Values).

3.1.3   Uptake

Arsenic and arsenic compounds are taken up mainly via the airways in the form of dust or fumes and through the gastrointestinal tract.

3.1.4   Biomonitoring

Information about biomonitoring may be found in Appendix 1 "Biomonitoring".

Exposure equivalents for carcinogenic substances (EKA: see the current List of MAK and BAT Values) give the relationships between the concentration of a substance in the workplace air and that of the substance or its metabolites in biological material. From these relationships, the body burden which results from uptake of the substance exclusively by inhalation may be determined. They are intended to provide the physician with a tool to help in the assessment of the analytical results. The EKA are not threshold values but data from occupational medical examinations.

Exposure equivalents for carcinogenic materials (EKA)[1] from the List of MAK and BAT Values

arsenic trioxide	
	Sampling time: end of exposure or end of shift
air arsenic (mg/m^3)	urine[2] arsenic (µg/l)
0.01	50
0.05	90
0.10	130

See also the section on BLW ("Biologischer Leit-Wert") in the List of MAK and BAT Values.

Biomonitoring should be carried out with reliable methods and meet quality control requirements (see Appendix 1 "Biomonitoring").

3.2   Functional disorders, symptoms

3.2.1   Mode of action (uptake, metabolism, elimination)

Arsenic and inorganic arsenic compounds can be taken up by inhalation or orally. They are rapidly distributed into all organs and accumulate especially in the liver, kidneys and lungs.

In the body, inorganic arsenic compounds are first reduced to arsenites. These are then methylated and yield dimethylarsinic acid (cacodylic acid) via monomethylarsonic acid. Dimethylarsinic acid is excreted as the main urinary metabolite of inorganic arsenic compounds.

Arsenic and arsenic compounds do not accumulate markedly; they are stored in the liver, kidneys, bones, skin and nails. Most of the dose has a half life of only 2 days. This is important for biomonitoring.

Small amounts of absorbed arsenic are eliminated via the skin, hair, nails and mother's milk. Even when the level of internal exposure is low, arsenic enters the placenta.

---

[1] Expositionsäquivalente für Krebserzeugende Arbeitsstoffe = exposure equivalents for carcinogenic materials
[2] volatile arsenic compounds by hydrogenation

3.2.2   Acute and subacute effects on health

There is little information available about adverse effects on health of grey metallic arsenic. It is assumed that the handling of pure metallic arsenic does not cause poisoning.

The toxic effects which are, however, often observed are ascribed by various authors to contamination with arsenic trioxide.

Yellow, non-metallic arsenic is, in contrast, highly toxic. Its properties are like those of yellow (white) phosphorus. But yellow arsenic is not very stable (metastable) and is rapidly converted to the metallic modification.

Exposure to arsenic compounds causes local irritation of the eyes, the upper respiratory tract and the skin. Conjunctival inflammation often develops with itching, burning, lacrimation and sensitivity of the eyes to light, occasionally also severe eye damage. Most reports describe severe airway damage with dyspnoea, coughing and pains in the chest. Acute inflammation of the skin can also develop.

In some cases gastrointestinal disorders and systemic effects on the peripheral and central nervous systems have also been reported after inhalation exposure.

Oral poisoning with arsenic trioxide can follow two courses:

paralytic form
severe cardiocirculatory and central nervous disorders with circulatory collapse/ shock, respiratory paralysis and death

gastrointestinal form
metallic, garlic-like taste, burning sensation in the mouth and on the lips, dysphagia, reflex vomiting, diarrhoea with drop in blood pressure, cardiac dysrhythmia, muscle spasms, functional disorders of the kidneys, etc.

After uptake of very high doses (>2 mg arsenic per kg body weight) subsequent damage is often observed in the peripheral nerves (peripheral neuropathy) and sometimes also CNS disorders (confusion, hallucinations, etc.). Also blood disorders (anaemia, leukopenia), functional liver disorders (hepatomegaly) and skin changes have been described.

3.2.3   Chronic effects on health

Little is known of long-term effects of pure metallic arsenic. Mostly people are exposed to mixtures of arsenic and arsenic trioxide.

Dusts containing arsenic (also in poorly soluble forms) cause irritation and tissue changes in the conjunctiva, the upper respiratory tract and the skin. Systemically induced skin damage (hyperpigmentation, hyperkeratosis) and damage to peripheral vessels (especially the arteries of the fingers) have been reported.

In addition, cardiovascular disorders, diabetes, peripheral nerve damage, disorders of vessels in the brain and encephalopathy have been observed.

Carcinomas of the skin, airways, urinary bladder and kidneys have been described.

G 16

4   References

Commission Recommendation 2003/670/EC concerning the European schedule of occupational diseases. Annex I

Council Directive 67/548/EEC on the approximation of the laws, regulations and administrative provisions relating to the classification, packaging and labelling of dangerous substances

Council Directive 98/24/EC on the protection of the health and safety of workers from the risks related to chemical agents at work

Deutsche Forschungsgemeinschaft (German Research Foundation, DFG) (ed) List of MAK and BAT Values 2007. Maximum Concentrations and Biological Tolerance Values at the workplace. Wiley-VCH, Weinheim

Deutsche Forschungsgemeinschaft (German Research Foundation, DFG) (ed) The MAK-Collection for Occupational Health and Safety. Wiley-VCH
      at: www.mrw.interscience.wiley.com/makbat

GESTIS-database on hazardous substances. BGIA
      at: www.dguv.de/bgia/gestis-database

GESTIS-international limit values for chemical agents. BGIA
      at: www.dguv.de/bgia/gestis-limit-values

G 19   Dimethylformamide

Committee for occupational medicine, working group "Hazardous substances", Berufsgenossenschaft der chemischen Industrie, Heidelberg

Preliminary remarks

The present guideline describes a scheme for occupational medical prophylaxis which aims to prevent or ensure early diagnosis of disorders which can be caused by dimethylformamide.

Schedule

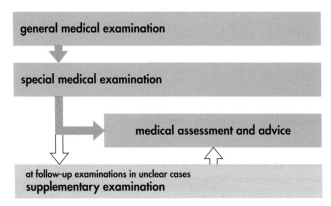

general medical examination

special medical examination

medical assessment and advice

at follow-up examinations in unclear cases
supplementary examination

1   Medical examinations

Occupational medical examinations are to be carried out for persons exposed at work to levels of dimethylformamide (DMF) which could have adverse effects on health (e.g. the occupational exposure limit value is exceeded) or for whom dermal absorption could endanger health.

1.1   Examinations, intervals between examinations

initial examination	before taking up the job
first follow-up examination	after 6–12 months
further follow-up examinations	after 12–24 months and when leaving the job
premature follow-up examination	• after an illness lasting for several weeks or when a physical handicap gives cause for concern about whether the work should be continued • in individual cases when the physician considers it necessary, e.g. when there is short-term concern about the person's health • when requested by an employee who suspects a causal association between his or her illness and work

1.2   Medical examination schedule

1.2.1   General medical examination

Initial examination

review of past history (general anamnesis, work anamnesis)

Follow-up examination

interim anamnesis (including work anamnesis)
Particular attention should be paid to: headaches, anorexia, nausea, vomiting, feeling of pressure in the epigastric region, sometimes colic-like abdominal pain, digestive disorders (diarrhoea, constipation), nausea and vomiting, weight loss, alcohol intolerance

1.2.2   Special medical examination

| **Initial examination** | **Follow-up examination** |

- urinalysis (multiple test strips)
- SGPT (ALT), γ-GT, SGOT (AST)
- biomonitoring (see Section 3.1.4) – but not at the initial examination

1.2.3   Supplementary examination

Follow-up examination

In unclear cases:
- further liver diagnostics, e.g. epigastric sonography

1.3   Requirements for the medical examinations

- competent doctor or occupational health professional
- laboratory analyses carried out with appropriate quality control (Good Laboratory Practice)

2   Occupational medical assessment and advice

An assessment is only possible when the workplace situation and the exposure of the individual are known. For this purpose a risk assessment as defined in Article 4 Council directive 98/24/EC must have been carried out; it must specify which technical, organizational and individual protective measures have been applied.

2.1   Assessment criteria

2.1.1   Long-term concern about health

| **Initial examination** | **Follow-up examination** |

Persons with
- chronic liver disorders
- addiction to alcohol, drugs or medication

2.1.2   Short-term concern about health

Initial examination

Persons with the disorders mentioned in Section 2.1.1, provided recovery is to be expected.

Follow-up examination

See initial examination.
Depending on the severity of the liver function disorder from which they have recovered, a period of several months without DMF-exposure should be considered for employees returning to work. At the end of this period and after a medical examination, the persons may return to their job.

2.1.3   No concern about health under certain conditions

Initial examination   **Follow-up examination**

If the illnesses or functional disorders mentioned in Section 2.1.1 are less severe, the doctor should establish whether or not it is possible for the person to start work or go on working under certain conditions. Such conditions could include
- technical protective measures
- organizational protective measures, e.g., limitation of exposure periods
- transfer to workplaces known to involve lower levels of exposure
- personal protective equipment which takes the individual's state of health into account
- more frequent follow-up examinations

2.1.4   No concern about health

Initial examination   **Follow-up examination**

All other persons, provided there are no restrictions on their employment.

2.2   Medical advice

The advice in an individual case should be commensurate with the workplace situation and the results of the medical examinations.

Employees should be informed about general hygienic measures and personal protective equipment. Because dimethylformamide can be absorbed through the skin, particular attention should be paid to the use of personal protective equipment including gloves (appropriate material for handling pure DMF: butyl rubber) which provide sufficient protection for the duration of the specific activity. Substance-specific protective measures are documented in the information system on hazardous substances (GESTIS) in the section "Handling and usage" (see Section 4).

Employees should be advised of the alcohol intolerance caused by the synergistic effects of dimethylformamide and alcohol. Medications which cause inhibition of aldehyde dehydrogenases can increase the risk of DMF-induced liver damage.

During the consultation the potential reproductive toxicity of dimethylformamide should be kept in mind (avoidance of exposure of pregnant women).

If during the course of his work in the company the occupational physician finds indications that the risk assessment should be brought up to date to improve health and safety standards, he is to inform the employer. When it is necessary to inform the employer, the interests of the employee are to be protected (medical confidentiality).

3   Supplementary notes

3.1   External and internal exposure

3.1.1   Occurrence, sources of hazards

Occurrence and hazards for specific substances are documented in the information system on hazardous substances (GESTIS) (see Section 4).

Dimethylformamide is used especially as a solvent for plant and animal fats and oils and for certain resins and waxes. It is used in the following industrial production areas:

- production of imitation leather
- the polyacrylonitrile (acrylic) fibre industry
- fine chemicals, pharmaceuticals, cosmetics
- plastic coatings (polyurethane)

3.1.2 Physicochemical properties, occupational exposure limit value and classification

At room temperature dimethylformamide is a clear liquid which is difficult to ignite, is miscible with water and has a faint amine odour. The vapour is heavier than air. At higher temperatures the vapour can form an explosive mixture with air.

N,N-Dimethylformamide
Formula C_3H_7NO
CAS number   68-12-2
MAK[1] value   5 ml/m^3, 15 mg/m^3

The information system on hazardous substances (GESTIS) provides details of classification, evaluation and other substance-specific information (see Section 4).

3.1.3 Uptake

The vapour is taken up readily and rapidly at the workplace by inhalation and through the skin. On direct contact with liquid DMF, the skin is penetrated rapidly. The amount of DMF absorbed when one hand is immersed in the pure liquid for 10 minutes is the same as that inhaled during 8 hours light work in an atmosphere containing a DMF vapour concentration of 30 mg/m^3.

3.1.4 Biomonitoring

Because DMF is so readily absorbed through the skin, biomonitoring is of particular significance for analysis and control of exposure.
Absorbed DMF is rapidly metabolized in the liver and excreted with the urine. There are a number of urinary metabolites including *N*-methylformamide (NMF) and the mercapturic acid, *N*-acetyl-*S*-(*N*-methylcarbamoyl)cysteine (AMCC) which can be used as biomarkers. In addition, it is possible to estimate DMF exposure by determination of haemoglobin adducts in the blood.
If NMF is used as biomarker, it should be remembered that this metabolite is broken down rapidly (half life about 4 hours). Thus accumulation in the organism does not take place.

---

[1] Maximale Arbeitsplatz-Konzentration = maximum workplace concentration

Biological tolerance value for occupational exposures

Substance	Parameter	BAT[2]	Assay material	Sampling time
dimethylformamide	N-methylformamide	35 mg/l	urine	end of exposure or end of shift

Biomonitoring should be carried out with reliable methods and meet quality control requirements.
Further recommendations may be found in Appendix 1 "Biomonitoring".

3.2   Functional disorders, symptoms

3.2.1   Mode of action

The critical target organ of dimethylformamide exposure is the liver. Absorbed DMF is rapidly distributed in the organism. In the liver it is oxidized by microsomal enzyme systems. There the result can be liver cell damage which is manifested histologically in deposits of mostly small fat droplets and parenchymal changes. Clinical symptoms often include a slight, uncharacteristic feeling of pressure or fullness on the right side, nausea and vomiting. The toxic effects on the liver are thought to be caused by metabolites of DMF such as methyl isocyanate.
DMF metabolism interacts with ethanol breakdown in the body and inhibits aldehyde dehydrogenases. If alcohol is consumed during exposure to DMF levels below the occupational exposure limit value, intolerance reactions such as facial flushing, dizziness, nausea and a feeling of tightness in the breast can develop. Such alcohol intolerance reactions are a clear indication of DMF exposure and can be observed for up to 4 days after the end of exposure.

3.2.2   Adverse effects on health

Inhaled DMF vapour can irritate the mucosa of the upper airways. Direct contact of the skin with the liquid can cause local irritation with itching and desquamation. Exposure of the eyes to DMF can cause reddening, a burning sensation, lacrimation or spasmic closure of the eyelids.
Especially in high doses, DMF is hepatotoxic and causes functional changes (increased levels of liver enzymes) and liver damage. Other gastrointestinal symptoms (abdominal pain, anorexia, nausea, vomiting, constipation or diarrhoea), pancreatitis and disorders of the CNS and the circulatory system can develop.

---

[2] Biologischer Arbeitsstoff-Toleranzwert = biological tolerance value for occupational exposures

Existing liver damage, alcohol consumption and the use of medication which inhibits aldehyde dehydrogenases increase the risk of DMF-induced liver damage. The prognosis in cases of hepatocellular damage is generally favourable after an exposure-free interval.

DMF is classified as embryotoxic and/or foetotoxic for man.

4   References

Council Directive 98/24/EC on the protection of the health and safety of workers from the risks related to chemical agents at work

Deutsche Forschungsgemeinschaft (German Research Foundation, DFG) (ed) List of MAK and BAT Values 2007. Maximum Concentrations and Biological Tolerance Values at the workplace. Wiley-VCH, Weinheim

Deutsche Forschungsgemeinschaft (German Research Foundation, DFG) (ed) The MAK-Collection for Occupational Health and Safety. Wiley-VCH
    at: www.mrw.interscience.wiley.com/makbat

GESTIS-database on hazardous substances. BGIA
    at: www.dguv.de/bgia/gestis-database

GESTIS-international limit values for chemical agents. BGIA
    at: www.dguv.de/bgia/gestis-limit-values

Kennedy GL (2001) Biological effects of acetamide, formamide, and their mono and dimethyl derivatives: an update. Crit Rev Toxicol 31: 139–222

G 20   Noise

Committee for occupational medicine, working group "Noise", Metall-Berufsgenossenschaft Nord Süd, Mainz

Preliminary remarks

The present guideline describes a scheme for occupational medical prophylaxis which aims to ensure early diagnosis of adverse effects on the sense of hearing caused by noise and to maintain adequate functioning of the sensory organ ear.
This guideline does not apply for persons without any useful residual hearing.
The working group on noise considers that employment in noisy areas is possible for persons who have been demonstrated by an ear, nose and throat specialist to be deaf in both ears and without useful residual hearing, provided that an increased risk of accidents could not result from their deafness.

Schedule

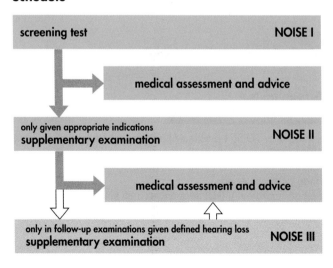

1   Medical examinations

Occupational medical examinations are to be carried out for persons working at places with noise levels which can cause hearing damage (the exposure attains or exceeds the upper exposure action values $L_{EX,8h}$ = 85 dB(A) or $L_{pC,peak}$ = 137 dB(C)). Preventive audiometric testing shall also be available for workers whose exposure exceeds the lower exposure action values $L_{EX,8h}$ = 80 dB(A) or $L_{pC,peak}$ = 135 dB(C).

1.1   Examinations, intervals between examinations

initial examination	before taking up the job
first follow-up examination	after 12 months
further follow-up examinations	within 36 months and when leaving the job within 60 months when $L_{EX,8h}$ < 90 dB(A) or $L_{pC,peak}$ < 137 dB(C)
premature follow-up examination	• in individual cases when the physician considers it necessary, e.g. when there is short-term concern about the person's health • when requested by an employee who suspects a causal association between his or her illness and work • on development of hearing disorders after an illness or accident (e.g. after craniocerebral trauma) and/or tinnitus

1.2   Medical examination schedule

1.2.1   Screening test

Initial examination	Follow-up examination

See the screening test NOISE I (Section 6) and the schedule of examinations and assessment in Section 5:
• brief anamnesis
• examination of the outer ear
• air-conduction audiometry (test frequencies 1–6 kHz)
• medical advice (see 2.2)

1.2.2   Supplementary examination

Initial examination	Follow-up examination

See the supplementary examination NOISE II (Section 6) and the schedule of examinations and assessment in Section 5:

G 20

- medical anamnesis
- otoscopy
- Weber's test
- air-conduction audiometry (test frequencies 0.5–8 kHz) and bone-conduction audiometry (test frequencies 0.5–4 kHz or 6 kHz, depending on the kind of instrument)
- SISI test (if indicated, see the extended supplementary examination NOISE III)
- individual medical advice on hearing protection (see Section 2.2)

The supplementary examination is necessary when
- in the screening test the initial examination
  - reveals a loss of air-conduction hearing in at least one ear for more than one test frequency (1 to 6 KHz) which is greater than the relevant hearing loss threshold value given in Table 1

Table 1: Threshold values for hearing loss at the initial examination.
The values apply in the screening test for air-conduction (AC) audiometry, in persons with sound conduction disorders (as defined in Section 3.4.5) the values in the table apply for bone-conduction (BC) audiometry

Age of person A in years	Frequency in kHz				
	1	2	3	4	6
	Hearing loss in dB				
A ≤ 30	15	15	20	25	25
30 < A ≤ 35	15	20	25	25	30
35 < A ≤ 40	15	20	25	30	35
40 < A ≤ 45	20	25	30	40	40
A > 45	20	25	35	45	50

- in the screening test of the follow-up examination
  - compared with the results of the previous test, hearing loss over a period of at most 3 years in at least one ear of more than 30 dB determined by air-conduction audiometry as the sum of the hearing losses at 2, 3 and 4 kHz
  - or the loss of hearing in at least one ear determined by air-conduction audiometry at 2 kHz is greater than or equal to 40 dB
  - or the sum of hearing losses determined by air-conduction audiometry at 2, 3 and 4 kHz exceeds the relevant threshold value shown in Table 2 in at least one ear

Table 2: Threshold values for hearing loss at the follow-up examinations.
The values apply for air-conduction (AC) audiometry, in persons with sound conduction disorders (as defined in Section 3.4.5) the values in the table apply for bone-conduction (BC) audiometry

Age of person A in years	Sum of hearing losses at 2, 3 and 4 kHz in dB
A ≤ 20	65
20 < A ≤ 25	75
25 < A ≤ 30	85
30 < A ≤ 35	95
35 < A ≤ 40	105
40 < A ≤ 45	115
45 < A ≤ 50	130
A > 50	140

- in the initial examination or for the first time in the follow-up examination there is evidence of
  - operations on the middle and/or inner ear
  - sudden deafness in the past
  - disorders of hearing or tinnitus together with attacks of dizziness
  - inflammation in the auditory canal or on the auricle

1.2.3   Extended supplementary examination

Follow-up examination

See the extended supplementary examination NOISE III (Section 6) and the schedule of examinations and assessment in section 5:
- otoscopy
- air-conduction and bone-conduction audiometry
- speech audiogram for both ears
  (hearing loss for numbers and understanding of single syllables at least at the speech intensities of 50, 65, 80 and 95 dB)

Only when indications make it justified:
- tympanometry (pressure in the auditory canal –300 to +300 daPa)
- stapedius reflex threshold (preferably contralateral, at least 4 frequencies in the range 0.5 to 4 kHz)

The extended supplementary examination is necessary when the hearing loss determined in the supplementary examination NOISE II is greater or equal to 40 dB in both ears at 2 kHz (see 3.4.5).

Note: The works physician can commission an ear, nose and throat specialist to carry out all or part of the extended supplementary examination.

If the hearing loss since the previous follow-up examination has not increased, the extended supplementary examination NOISE III need not be repeated.

1.2.3.1 Determination of acoustic impedance of the eardrum

When justified by the following indications:
- generally unclear audiometric findings
- when a sound conduction disorder has been excluded objectively
- to differentiate between damage to the auditory cells and the auditory nerves

the works physician can have the acoustic impedance of the eardrum determined, provided that the ear, nose and throat specialist approves.

1.3   Requirements for the medical examinations

- competent doctor or occupational health professional
- experience in performing and assessing the results of audiometric tests
- appropriate equipment (see Sections 3.4.1 and 3.4.2)

2   Occupational medical assessment and advice

An assessment is only possible when the workplace situation and the exposure of the individual are known. For this purpose a risk assessment as defined in Article 9 Council directive 89/391/EEC must have been carried out; it must specify which technical, organizational and individual protective measures have been applied.

2.1   Assessment criteria

2.1.1   Long-term concern about health

Initial examination	Follow-up examination

Persons for whom general occupational medical and otologic experience suggests that the results of the medical examinations indicate an increased individual risk of hearing damage caused by noise.
Such a conclusion may be based on the following findings and anamnestic data:

Initial examination

- bone-conduction hearing loss in at least one ear for more than one test frequency (1 to 6 KHz) greater than the relevant hearing loss threshold value given in Table 1

Initial examination	Follow-up examination

- Meniere's disease even without exceeding of the hearing loss threshold values in Table 1 or Table 2
- previous disorders of the inner ear, e.g. sudden deafness, even without exceeding of the hearing loss threshold values in Table 1 or Table 2
- deafness due to inner ear or auditory nerve defects resulting from cranial trauma (hearing loss threshold values of Table 1 exceeded and/or secondary increase in deafness after the accident)
- after an operation for otosclerosis even without exceeding of the hearing loss threshold values in Table 1 or Table 2
- therapy-resistant eczema of the outer auditory canal, secretion from the middle ear which does not respond to therapy, inflammatory skin reactions on or around the auricle which make it impossible to use hearing protectors

Follow-up examination

- long-term concern about health is to be reported when, in spite of exclusion of a middle ear contribution,
  - the hearing loss in both ears is greater than or equal to 40 dB at 2 kHz (see 3.4.5)
  - and, in addition, the plot of proportion of single syllables understood against loudness lies entirely in the hatched area (see the extended supplementary examination NOISE III)

2.1.2   Short-term concern about health

Initial examination	Follow-up examination

Persons who cannot use hearing protectors in the short term because of a transient problem such as acute inflammation of the auditory canal or auricle.

2.1.3   No concern about health under certain conditions

Initial examination	Follow-up examination

Persons as for Section 2.1.1 for whom an increase in hearing loss above 1 kHz is not to be expected provided certain conditions are observed. This applies especially for persons older than 55 years.

G 20

Follow-up examination

Persons for whom a supplementary examination NOISE II or NOISE III has demonstrated that
- the sum of bone-conduction hearing loss at the frequencies 2, 3 and 4 kHz exceeds the threshold values of Table 2 in at least one ear

  or
- the hearing loss has increased by more than 30 dB in at least one ear over a period of at most 3 years

Conditions:
- reduced interval between follow-up examinations (preferably 12 or 24 months)
- provision and use of specially selected hearing protectors (see Section 2.2)
- particular supervision of the use of hearing protectors at the workplace
- if necessary, in agreement with the firm, measures to reduce the daily noise exposure level

2.1.4   No concern about health

Initial examination   **Follow-up examination**

All other persons, provided there are no restrictions on their employment.

2.2   Medical advice

The advice in an individual case should be commensurate with the workplace situation and the results of the medical examinations. Of particular significance is the medical advice as to choice and use of hearing protectors. The employee has to take his or her hearing protectors to the medical examination.

If the results of occupational medical examinations indicate focal cumulation of health risks, the physician, while observing medical confidentiality, is to inform and advise the employer.

The medical advice can, for example, also cover the following points:
- communication difficulties resulting from hearing loss
- increased risk of accidents
- contributions to noise reduction which the employee can make
- recovery of hearing away from the workplace
- causes, effects and treatment of tinnitus
- use of hearing aids

In the consultation with the employer the physician is subject to the rules of medical discretion. The important points to be discussed could include:
- reduction of noise exposure of the employees by means of technical, organizational and individual measures
- content of the general medical advice given to employees on health risks associated with noise

- selection of quiet equipment and processes
- selection of appropriate personal hearing protection

Instruction and information of the employees to motivate them to keep noise to a minimum and to use their personal hearing protectors at work.

3   Supplementary notes

3.1   Exposure

3.1.1   Occurrence, sources of hazards

Fundamentally, whenever persons are employed in noisy areas, there is a risk of hearing damage. Noisy areas are work areas in which the upper exposure action values of the EU guideline ($L_{EX,8h}$ = 85 dB(A) or $L_{C,peak}$ = 137 dB(C)) are attained or exceeded. Such noisy areas must be marked with appropriate signs.

Noisy workplaces are found in most branches of industry, especially often in mining, in the iron and metal industries, stone and other raw material production, woodworking, textile and leather, building and construction, and printing and paper industries.

3.1.2   Risk of hearing damage caused by exposure to noise
         – noise exposure level and exposure duration

The daily noise exposure level and the duration of noise exposure are the external parameters which determine the risk of hearing damage.

Hearing damage may be caused by exposure to daily noise exposure levels of 85 dB(A) or more. Whereas daily noise exposure levels of 85 to 89 dB(A) can cause hearing damage only after long periods of exposure, at levels of 90 dB(A) and more the risk of damage is markedly higher. Daily noise exposure levels of less than 85 dB(A) are unlikely to cause noise-related hearing damage.

It may in general be assumed that noise-related hearing damage will not develop in persons with healthy ears at a daily noise exposure level of 90 dB(A) if the duration of exposure does not exceed 6 years, at 87 dB(A) if it does not exceed 10 years and at 85 dB(A) if it does not exceed 15 years. If hearing damage does develop although the noise level was not higher nor the exposure period longer, the occupational physician is to obtain an anamnesis with the object of discovering the reasons for the damage.

3.2   Functional disorders, clinical picture

3.2.1   Noise-related hearing loss

Noise-related hearing loss is audiometrically detectable loss of hearing acuity which usually develops at frequencies above 1 kHz. Characteristic is an audiometric minimum between 3 and 6 kHz. Later the hearing loss involves also higher frequencies and finally the middle frequency range as well. Noise-related hearing loss is a functional disorder of the inner ear. Workplace exposure to ototoxic substances or vibration can have adverse effects on noise-induced hearing disorders.

3.2.2   Temporary threshold shift

Temporary threshold shift (TTS) is a change in the hearing threshold which is reversible after the end of the daily noise exposure.

3.2.3   Permanent threshold shift

Permanent threshold shift (PTS) is a change in the hearing threshold which is not reversible.

3.2.4   Recovery of hearing

Recovery of hearing is the regression of the hearing loss. The lower the noise level during the recovery period and the longer the recovery period lasts, the greater is the degree of recovery of hearing. In general, sufficient recovery of hearing requires that the average sound pressure level during the recovery period is not greater than 70 dB and that the recovery period lasts at least 10 hours. Much higher sound pressure levels prevent recovery of hearing and thus can contribute to the development of permanent hearing loss or hearing damage.

3.3   Noise-related hearing damage

Noise-related hearing damage is noise-induced hearing loss with audiometrically detectable symptoms of hair cell damage; the hearing loss exceeds 40 dB at 3 kHz.

3.3.1   Acute hearing damage

At extremely high sound pressure levels, $L_{C,peak}$ of more than 137 dB(C), hearing damage can be caused by a single noisy event (e.g. bang, explosion).

3.3.2   Chronic hearing damage

Chronic hearing damage can develop as a result of long-term noise exposure.

3.4   Methods (audiometry, medical examination)

3.4.1   Audiometer
- pure tone audiometer (EN 60645-1)
- speech audiometer (EN 60645-2)

3.4.2   Medical examination room

The level of extraneous noise in the examination room must be so low that all test tones can be heard at the normal threshold level (hearing loss = 0 dB). To test whether a room is suitable for this purpose, it is expedient to record the audiogram of a young test person with no hearing impairment. This audiogram must not differ significantly from one recorded in the absence of extraneous noise (e.g. one recorded after working hours).

These requirements may be met if necessary by sound-proofed cubicles or, for air-conduction audiometry, by sound-proofed audiometer earphones (constructed like earmuff hearing protectors).

3.4.3   Times of the medical examinations

For at least 14 hours before the examination the person's hearing should not have been exposed to average noise levels of $L_{Aeq} \geq 80$ dB(A). Generally this can be ensured if the person wears adequate hearing protectors during any noisy working periods before the medical examination.

No audiometry should be carried out if the person has been exposed before the examination to average noise levels of $L_{Aeq} \geq 85$ dB(A) followed by a recovery period of less than 30 minutes at $L_{Aeq} < 75$ dB(A).

3.4.4   Erroneous audiometric data

Increased numbers of false positive findings as defined in this guideline are obtained especially if audiometry is carried out too quickly. The standards EN 26189 (ISO 6189) for the screening test and ISO 8253 for the supplementary examination should be observed (see Section 4). In addition, if the conditions described in Sections 3.4.1 to 3.4.3 are not observed, erroneous results will be obtained.

3.4.5   Sound conduction disorders

A sound conduction disorder is reflected in the audiogram by a difference between the hearing loss determined by air-conduction and that determined by bone-conduction of more than 15 dB at more than one frequency. If there is no sound conduction disorder, the bone-conduction hearing loss should be estimated from the air-conduction hearing threshold.

4   References

Commission recommendation 2003/670/EC concerning the European schedule of
   occupational diseases
Directive 89/391/EEC on the introduction of measures to encourage improvements
   in the safety and health of workers at work
Directive 2003/10/EC on the minimum health and safety requirements regarding
   the exposure of workers to the risks arising from physical agents (noise)
EN 26189 Acoustics: Pure tone air conduction threshold audiometry for hearing con-
   servation purposes (identical with ISO 6189)
EN 60645-1 Audiometers – Part 1: Pure-tone audiometers
EN 60645-2 Audiometers – Part 2: Equipment for speech audiometry
ISO 8253 Acoustics: Audiometric test methods; part 1: Basic pure tone air and bone
   conduction threshold audiometry; part 3: Speech audiometry
ISO 1999:1990: Acoustics: Determination of occupational noise exposure and esti-
   mation of noise-induced hearing impairment

G 20

5   Examination schedules

Screening test NOISE I:
schedule for the initial examination

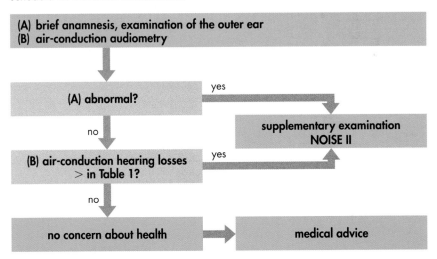

Screening test NOISE I:
Schedule for the follow-up examination

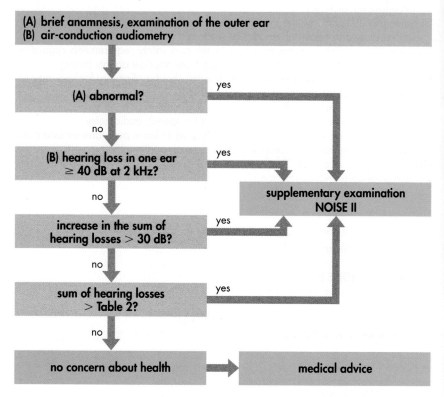

Supplementary examination NOISE II:
schedule for the initial examination

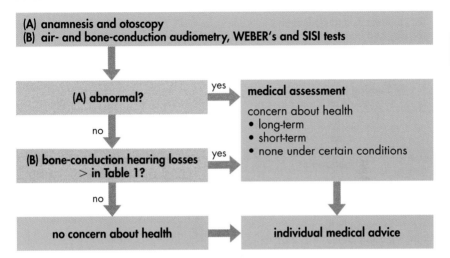

Supplementary examination NOISE II:
schedule for the follow-up examination

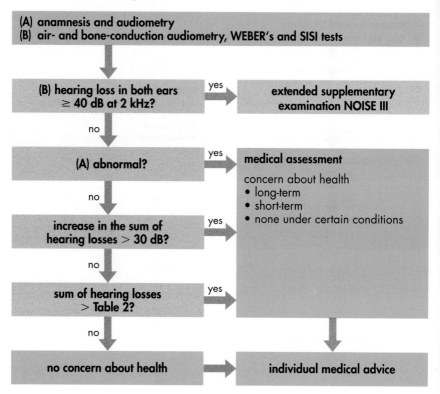

Extended supplementary examination NOISE III:
schedule of examination and assessment

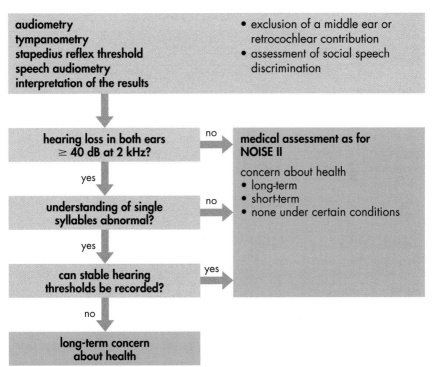

G 20

audiometry **tympanometry** **stapedius reflex threshold** **speech audiometry** **interpretation of the results**	• exclusion of a middle ear or retrocochlear contribution • assessment of social speech discrimination

hearing loss in both ears ≥ 40 dB at 2 kHz? — no → **medical assessment as for NOISE II**

yes ↓

concern about health
• long-term
• short-term
• none under certain conditions

understanding of single syllables abnormal? — no →

yes ↓

can stable hearing thresholds be recorded? — yes →

no ↓

long-term concern about health

6   **Forms**
• Screening test NOISE I,
• Supplementary examination NOISE II,
• Extended supplementary examination NOISE III

G 20 Screening test NOISE I

Surname	First name
Address: street	
Postcode, town	
Employer	
Address: street	
Postcode, town	

☐ Initial examination   ☐ Follow-up examination   ☐ Examination when leaving the job

Details of workplace

Place of work   _____

Kind of job   _____

Work in noisy areas   ☐ mainly   ☐ occasionally   ☐ changes with the job

Level of noise exposure   ☐ >80–84   ☐ 85–89   ☐ 90–94   ☐ 95–100   ☐ >100 dB(A)

Peak sound pressure   [＿＿] dB(C)

The noise is   ☐ medium to high frequency   ☐ very low frequency

Simultaneous exposures   ☐ whole body vibration   ☐ hand-arm vibration

☐ ototoxic substances: _____

Hearing protectors   ☐ ear plugs   ☐ ear muffs   ☐ no answer

Type, manufacturer   _____

Anamnesis

1. Duration of noise-free period before the hearing test	[＿＿] hours or [＿＿] minutes		
2. For how many years all together have you worked in noisy areas?	[＿＿] years		
3. Have you had an operation on an ear?	☐ I don't know	☐ no	☐ yes, in the year _ _ _ _
4. Have you ever had hearing problems together with attacks of dizziness and buzzing in the ears?	☐ I don't know	☐ no	☐ yes, last in the year _ _ _ _
5. Do you have buzzing in the ears?	☐ yes	☐ no	
6. Do you ever suffer from inflammation in the acoustic canal or on the outer ear?	☐ I don't know	☐ no	☐ yes, in the year _ _ _ _
7. Have you ever suffered from sudden deafness?	☐ I don't know	☐ no	☐ yes, in the year _ _ _ _

Advice about hearing protection

Hearing protectors present	☐ yes	☐ no
should go on being used?	☐ yes	☐ no
Defects detected		
Use of the following hearing protectors	Type:	Manufacturer:

Results

	right		left
Inspection of the auricle	☐	normal	☐
and external acoustic meatus	☐	abnormal	☐

Evaluation - follow-up examination

Hearing loss at 2 kHz in at least one ear is 40 dB or more?   ☐ yes

abnormal?   Increase in the sum of hearing losses within 3 years more than 30 dB?   abnormal?

☐ yes   [   ] dB   Values from last check-up right and left   [   ] dB   ☐ yes

Calculate sum of hearing losses at 2, 3 and 4 kHz and compare with threshold value (G 20 Table 2)

☐ yes   [   ] dB   threshold value [   ]   [   ] dB   ☐ yes

[   ]   Difference between new and previous results   [   ]

G 20

AC [   ][   ][   ][   ][   ][   ]   measured values (air conduction)   AC [   ][   ][   ][   ][   ][   ]

right ear   left ear

☐
Test disturbed by noise

☐
Person gave uncertain responses

Evaluation - initial examination
Measured values
Threshold values from Table 1
Mark values above the threshold!

Comments

Assessment   Previous check-up was on [   ]

☐ no concern about health   next check-up in __ __ months
☐ no concern about health under certain conditions*
* Details _____

☐ Supplementary examination required

Reasons:
☐ Increase in the sum of hearing losses of more than 30 dB in 3 years   ☐ excessive hearing loss at 2 kHz
☐ Hearing loss greater than given in Table 1 or 2   ☐ Anamnesis question no. __ __
☐ External ear abnormal

Date, stamp, signature of the physician

G 20 Supplementary examination NOISE II

Surname	First name
Address: street	
Postcode, town	
Employer	
Address: street	
Postcode, town	

☐ Initial examination   ☐ Follow-up examination   ☐ Examination when leaving the job

Details of workplace

Place of work

Kind of job

Work in noisy areas   ☐ mainly   ☐ occasionally   ☐ changes with the job

Level of noise exposure   ☐ >80–84   ☐ 85–89   ☐ 90–94   ☐ 95–100   ☐ >100 dB(A)

Peak sound pressure   [ ] dB(C)

The noise is   ☐ medium to high frequency   ☐ very low frequency

Simultaneous exposures   ☐ whole body vibration   ☐ hand-arm vibration

☐ ototoxic substances:

Hearing protectors   ☐ ear plugs   ☐ ear muffs   ☐ no answer

Type, manufacturer

Anamnesis

1. Duration of noise-free period before the hearing test		hours or		minutes
2. Previous period of exposure to noise	at work	years	other	years
			kind	

3. Ear operation   ☐ no   ☐ yes, in the year _ _ _ _   kind

4. Suspected Menière's disease   ☐ no   ☐ yes

5. Recurring inflammation of outer ear?   ☐ no   ☐ yes   kind

6. Sudden deafness   ☐ no   ☐ yes, in the year _ _ _ _

7. Buzzing in the ears   ☐ no   ☐ yes, in the year _ _ _ _

8. Subjective loss of hearing   ☐ no   ☐ yes, in the year _ _ _ _

9. Genesis and development of the hearing problems, beginning after   ☐ bang, explosion   ☐ noise of shooting   ☐ skull injury   ☐ ear operation   ☐ infection   ☐ other:

Advice about hearing protection

Hearing protectors present   ☐ yes   ☐ no   should go on being used?   ☐ yes   ☐ no

Defects detected

Use of the following hearing protectors   Type: Manufacturer:

Otoscopy

external auditory canal			eardrum		
right		left	right		left
☐	normal	☐	☐	normal	☐
☐	very narrow	☐	☐	central defect	☐
☐	moist	☐	☐	defect at the edge	☐
			☐	state after an operation	☐
			☐	not assessable	☐

Evaluation - follow-up examination

Hearing loss at 2 kHz in at least one ear is 40 dB or more?   ☐ yes

abnormal?   Increase in the sum of hearing losses within 3 years more than 30 dB?   abnormal?

☐ yes   ☐ dB   Values from last check-up right and left   ☐ dB   ☐ yes

Calculate sum of hearing losses at 2, 3 and 4 kHz and compare with threshold value (G 20 Table 2)

☐ yes   ☐ dB   threshold value ☐   ☐ dB   ☐ yes

☐   Difference between new and previous results   ☐

G 20

BC ☐   measured values (bone conduction)   BC ☐
AC ☐   (air conduction)   AC ☐

right ear   left ear

	0,5	1	2	3	4	6	8 kHz

☐ Person gave uncertain responses

Hearing level in dB: -10, 0, 10, 20, 30, 40, 50, 60, 70, 80, 90

SISI at 1 dB	
right	left
kHz	
%	

WEBER at 500 Hz		
right	med	left
☐	☐	☐

Frequency   0,5   1   2   3   4   6   8 kHz

Evaluation - initial examination

Measured values
Threshold values from Table 1
Mark values above the threshold!

Comments

Assessment   Previous check-up was on ☐

Examination NOISE III necessary   ☐ no   ☐ yes

☐ no concern about health
next check-up in _ _ months as   ☐ screening test   ☐ supplementary examination

☐ no concern about health under certain conditions
next check-up prematurely in _ _ months as   ☐ screening test   ☐ supplementary examination
☐ use recommended hearing protection (pto)   ☐ use of hearing protection to be checked
Other stipulations: ————————————————————————————————————

☐ short-term concern about health for a period of _ _ months   ☐ long-term concern about health

Reasons:
☐ marked loss of hearing   ☐ excessive loss of hearing   ☐ speech audiogram not normal
☐ Menière's disease   ☐ sudden loss of hearing   ☐ skull injury
☐ state after an operation   ☐ disease of the external ear

Date, stamp, signature of the physician

G 20 Extended supplementary examination NOISE III

Surname | First name

Address: street

Postcode, town

Date of birth | Nationality

Patient referred for the examination NOISE III on ___.___.___ ___ ___

Determination of acoustic impedance of the eardrum suggested, provided that it does not seem inadvisable to the ENT specialist   ☐ yes   ☐ no

Indications: generally unclear audiometric findings; objective exclusion of a sound conduction disorder; differentiation between damage to the auditory cells and the auditory nerves

Date, stamp, signature of the physician[1]

Examination completed on ___.___.___ ___ ___   Results sent to[1] on ___.___.___ ___ ___

Signature, stamp of the examining physician (unless identical with[1])

1 Findings (summary)

1 On the basis of audiometric and perhaps ear drum impedance measurements, a sound conduction disorder (a difference between the hearing losses determined by air-conduction and by bone-conduction of more than 15 dB at more than one frequency) has been

    right ☐   excluded   ☐ left   right ☐   confirmed   ☐ left

2 Cochlear sensorineural hearing loss is

    right ☐   unlikely   ☐ left   right ☐   likely   ☐ left

3 Hearing loss for numbers determined audiometrically especially for the frequencies 500, 1.000 und 2.000 Hz was

    right ☐   not confirmed   ☐ left   right ☐   confirmed   ☐ left

4 The plot of proportion of single syllables understood against loudness lies in the abnormal hatched area

    right ☐   no   ☐ left   right ☐   partially   ☐ left

    right ☐   entirely   ☐ left

    The understanding of single syllables could not be determined because the patient does not speak the local language sufficiently well. The other examination results, especially the audiogram and the loss of hearing for numbers, suggest that the results of the test for understanding of single syllables would also be abnormal

    right ☐   no   ☐ left   right ☐   yes   ☐ left

5 Given continued exposure to noise, even if hearing protection is worn, a further noise-induced increase in hearing loss is

    ☐ unlikely

    ☐ likely because

6 Diagnosis

7 Notification of an occupational disease   ☐ no   ☐ yes   Date of notification ___.___.___ ___ ___

2 Otoscopy

external auditory canal			eardrum	
right		left	right	left
☐	normal	☐	☐ normal	☐
☐	very narrow	☐	☐ central defect	☐
☐	moist	☐	☐ defect at the edge	☐
			☐ state after an operation	☐
			☐ scarring	☐
			☐ other findings	☐
			(see comments)	

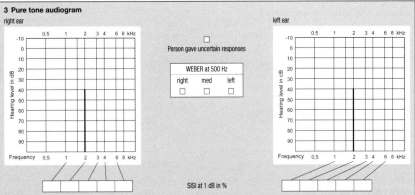

3 Pure tone audiogram

right ear

left ear

Person gave uncertain responses

WEBER at 500 Hz

right   med   left

SISI at 1 dB in %

G 20

4 Speech audiogram (only when the bone-conduction hearing loss at 2 kHz is already 40 dB or more in both ears)

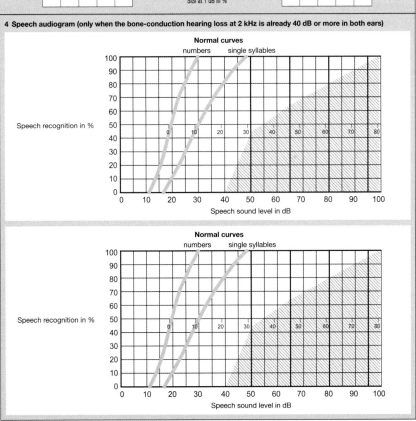

Normal curves

numbers   single syllables

Speech recognition in %

Speech sound level in dB

Normal curves

numbers   single syllables

Speech recognition in %

Speech sound level in dB

5 Acoustic impedance of the eardrum (if indicated)

1 Tympanometry

	right	type of tympanogram	left		right	no compliance	left
	☐	normal	☐		☐	eardrum defect	☐
	☐	increased amplitude	☐		☐	auditory canal not sealed	☐
	☐	negative pressure	☐				
	☐	curve flattened	☐				
	☐	completely flat curve	☐		[ ] middle ear pressure in mm H_2O [ ]		

2 Impedance changes in the monitored ear

	monitored ear right				stapedius reflex	monitored ear right				
stimulus left					contralateral					stimulus left
kHz	0.5	1	2	4		0.5	1	2	4	kHz
stimulus right					ipsilateral*					stimulus right

(* only if contralateral is not possible)

Comments

Explanations

The examination NOISE III is, according to G 20, necessary for persons for whom the occupational medical assessment "long-term concern about health" is being considered. It provides the basis for a more extensive otological diagnosis than is possible with the examination NOISE II.

If the responsible physician is not in a position to do the examination himself, he is to commission an ear, nose and throat specialist to carry it out.

The examination must be immediately preceded by a noise-free period (for recovery of hearing) of at least 12 hours.

Point 1.3 The hearing loss (HL) for numbers is considered to confirm the air-conduction audiogram if (HL_{500Hz} + HL_{1000Hz} + HL_{2000Hz}) x 1/3 ≈ hearing loss for numbers

Point 1.4 Whereas the understanding of single syllables can rarely be determined when carrying out speech audiometry of foreigners, apart from those with a very good knowledge of the local language, the hearing loss for numbers can often be determined successfully. In such cases, the plot of the proportion of single syllables understood against loudness may be assumed to lie in the hatched area for the ear in question if

☐ the bone-conduction hearing loss at 2 kHz is more than 40 dB and

☐ the hearing loss for numbers is more than 25 dB and the pure tone audiogram reveals a local loss of hearing at high frequencies (valley or drop at high frequencies)

Point 3 The pure tone audiometer should meet the requirements of DIN EN 60645-1 class 2 and requires regular servicing. It is expedient to carry out the SISI test at the frequency for which the bone-conduction hearing loss is about 60 dB. Note: careful determination of the air-conduction hearing threshold is necessary **before** setting the listening level to 20 dB above the hearing threshold.

Point 4 The speech audiometer should meet the requirements of DIN EN 60645-2 class 2 and requires regular servicing. The test material should meet recognized quality control standards.

Point 5 The tympanogram or a copy of it should be included with this form. The range of auditory canal pressures used in the measurements is between –300 daPa and +300 daPa.

G 21   Cold working conditions

Committee for occupational medicine, Berufsgenossenschaft Nahrungsmittel und
Gaststätten, Mannheim

G 21

Preliminary remarks

The present guideline describes a scheme for occupational medical prophylaxis
which aims to prevent or ensure early diagnosis of disorders which can be caused
by cold while working in rooms at temperatures below –25°C.

Schedule

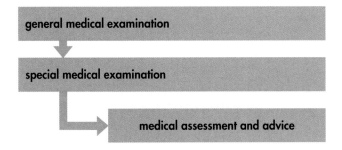

1   Medical examinations

Occupational medical examinations are to be carried out for persons working at temperatures below –25°C.

1.1   Examinations, intervals between examinations

initial examination	before taking up the job
first follow-up examination	• within 6 months for persons working at low temperatures between –25°C and –45°C • within 3 months for persons working at low temperatures below –45°C
further follow-up examinations	• within 12 months for persons working at low temperatures between –25°C and –45°C • within 6 months for persons working at low temperatures below –45°C
premature follow-up examination	• for persons working at low temperatures below –25°C after illnesses lasting more than 6 weeks or after repeated brief illnesses within 6 months which give rise to concern as to whether this kind of work should be continued: medical advice and perhaps follow-up examination • when requested by an employee who suspects a causal association between his or her illness and work

1.2   Medical examination schedule

1.2.1   General medical examination

Initial examination	Follow-up examination

review of past history (general anamnesis, work anamnesis, symptoms)

1.2.2   Special medical examination

Initial examination	Follow-up examination

urinalysis (multiple test strips)

1.3   Requirements for the medical examinations

competent doctor or occupational health professional

2   Occupational medical assessment and advice

An assessment is only possible when the workplace situation and the exposure of the individual are known. For this purpose a risk assessment as defined in Article 9 Council directive 89/391/EEC must have been carried out; it must specify which technical, organizational and individual protective measures have been applied.

G 21

2.1   Assessment criteria

2.1.1   Long-term concern about health

Initial examination	Follow-up examination

Persons with chronic disorders of
- the heart and circulatory system
- the respiratory organs
- the blood
- the skin if the circulation is affected
- the kidneys and lower urinary tract
- rheumatic type and related conditions

Persons with
- chronic disorders of the anterior eye
- seizures – depending on their kind, frequency, prognosis and state of treatment
- tendency to hypersensitivity reactions to cold (e.g. cold urticaria, cold haemo-globinuria)
- incompletely healed skull and brain injuries
- tendency to alcohol abuse, drug addiction and other addictions

2.1.2   Short-term concern about health

Initial examination	Follow-up examination

Persons with the disorders mentioned in Section 2.1.1, provided recovery is to be expected.

2.1.3   No concern about health under certain conditions

Initial examination	**Follow-up examination**

For persons with less severe illnesses of the kind mentioned in the first paragraph of Section 2.1.1, the doctor should establish whether or not it is possible for the person to begin work or go on working under certain conditions, e.g. shorter intervals between follow-up examinations.

2.1.4   No concern about health

Initial examination	**Follow-up examination**

All other persons, provided there are no restrictions on their employment.

2.2   Medical advice

The advice in an individual case should be commensurate with the workplace situation and the results of the medical examinations.

The employee should be told about technical and organizational protective measures and personal protective equipment appropriate for the individual's state of health.

If the results of occupational medical examinations indicate focal cumulation of health risks, the physician, while observing medical confidentiality, is to inform and advise the employer.

3   Supplementary notes

3.1   Exposure

3.1.1   Occurrence, sources of hazards

A person may be assumed to be exposed to cold stress when working in rooms cooled technologically to temperatures below –25°C, unless the exposure to the low temperature is brief. Cold stress may be expected during work (including repair jobs) in cold rooms, freezer rooms, freeze-drying rooms and low temperature research cabinets.

Brief exposures are those which involve going into such rooms for control purposes or to give instructions for periods of less than 15 minutes. This assumes that insulating clothing is worn.

At workplaces where wind or draughts increase the cooling effect on the body, employees are at particular risk.
Local cooling caused by direct contact with evaporating coolants or brief contact with cold surfaces can cause frostbite.

3.2   Functional disorders, symptoms

G 21

3.2.1   Mode of action

general:
reflex and – given reduced body core temperature – also direct effects on the regulation of cardiac action and the circulatory system, on breathing and metabolism
local:
adverse effects on circulation and metabolism in the skin and mucous membranes caused by local cooling; cold stimulation of thermoreceptors.

3.2.2   Symptoms

general:
- reflex induction of angina pectoris or bronchospasm, in persons suffering from hypothermia first subjective chills, shivering or stiffening of the muscles,
- then reduction of the body core temperature
- tiredness
- slowing and weakening of respiratory and cardiac activity
- danger of collapse
- on further cooling, cardiac arrhythmia or even ventricular fibrillation, adverse effects on blood and tissue electrolyte balance, unconsciousness and finally death

local:
- frostbite on exposed skin
- catarrhal or inflammatory reactions of the mucosa

4   References

DIN 33403: Climate at the workplace and its environments – Part 5: Ergonomic design of cold workplaces

Directive 89/391/EEC on the introduction of measures to encourage improvements in the safety and health of workers at work

Giesbrecht GG (1995) The respiratory system in a cold environment. Aviat Space Environ med 66: 890–902

Hassi J (1994) Cold related diseases and cryopathics. In: Holmer J: Work in cold environments. Arbetsmiljöinstitutet/NIVA, Solna, 33–40

Hassi J, Raatikka VP, Huurre M (2003) Health-check questionnaire for subjects exposed to cold. Int J Circumpolar Health 62(4): 436–43

ISO/DIS 15743: Ergonomics of the thermal environment – Cold workplaces – Risk assessment and management

Parsons KC (2003) Human Thermal Environments. The effects of hot, moderate and cold environments on human health, comfort and performance. Taylor & Francis, London

Risikko T, Makinen TM, Pasche A, Toivonen L, Hassi J (2003) A model for managing cold-related health and safety risks at workplaces. Int J Circumpolar Health 62(2): 204–15

G 23   Obstructive airway disorders

Committee for occupational medicine, working group "Obstructive airway disorders", Berufsgenossenschaft Nahrungsmittel und Gaststätten, Mannheim

G 23

Preliminary remarks

The present guideline describes a scheme for occupational medical prophylaxis which aims to prevent if possible or to ensure early diagnosis of obstructive airway disorders which can be caused or exacerbated by allergenic, chemically irritative or toxic substances at the workplace or to prevent further deterioration in persons with existing airway damage.

If the exposures are to respirable or inhalable dust in general or to substances with germ cell mutagenic, carcinogenic, fibrogenic or other toxic effects, the relevant Guidelines for Occupational Medical Examinations should be consulted.

Schedule

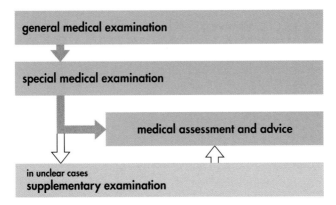

1   Medical examinations

Occupational medical examinations are to be carried out for persons at whose work-places the occupational exposure limit value for cereal flour dusts or for platinum compounds is exceeded, for persons exposed at work to concentrations of cereal and feedstuff dusts above 4 milligrams inhalable dust per cubic metre of air, for persons whose work involves exposure to dust from laboratory animals in animal houses and facilities, for persons using natural rubber latex gloves containing more than 20 microgram protein per gram glove material, and for persons exposed by inhalation to incompletely polymerized epoxide resins.

In addition, occupational medical examinations should be offered to persons at whose workplaces an increased incidence of obstructive airway disorders caused by exposure to allergens, chemical irritants or toxic substances is to be expected.

1.1   Examinations, intervals between examinations

initial examination	before taking up the job
first follow-up examination	after 6–12 months
further follow-up examinations	after 12–36 months and when leaving the job
premature follow-up examination	• when symptoms indicative of airway obstruction caused by allergens, chemical irritants or toxic substances develop and after airway disorders lasting several weeks which give rise to concern as to whether the work should be continued • in individual cases when the physician considers it necessary, e.g. when there is short-term concern about the person's health • when requested by an employee who suspects a causal association between his or her illness and work

1.2   Medical examination schedule

1.2.1   General medical examination

Initial examination

- review of past history (general anamnesis including smoking anamnesis)
- work anamnesis
  - previous jobs (times/exposures)
  - current work/substances occurring at the workplace
- specific allergological anamnesis
  - seasonal rhinitis or rhinitis of manifestly allergic genesis, conjunctivitis and/or bronchial asthma
  - workplace-related symptoms (e.g. runny nose, sneezing, burning of the eyes, respiratory symptoms, skin symptoms such as urticaria)
  - medically diagnosed atopic eczema (neurodermatitis)

Particular attention is to be paid to disorders which cause concern about health (see Section 2.1).

Follow-up examination

Interim anamnesis (including work anamnesis), especially questions about current jobs, substances occurring at the workplace, and workplace-related symptoms (runny nose, sneezing, burning of the eyes, respiratory symptoms, urticaria)

1.2.2   Special medical examination

Initial examination   **Follow-up examination**

Extensive examination of the respiratory organs, spirometry.

1.2.3   Supplementary examination

Initial examination

The necessity for supplementary examinations may be concluded from the work anamnesis, respiratory symptoms and medical indications.

Generally it is not necessary to carry out all the examinations listed below.

- extended lung function tests
  - where indicated, determination of the airway resistance, if possible by whole body plethysmography
  - tests for bronchial hyperreactivity
- large format posterior-anterior thorax radiograph taken with high kilovolt technique for specific diagnostic purposes

G 23

Follow-up examination

As for the initial examination. Given any of the workplace-related symptoms listed in Section 1.2.1, more extensive tests are to be carried out by a physician with experience in occupational medicine, allergology and pneumology:
* workplace or job-specific diagnosis
  * workplace or job-specific allergy diagnosis
  * determination of the peak expiratory flow or timed vital capacity in one second during a period of 3–6 weeks at least 4 times daily during and after work (also in an analogous way on exposure-free days). Documentation of the measured values, exposure, symptoms and therapy is necessary.

1.3 Requirements for the medical examinations
* competent doctor or occupational health professional

2 Occupational medical assessment and advice

An assessment is only possible when the workplace situation and the exposure of the individual are known. For this purpose a risk assessment as defined in Article 4 Council directive 98/24/EC must have been carried out; it must specify which technical, organizational and individual protective measures have been applied.

2.1 Assessment criteria

2.1.1 Long-term concern about health

Initial examination

Persons with
* manifest obstructive airway disease, especially bronchial asthma with persistent symptoms and/or chronic obstructive bronchitis
* severe lung disease such as advanced diseases of the lung architecture and pulmonary emphysema
* symptomatic type I sensitization of the upper and/or lower airways to the specific workplace allergens

Follow-up examination

Persons with
- manifest obstructive airway disease, especially bronchial asthma with persistent symptoms and/or chronic obstructive bronchitis, which does not respond to the measures described in Section 2.1.3 with remission or disappearance of symptoms
- existing clinically relevant type I sensitization of the upper and/or lower respiratory tract to the specific workplace allergens which does not respond to the measures described in Section 2.1.3 with remission or disappearance of symptoms
- severe lung disease such as advanced disorders of lung architecture and pulmonary emphysema

2.1.2   Short-term concern about health

Initial examination   **Follow-up examination**

Persons with transient hypersensitivity of the upper and/or lower respiratory tract for whom a worsening of symptoms is to be expected on exposure to even relatively low concentrations of inhalable agents (e.g. during a bronchopulmonary infection).

2.1.3   No concern about health under certain conditions

Initial examination   **Follow-up examination**

If the illnesses or functional disorders mentioned in Section 2.1.1 are less severe, the doctor should establish whether or not it is possible for the person to start work or go on working under certain conditions. Such conditions could include
- special technical and organizational protective measures, e.g. transfer to workplaces where the concentrations of allergens or chemical irritants or toxic substances have been shown to be lower
- personal protective equipment
- participation in special preventive programs
- more frequent follow-up examinations.
Such measures are to be considered especially for persons with
- atopic diseases
- type I sensitization to job-specific allergens or cross-reacting environmental allergens (e.g. cereal pollen or animal hair)
- unspecific bronchial hyperreactivity
- chronic conjunctivitis or rhinitis

2.1.4   No concern about health

Initial examination	**Follow-up examination**

All other persons.

2.2   Medical advice

Individual advice (e.g. as to the use of personal protective equipment) should take into account the risk assessment and the results of the medical examination.

If there are indications of airway or lung disease, the employee should be told that specific medical treatment can be advisable and possible. Cigarette smoking is the most common cause of chronic obstructive pulmonary disease (COPD).

Giving up inhalative smoking of tobacco has been shown to result in an improvement in lung function and so to a more favourable course of the disease. The physician is to inform the smoker about the position and that treatment can successfully help him or her to stop smoking.

3   Supplementary notes

3.1   Exposure

3.1.1   Occurrence, sources of hazards[1]

These substances are ones which can cause biological reactions even in very small quantities. Even when workplace threshold limit values are observed, sensitizing substances can cause sensitization or clinically manifest allergic reactions in individuals of appropriate disposition.

High molecular weight allergens

The vast majority of allergenic substances are naturally existing high molecular weight proteins found, e.g. in flour dust, cereal dusts, feedstuffs, enzyme preparations, saliva, urine, skin and hair of laboratory and farm animals, and natural rubber latex.

---

[1] The list of substances provides examples; it does not claim to be complete. The potential of a substance or a formulation to have adverse effects on health is determined by the factors potential effects of the substance (see R-phrases), workplace concentration and the work process being used in the particular case.

Low molecular weight allergens
Low molecular weight substances can often be not only allergens but also chemical irritants. Of particular importance are dicarboxylic acid anhydrides, persulfates (used in hairdressing), isocyanates (see G 27) and metal compounds (e.g. platinum compounds).

Chemical irritants and toxic substances
Depending on the occupational hygiene at the particular workplace, chemical irritants and toxic substances can occur in the form of vapour, gas, dust or fumes. Of particular importance are aerosols of acids and alkalis (e.g. caustic potash solution, caustic soda solution, nitric acid, hydrochloric acid, sulfuric acid), dicarboxylic acid anhydrides, incompletely polymerized epoxide resins, formaldehyde, isocyanates (see G 27), metal dusts or fumes, irritant gases (e.g. acrolein, ammonia, hydrogen chloride, halogens, nitrous gases, phosgene, sulfur dioxide).
In addition, a large number of substances with weaker irritant effects (e.g. a variety of solvents) can exacerbate existing bronchial hyperreactivity by inducing symptoms.

G 23

3.1.2   Uptake
The substances are taken in by inhalation; allergens are less often also absorbed by mouth and through the skin.

3.1.3   Dose-effect relationships
Dose-effect relationships[2] are dependent on the potential effects of the particular substance and in many cases are not known in detail.
For allergenic substances on the one hand and chemical irritants or toxic substances on the other quite different dose-effect relationships must be expected because of the different pathomechanisms involved.
For allergies it is necessary to distinguish between induction of the allergy and provocation of symptoms.
Primary preventive measures in the form of reduction of exposure concentrations can reduce the risk of sensitization (induction). The question as to whether such measures are sufficient during tertiary prevention for persons with already existing allergies cannot be answered satisfactorily to date. A progression of the disorder must be expected in spite of improvements in occupational hygiene.

---

[2] Peak concentrations can be of particular significance.

3.2   Functional disorders, symptoms

Pathomechanism

Allergic airway disorders are seen only in some of the persons exposed in a given job. In addition to the substance-specific potential for causing sensitization, the amount of the allergen, the exposure period and the genetically determined or acquired disposition of the exposed person play a decisive role. After exposure to high molecular weight allergens (e.g. plant, microbial and animal allergens), atopic persons have a higher risk of developing an allergy, but persons who are not atopic can also become sensitized. There is evidence that, in persons with allergic obstructive airway diseases, allergic symptoms and sensitization are more sensitive indicators and develop earlier than the impairment of lung function. Thus the intervals between follow-up examinations should be short for persons with work-related symptoms (given continual exposure). If exposure is avoided early, the prognosis is favourable.

Obstructive airway disorders can also be caused by repeated or continual inhalation of chemical irritants or toxic substances (i.e. without accidental high level inhalative exposure of the kind causing reactive airways dysfunction syndrome (RADS)). The effects are known to depend on the quality (e.g. water-soluble substances have more effect in the upper airways) and quantity of exposure. Atopic persons with or without existing symptoms of bronchial hyperreactivity are particularly at risk. Here too, as for the allergic obstructive airway diseases, the period of exposure after appearance of symptoms should be kept as short as possible.

Symptoms

Symptoms of an obstructive airway disease caused by allergenic substances are mostly a combination of runny nose, attacks of sneezing, conjunctival reactions and/or respiratory distress after exposure to an allergen. Exposure-dependence of the symptoms with improvement after an exposure-free interval (e.g. free weekend, holiday) suggests that they are caused by a work-related inhalation allergy. Even low concentrations of the inhaled allergen are sufficient to induce symptoms in persons who are already sensitized. In persons with obstructive airway diseases caused by chemical irritants or toxic substances, rhinoconjunctival symptoms are generally less common and with some noxious substances there may also be no association of the symptoms with work.

Diagnosis

That asthma is first manifested in an adult is in general a rather rare occurrence but poorly reversible obstructive airway diseases in the sense of COPD develop frequently in smokers aged 40 years and more. Therefore the first manifestation of an obstructive airway disease in a non-smoker or its frequent occurrence at the workplace is a ground for more extensive diagnostic tests. These may include skin tests or *in vitro* tests for sensitization (when available), lung function tests at work and on work-free days (mostly PEF or FEV1, but also serial methacholine provocation tests). Workplace-related inhalation tests should be carried out by persons with experience in the field because they are complex to carry out and interpret.

4   References

Commission Recommendation 2003/670/EC concerning the European schedule of
    occupational diseases. Annex I
Council Directive 98/24/EC on the protection of the health and safety of workers
    from the risks related to chemical agents at work
Deutsche Forschungsgemeinschaft (German Research Foundation, DFG) (ed) List of
    MAK and BAT Values 2007. Maximum Concentrations and Biological Tolerance
    Values at the workplace. Wiley-VCH, Weinheim
Deutsche Forschungsgemeinschaft (German Research Foundation, DFG) (ed) The
    MAK-Collection for Occupational Health and Safety. Wiley-VCH
    at: www.mrw.interscience.wiley.com/makbat
GESTIS-database on hazardous substances. BGIA
    at: www.dguv.de/bgia/gestis-database
GESTIS-international limit values for chemical agents. BGIA
    at: www.dguv.de/bgia/gestis-limit-values
World Health Organization (WHO): www.who.int/respiratory/asthma/en/ and
    www.who.int/respiratory/copd/en

G 23

G 24   Skin disorders (not including skin cancer)

Committee for occupational medicine, working group "Occupational risks for the skin", Berufsgenossenschaft Nahrungsmittel und Gaststätten, Mannheim

Preliminary remarks

The present guideline describes a scheme for occupational medical prophylaxis which aims to prevent or ensure early diagnosis of skin disorders.

It is still not possible before the first exposure to a given substance to identify those persons who are predisposed to become sensitized to that substance. So-called prophetic allergy tests are therefore not indicated.

G 24

Schedule

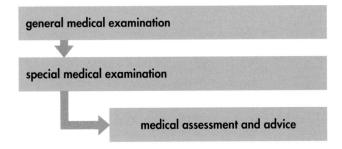

1.   Medical examinations

Occupational medical examinations are to be carried out for persons whose work can cause skin disorders. This applies in particular to

- work involving contact with water (wet work) for 4 hours or more each day
- work involving exposure to isocyanates where frequent skin contact cannot be avoided
- work involving the wearing of natural rubber latex gloves containing more than 30 µg protein per gram glove material
- work in which the skin is exposed to incompletely cured epoxy resins

1.1   Examinations, intervals between examinations

initial examination	before taking up the job
first follow-up examination	within 24 months
further follow-up examinations	within 60 months and when leaving the job
premature follow-up examination	• when workplace-related changes and/or symptoms appear on the skin • when there is cause for concern about the person's health in the short term (see Section 2.1.2) • in individual cases when there is no cause for concern about the person's health under certain conditions (see Section 2.1.3) when the physician considers it necessary • when requested by an employee who suspects a causal association between his or her skin disorder and work

1.2   Medical examination schedule

1.2.1   General medical examination

Initial examination

Review of past history (general anamnesis, work anamnesis, symptoms)
Particular attention is to be given to:
- eczema on the hands, symmetrical eczema of the flexures, dyshidrotic eczema, white dermographia, existing allergies
- and other disorders and dispositions such as psoriasis, ichthyosis, xerosis cutis, increased sensitivity to light
- and in the work anamnesis: tolerance of skin exposures in previous jobs, occupational skin disorders

G 24

Follow-up examination

Interim anamnesis (work anamnesis, anamnesis of illnesses); establish by questioning and document preventive measures which have been used such as the wearing of gloves, use of protective skin creams, skin cleaning agents, skin disinfectants and skin care preparations. The person should be asked about the acceptability, tolerability and ease of use of these measures in practice.

1.2.2   Special medical examination

Initial examination   **Follow-up examination**

Examination of exposed skin, generally hands, forearms and face, especially for dry skin, hyperhidrosis and eczematous foci.
In unclear cases: extend the physical examination, take into account available results of medical examinations and current exposure data, if necessary organize specialist dermatological diagnosis.

1.3   Requirements for the medical examinations
- competent doctor or occupational health professional
- experience in the assessment of occupational dermatosis and advising workers about preventive measures

2   Occupational medical assessment and advice

An assessment is only possible when the workplace situation and the exposure of the individual are known. For this purpose a risk assessment as defined in Article 4 Council directive 98/24/EC must have been carried out; it must specify which technical, organizational and individual protective measures have been applied.

2.1   Assessment criteria

2.1.1   Long-term concern about health

Initial examination

Persons with
- allergic disorders of the skin caused by unavoidable workplace exposure to the allergen
- severe or recurring eczema of exposed skin areas, especially the hands, forearms (also anamnestic)
- extremely sensitive skin (e.g. atopic eczema of the exposed skin, psoriasis with Köbner's phenomenon, UV-induced dermatosis in persons exposed unavoidably to ultraviolet radiation). See especially Section 2.1.3

Follow-up examination

Persons with
- allergic disorders of the skin caused by workplace exposure to an allergen which cannot be avoided sufficiently
- severe or recurring eczema of exposed skin areas, especially the hands, forearms, for which preventive measures have not been successful

2.1.2   Short-term concern about health

Initial examination   **Follow-up examination**

Persons with
- therapy-requiring skin disorders the healing of which is prevented by workplace conditions (e.g. fungal infections and occlusion)
  or
- skin disorders which increase the risk for the person at work (e.g.: increased absorption of noxious substances)

provided that these skin disorders are known not to lead to long-term concern about the person's health.

The occupational medical assessment is to be repeated when the person has recovered from the disorder.

2.1.3   No concern about health under certain conditions

Initial examination	Follow-up examination

Persons with skin disorders or sensitive skin and persons not covered by Sections 2.1.1 or 2.1.2 for whom the normal workplace preventive measures must be changed to suit the individual.

Such changes could include
- special technical and organizational protective measures
- individual personal protective equipment and skin protection (e.g.: a different protective skin cream for persons allergic to a component of the usual skin cream)

2.1.4   No concern about health

Initial examination	Follow-up examination

All other persons.

2.2   Medical advice

The medical advice covers general preventive measures for the skin and any particular points necessary in an individual case. The advice about skin protection should take into account the situation at the workplace, the individual's way of working and his or her skin constitution.

On the basis of the results of the medical examination (Section 1.2.1) any protective gloves, protective skin cream, disinfectant and skin care preparation should be selected for the individual, who should be advised as to way of working and behaviour.

Examples:
- avoidance of direct skin contact, use of aids such as tongs or sieves
- skin cleaning should be as gentle as possible and be appropriate for the kind of dirt and the state of the skin
- combined skin cleaning and skin disinfection should be avoided whenever possible
- change to different protective gloves, e.g., in cases of intolerance, lack of sensitivity
- use of absorbent under-gloves for long periods of glove wearing

G 24

3   Supplementary notes

3.1   Exposure

3.1.1   Occurrence, sources of hazards

The skin can be damaged by substances with irritative, sensitizing or acnegenic potency, by physical agents and microorganisms.

irritating substances, e.g.
- solvents
- petrol, kerosene
- alkaline substances
- metal-working fluids
- industrial oils and fats
- aqueous solutions of detergents

sensitizing substances, e.g.
incompletely cured epoxy resins, permanent-wave preparations, para-substituted amines (colourants), latex and rubber components, disinfectants and preservatives, acrylates, proteins, emulsifiers, amine curing agents, colophonium, bleaches, plant fragments, isocyanates, metal ions (chromium, cobalt, nickel, etc.)

The information system on hazardous substances (GESTIS) provides further substance-specific information (see Section 4).

physical agents, e.g.:
contact with mineral and ceramic fibres, metal shavings, abrasive particles, rough surfaces, hairs, irradiation, heat and cold

other exposures
- microorganisms which are pathogenic for the skin are of less importance in terms of the number of cases involved
- acnegenic substances e.g. chlorinated polycyclic hydrocarbons

3.1.2   Uptake

Occupational skin diseases are generally caused by exogenous agents. The present guideline does not apply for substances which are absorbed through the skin but have systemic effects in other organs.

3.1.3   Mode of action

Allergenic, toxic irritating, microtraumatic or infectious exogenous agents can regularly or occasionally cause skin disorders or make existing disorders worse. Mainly the skin areas in contact with the damaging agents are affected; spread to other parts of the body and generalization are also possible. Often the skin disorders only develop when several factors are involved, e.g. because of a combination of mechanical, chemical and physical effects (the last include the indoor climate, humidity, the wearing of protective clothing, rubber gloves, boots, etc.) and simultaneous defects in the epidermal barrier.

3.2   Functional disorders, symptoms

G 24

The vast majority of cases of occupational dermatosis involve disorders of eczema type (more than 95 %)
Putting it simply, they may be subdivided into
*   atopic eczema, due to individual disposition but made worse by workplace conditions
*   cumulative subtoxic eczema
*   allergic contact eczema or contact urticaria
These can occur on their own or in the form of two-phase or three-phase eczema in sequence. Mixed forms are very frequent.

4   References

Adams RM (1999) Occupational Skin Diseases (3rd edition). WB Saunders, Philadelphia

Agner T, Held E (2002) Skin protection programmes. Contact Dermatitis (Denmark) 47(5): 253–6

Commission Recommendation 2003/670/EC concerning the European schedule of occupational diseases. Annex I

Council Directive 89/391/EEC on the introduction of measures to encourage improvements in the safety and health of workers at work

Council Directive 98/24/EC on the protection of the health and safety of workers from the risks related to chemical agents at work

Cvetkovski RS, Rothman KJ, Olsen J, Mathiesen B, Iversen L, Johansen JD, Agner T (2005) Relation between diagnoses on severity, sick leave and loss of job among patients with occupational hand eczema. Br J Dermatol 152(1): 93–8

Diepgen TL (2003) Occupational skin-disease data in Europe. Int Arch Occup Environ Health 76(5): 331–8. Epub 2003 Apr 11

GESTIS-database on hazardous substances. BGIA
    at: www.dguv.de/bgia/gestis-database

Harries MJ, Lear JT (2004) Occupational skin infections. Occup Med (Lond) 54 (7): 441–9

Jungbauer F (2004) Wet work in relation to occupational dermatitis. Dissertation University Groningen

Kanerva L, Elsner P, Wahlberg JE, Maibach HI (eds) (2000) Handbook of Occupational Dermatology. Springer Verlag Berlin Heidelberg New York

Morris-Jones R, Robertson SJ, Ross JS, et al. (2002) Dermatitis caused by physical irritants. Br J Dermatol 147 (2): 270–5

Ring J, Darsow U, Behrendt H (2001) Atopic eczema and allergy. Curr Allergy Rev 1: 39–43

G 25   Driving, controlling and monitoring work

Committee for occupational medicine, working group "Driving, controlling and monitoring work", Berufsgenossenschaft der Straßen-, U-Bahnen und Eisenbahnen, Hamburg

Preliminary remarks

The present guideline describes a scheme for occupational medical prophylaxis which aims to prevent accidents and avoid health risks for persons involved in driving, controlling and monitoring work and for third parties.

Schedule

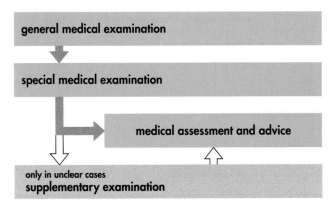

1   Medical examinations

1.1   Examinations, intervals between examinations

initial examination	before beginning driving, controlling and monitoring work	
further follow-up examinations	• until age 40 years	after 36 to 60 months[1]
	• from age 40 to 60 years	after 24 to 36 months
	• from age 60 years	after 12 to 24 months
premature follow-up examination	• after a prolonged period of being unfit for work (an illness lasting for several weeks) or when a physical handicap gives cause for concern about whether the work should be continued	
	• when beginning a new job	
	• in individual cases when the physician considers it necessary, (e.g. when there is short-term concern about the person's health)	
	• when requested by an employee who feels that continuing to work in the job is dangerous for health reasons	
	• if there are other indications which cause concern as to whether this kind of work should be continued	

1.2   Medical examination schedule

1.2.1   General medical examination

Initial examination	Follow-up examination

• review of past history (general anamnesis, work anamnesis)
• job-related examinations
Particular attention should be paid to
• cardiocirculatory disorders
• neurological and mental abnormalities
• sleep-related breathing disorders

---

[1] Depending on the risk assessment and the opinion of the occupational physician

1.2.2   Special medical examination

Initial examination	Follow-up examination

- visual acuity and hearing acuity
  see Tables 1 and 2
- urinalysis (multiple test strips)

1.2.3   Supplementary examination

Initial examination	Follow-up examination

In unclear cases, especially if physiological and psychological job requirements must be taken into consideration.
If necessary, also blood parameters and additional urine parameters.

G 25

1.3   Requirements for the medical examinations

- competent doctor or occupational health professional

1.3.1   Equipment required

see Table 3

1.3.2   Methods required

- visual acuity in the far range
- visual acuity in the near range
- three-dimensional vision
- colour vision
- visual field
- hearing (whispering and normal speech)
- scotopic vision, susceptibility to dazzle
- laboratory analyses carried out with appropriate quality control (Good Laboratory Practice)

2   Occupational medical assessment and advice

An assessment is only possible when the workplace situation and the exposure of the individual are known. For this purpose a risk assessment as defined in Article 9 Council directive 89/391/EEC must have been carried out; it must specify which technical, organizational and individual protective measures have been applied.

2.1   Assessment criteria

2.1.1   Long-term concern about health

Initial examination

Persons who do not fulfil the requirements given in Tables 1 and 2 and persons with
- disorders of consciousness or balance and any convulsive disorders, depending on the kind and frequency of the fits, the prognosis and the response to therapy
- untreated sleep-related breathing disorders (sleep apnoea) and the associated marked impairment of vigilance
- diabetes mellitus with marked variation in blood sugar levels, especially persons tending to hypoglycaemia
- chronic alcohol misuse, drug-dependence or other addictions
- long-term treatment with medicines which reduce the fitness to drive
- disorders or alterations of the heart or circulatory system which result in greatly reduced performance or impaired regulation, marked blood pressure changes
- severe restriction of mobility, loss of or loss of the strength of a limb which is important for the job
- diseases of or damage to the central or peripheral nervous system with disturbance of essential functions, especially organic brain or spinal cord diseases and their sequelae, functional disorders resulting from skull or brain injuries, disorders of cerebral blood flow
- emotional or mental disorders, even when these are in the past, if the possibility of recurrence cannot be excluded with sufficient certainly, abnormal mentality or highly abnormal behaviour

Follow-up examination

As for the initial examination if recovery or sufficient improvement in health is not to be expected.

2.1.2   Short-term concern about health

| **Initial examination** | **Follow-up examination** |

Persons with the disorders mentioned in Section 2.1.1, provided recovery or sufficient improvement is to be expected.

2.1.3   No concern about health under certain conditions

| **Initial examination** |

Persons who suffer from disorders or weaknesses of the kind listed in Section 2.1.1 but for whom, provided that certain conditions are fulfilled (e.g. situation at the workplace, shorter intervals between follow-up examinations, specific requirements) and the risk assessment indicates it need not be feared that they are a danger to themselves or others.

| **Follow-up examination** |

As for the initial examination if the persons have proved competent in the job for many years.

G 25

2.1.4   No concern about health

| **Initial examination** | **Follow-up examination** |

All other persons, provided there are no restrictions on their employment.

2.2   Medical advice

The advice in an individual case should be commensurate with the results of the medical examinations, should take into account the risk assessment, the workplace situation and the specific job involved.

If the results of occupational medical examinations indicate focal cumulation of work-related disorders, the physician, while observing medical confidentiality, is to inform and advise the employer with the aim of optimization of technical, organizational and individual protective measures.

3   Supplementary notes

3.1   Methods (visual acuity determination, medical examination)

Examples of the methods and equipment to be used are shown in Table 3.

4   References

DIN 58220: Visual acuity testing

Directive 89/391/EEC on the introduction of measures to encourage improvements
    in the safety and health of workers at work

Table 1: Minimum requirements for visual and hearing acuity

Parameter	Requirement level 1	Requirement level 2
visual acuity in the far range* – at the initial examination – at the follow-up examination persons with one eye	0.7/0.5 or both eyes 0.8 0.7/0.5 (0.2**) or both eyes 0.8 only after a job-specific assessment 0.7	0.5/0.5 (0.2**) or both eyes 0.6 0.4/0.4 (0.2**) or both eyes 0.6 0.6
visual acuity in the near range*	0.8/0.8	0.5/0.5
three-dimensional vision	three-dimensional vision sufficient for the job in question	
colour vision	colour vision sufficient for the job in question; if necessary, abnormalities to be investigated with the anomaloscope: no disorder in the red spectral range with an anomalo- scope quotient less than 0.5***	
visual field	normal visual field perimetry at the initial examination; in persons more than 40 years old at every second examination at least	visual field adequate for the job perimetry given evidence of visual field defects
scotopic vision suspectibility to dazzle	only when requirements are above average without dazzle: contrast 1 : 2.7 | contrast 1 : 5 luminance of surroundings 0.032 cd/m^2 with dazzle: contrast 1 : 2.7 | contrast 1 : 5 luminance of surroundings 0.1 cd/m^2	
hearing acuity	whispered speech 5 m	normal speech 5 m

G 25

*   If the given threshold values are attained with or without corrective appliances the
     appropriate occupational medical certificate is to be issued. However, if the examination
     does not reveal that the person has normal sight, he or she should be advised to see an
     ophthalmologist (not as part of the occupational medical prophylaxis) to establish
     whether optimal visual acuity could be achieved by correction. If the required visual
     acuity is only to be achieved with corrective appliances, this should be recorded in the
     certificate.
** Visual acuity of 0.2 in the eye with poorer sight only acceptable when permitted by the
     workplace assessment.
*** For driving jobs not involving transport of persons which are covered by the Road Traffic
     Act, the stipulations of this Act apply unless the special internal company requirements
     for colour vision exceed those required by the Act.

Table 2: Minimum requirements for visual and hearing acuity
at the initial examination (I) and follow-up examinations (F)

Driving, controlling and monitoring work*	Visual acuity in the far range		Visual acuity in the near range	
	I	F	I	F
driving of motor vehicles, provided no national/ international traffic regulations apply				
• cars, motorcycles, tractors	2	2	–	–
• goods vehicles (above 3.5 t maximum laden weight)	1	1	–	–
• buses, other motor vehicles for transporting persons	1	1	–	–
driving of track vehicles, provided national/ international traffic regulations do not apply				
• driving motive power units of long distance railways, urban railways (incl. tramways) and railways for transport of material	1	1	–	–
driving of industrial trucks with a driver's seat or stand and with a lifting mechanism, e.g. fork lift trucks	1	1	–	–
driving of industrial trucks with a driver's seat or stand without a lifting mechanism	2	2	–	–
operating "walk-along" industrial trucks with a lifting mechanism	1	1	–	–
operating devices for loading and unloading shelves	1	1	–	–
operating vehicle lifts, e.g. cranes, hydraulic ramps	1	1	2	2
driving of earth-moving machines, mobile machinery	1	2	–	–
operating motorized aircraft ground support equipment	1	1	2	2
driving of snow grooming equipment	1	1	–	–
control of shaft winding installations and cableway power units	1	1	1	2
control of charging machines and ladle transfer vehicles	1	1	1	2
control of load manipulating devices	1	1	1	2
control jobs requiring special abilities, e.g. controlling mobile elevating work platforms and winches	1	1	1	2
control jobs not requiring special abilities, e.g. controlling mechanical conveyor systems, hoists for building purposes	1	1	1	2
monitoring jobs requiring special abilities, e.g. at large switchboards, monitoring stations, control rooms, control centres, signal boxes, for work near railway tracks	1	1	1	1
monitoring jobs not requiring special abilities, e.g. at cableways and ski-lifts, monitoring equipment for non-destructive testing	1	1	1	2

* The requirement levels are described in Table 1. The workplace conditions are subject to change with technological developments Therefore jobs listed as having requirement level 1 can, in individual cases, be assigned to requirement level 2 if the risk assessment indicates that this is appropriate.

Three-dimensional vision		Colour vision		Visual Field		Scotopic vision, suspectibility to dazzle		Hearing acuity	
I	F	I	F	I	F	I	F	I	F
–	–	yes	yes	2	2	2	2	2	2
yes	–	yes	yes	1	1	1	1	2	2
yes	yes	yes	yes	1	1	1	1	2	2
–	–	yes**	yes**	1	1	–	–	2	2
yes	yes	–	–	1	1	–	–	2	2
–	–	–	–	2	2	–	–	2	2
yes	yes	–	–	2	2	–	–	2	2
yes	yes	–	–	2	2	–	–	2	2
yes	yes	–	–	1	1	2	2	2	2
–	–	yes**	yes**	2	2	2	2	–	–
yes	yes	yes**	yes**	1	1	1	2	2	2
–	–	–	–	1	1	1	2	2	2
–	–	–	–	2	2	–	–	2	2
–	–	–	–	2	2	2	2	2	2
yes	yes	–	–	2	2	–	–	2	2
yes	yes	yes	yes	1	1	–	–	2	2
–	–	–	–	2	2	–	–	2	2
–	–	yes	yes	1	1	–	–	1	1
–	–	yes	yes	1	2	–	–	2	2

** if coloured signals must be recognized

Table 3: Review ot test methods and devices for visual acuity tests

Parameter	Examples of methods and devices
visual acuity in the far range	methods as given in DIN 58220
visual acuity in the near range	vision-testing chart (e.g. Nieden, Birkhäuser) or vision testing devices
three-dimensional vision	Titmus test, TNO test, Lang stereo test, vision testing devices
colour vision	Velhagen and Ishihara colour test plates, vision testing devices, anomaloscope
visual field	perimeter*
scotopic vision, susceptibility to dazzle	nyctometer, mesotest, contrastometer

---

* Automatic hemispherical perimeter which uses a suprathreshold test method to examine the visual field in the range up to 70° to the right and left and 30° up and down. Alternatively the examination may be carried out with a manual Goldmann perimeter with at least four test points (e.g. III/4, I/4, I/2 and I/1) at 12 positions per test point at least.

G 26   Respiratory protective equipment

Committee for occupational medicine, working group "Respiratory protection", Bergbau-Berufsgenossenschaft, Hohenpeißenberg

Preliminary remarks

The present guideline describes a scheme for occupational medical prophylaxis which aims to establish whether in an individual case there is any medical cause for concern about the wearing of respiratory protective equipment.

Schedule

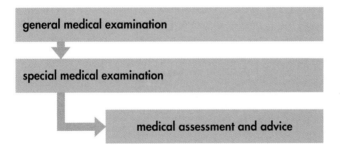

1   Medical examinations

Occupational medical examinations are to be carried out for persons at workplaces where the working conditions make it necessary to wear respiratory protective equipment (see Section 3.1.1).

1.1   Examinations, intervals between examinations

initial examination	before starting work in a job involving the use of respirators of classes 1–3[1]
first follow-up examination	• persons up to 50 years old: within 36 months • persons over 50 years old: within 24 months if devices weighing up to 5 kg are used within 12 months if devices weighing more than 5 kg are used
further follow-up examinations	• persons up to 50 years old: within 36 months • persons over 50 years old: within 24 months if devices weighing up to 5 kg are used within 12 months if devices weighing more than 5 kg are used
premature follow-up examination	• after an illness lasting for several weeks or when a physical handicap gives cause for concern about whether the work should be continued • in individual cases when the physician considers it necessary, e.g. when there is short-term concern about the person's health • when requested by an employee who suspects a causal association between his or her illness and work

---

[1] For the different classes of respiratory protective equipment (respirators) see Section 3.1.1

1.2   Medical examination schedule

1.2.1   General medical examination

Initial examination

The examination should take into account the workplace situation and the occupational medical criteria for evaluating respiratory protective equipment listed in Section 2.1.

Review of past history especially with respect to the

- workplace
- job
- training
- working hours

The working conditions, e.g. climatic conditions, physical effort involved in the work, and the period for which the respirator is to be used, should be taken into consideration.

G 26

Follow-up examination

Particular attention should be paid to the interim anamnesis, especially with respect to cardiac or pulmonary changes and any health problems associated with the wearing of respirators.

1.2.2   Special medical examination

Initial examination	Follow-up examination

<table>
<tr><th></th><th colspan="3">Class of device**</th></tr>
<tr><th></th><th>1</th><th>2</th><th>3</th></tr>
<tr><td>• large or medium sized thorax radiogram (not smaller than 10 x 10 cm) or use of an x-ray diagnosis which is less than 2 years old (see Table "Radiographic examination")</td><td></td><td></td><td></td></tr>
<tr><td>• spirometry</td><td>−</td><td>+</td><td>+</td></tr>
<tr><td>• blood count</td><td>(+)</td><td>+</td><td>+</td></tr>
<tr><td>• urinalysis</td><td>(+)</td><td>+</td><td>+</td></tr>
<tr><td>• ALAT (GPT)</td><td>(+)</td><td>+</td><td>+</td></tr>
<tr><td>• γ-GT</td><td>(+)</td><td>+</td><td>+</td></tr>
<tr><td>• fasting blood sugar</td><td>−</td><td>+</td><td>+</td></tr>
<tr><td>• resting ECG</td><td>−</td><td>+</td><td>+</td></tr>
<tr><td>• ergometry to assess physiological performance, taking into account the clinical findings, effort and age for persons using class 2 respirators</td><td>−</td><td>(+)</td><td>+</td></tr>
</table>

Note: ergometry for persons doing heavy work (e.g. in the fire brigade):
for persons up to 39 years old:
expected value (W 170) for men: 3.0 watt/kg body weight
women: 2.5 watt/kg body weight
from age 40 years
expected value (W 150) for men: 2.1 watt/kg body weight
women: 1.8 watt/kg body weight

	1	2	3
• visual acuity in the far range	−	+	+
• air-conduction audiometry (test frequencies 1–6 kHz), for persons using devices of classes 2 and 3 with acoustic warning signals (whistling tone)	−	+	+
• otoscopy in cases where the uptake of gases or vapours via the auditory canal is conceivable	+	+	+

** + means that the medical examination is necessary
   (+) means that whether or not the medical examination is necessary depends on the anamnesis or the exposure conditions
   − means that the medical examination is not necessary

Radiographic examinations	
• at the initial examination of persons using devices of classes 2 and 3	• at every second follow-up examination of persons less than 50 years old who use respirators of classes 2 and 3 (at 72-month intervals) • at every second follow-up examination of persons more than 50 years old who use respirators of class 2 (at 48-month intervals) • at every third follow-up examination of persons more than 50 years old who use respirators of class 3 (at 36-month intervals)

1.2.3   Other medical examinations

In unclear cases depending on the situation.

G 26

1.3   Requirements for the medical examinations
- competent doctor or occupational health professional
- regular participation in advanced training courses to stay up to date
- equipment required:
  own equipment:
  - lung function test device, preferably with documentation of the flow-volume curve
  - ECG (at least 3 channels)
  - ergometry equipment with 12-channel ECG and equipment for setting physically defined and reproducible work levels (bicycle ergometer)
  - for eyesight tests an optical instrument or vision testing charts for the far range
  - audiometer
  - otoscope
    own equipment or that of other physicians:
  - laboratory
  - x-ray apparatus for large or medium format radiographs

2   Occupational medical assessment and advice

An assessment is only possible when the workplace situation and the exposure of the individual are known. For this purpose a risk assessment as defined in Article 9 Council directive 89/391/EEC must have been carried out; it must specify which technical, organizational and individual protective measures have been applied.

2.1   Assessment criteria

2.1.1   Long-term concern about health

Initial examination	Follow-up examination

- for persons less than 18 years old who use respirators during rescue work and for those who use class 3 respirators; in general for persons more than 50 years old who use respirators during rescue work and for those who use class 3 respirators (but see Section 2.1.3)

Persons with	Class of device***		
	1	2	3
• general physical weakness	+	+	+
• disorders of consciousness or balance	+	+	+
• seizures, depending on their kind, frequency, prognosis and state of treatment	(+)	+	+
• disorders or damage of the central or peripheral nervous system with significant functional impairment and their sequelae, functional disorders after head or brain injuries, circulatory disorders in the brain	+	+	+
• emotional or mental disorders, even when these are in the past, if the possibility of recurrence cannot be excluded with sufficient certainly	+	+	+
• extremely abnormal behaviour (e.g. claustrophobia)	+	+	+
• addiction to alcohol, drugs or medication	+	+	+
• perforation of the tympanic membrane if there is a danger that gases and vapours can be taken up via the auditory canal	+	+	+
• complete dentures, for persons wearing respirators with a mouthpiece	+	+	+
• disorders or alterations of the respiratory organs which have severe effects on function, such as pulmonary emphysema, chronic obstructive lung disease, bronchial asthma	+	+	+
• persons whose vital capacity and/or timed vital capacity are decreased significantly or whose other lung parameters lie outside the normal range	+	+	+
• disorders or alterations of the heart or circulatory system which result in reduced performance or impaired regulation, e.g. condition after a heart attack, severe blood pressure changes	(+)	+	+

Persons with	Class of device***		
	1	2	3
• disorders or alterations of the thorax with marked effects on function	+	+	+
• disorders or alterations of the postural or locomotor system with marked functional impairment	–	+	+
• skin disorders which tend to exacerbation	(+)	+	+
• alterations which prevent the respirator seal fitting properly, e.g. scars	+	+	+
• disorders or alterations of the eyes which could cause acute impairment of sight, e.g. disorders of eyelid function	+	+	+
• corrected visual acuity below 0.7/0.7 (below 0.8 for persons who have had only one eye for many years) for persons doing rescue work	–	+	+
• hearing loss of more than 40 dB at 2 kHz in the better ear for persons doing rescue work	–	+	+
• established deafness, for persons using respirators of classes 2 or 3 with acoustic warning signals (whistling tone) if the deafness can prevent the person hearing the warning signal	–	+	+
• body weight more than 30 % above the normal weight determined by Broca's formula (height in cm minus 100 = normal weight in kg) or by other indices (e.g. BMI > 30)	–	+	+
• metabolic disorders, especially diabetes, or other disorders of endocrine glands, especially the thyroid, parathyroid or adrenal glands, if the disorders reduce the person's performance capacity markedly	–	+	+
• hernia	–	+	+

G 26

*** + means that persons who meet this criterion should be disqualified from doing work requiring the use of respirators of the given class

(+) means that the decision as to whether persons who meet this criterion should or should not do work requiring respirators of the given class depends on the exposure conditions

– means that the criterion is no reason to disqualify the person

2.1.2   Short-term concern about health

| **Initial examination** | **Follow-up examination** |

Persons with the disorders mentioned in Section 2.1.1, provided recovery is to be expected.

2.1.3   No concern about health under certain conditions

| **Initial examination** | **Follow-up examination** |

Persons who suffer from disorders like those listed in Section 2.1.1 but for whom no concern about health is necessary provided that follow-up examinations are carried out more frequently and
- the persons have many years of experience in the job and/or
- no risk for the person or for others is to be expected during the work in question or
- the person can be transferred to a job where a respirator which makes less physical demands on the wearer can be used or to a monitoring job.

2.1.4   No concern about health

| **Initial examination** | **Follow-up examination** |

All other persons, provided there are no restrictions on their employment.

2.2   Medical advice

The physician is to advise the employee about the special conditions of work carried out while using a respirator, taking into account the risk assessment for the particular workplace.

Especially persons working with the fire brigade must be physically very fit because people who need their help in emergencies must be able to depend on them. This kind of help must be provided without loss of time under very difficult conditions. The regular medical examination should take into account the high level of performance required.

3   Supplementary notes

3.1   Exposure

The use of respirators makes physical demands on the user, for example, because of the
- weight of the device
- resistance to breathing/work involved in breathing
- increased dead space
- device technology
- duration of use

Additional demands on the user can result from use of respirators together with other personal protective equipment, e.g. isolating protective clothing.
More detailed information may be found in the appropriate published standards. Information is also obtainable from the producer of the device being used.

3.1.1   Classification of respirators

G 26

Respiratory protective equipment is classified according to the weight of the device
and the pressure differences during inhalation and exhalation (inspiration resistance,
exhalation resistance). A respirator is placed in a certain class when at least one of
the two threshold values (weight of device or breathing resistance) is exceeded. The
physical demands on the user increase in the order class 1 to class 3.
- Class 1: weight of device up to 3 kg
  The breathing resistance during inhalation and exhalation is low (up to 5 mbar
  for a respiratory minute volume of 20×1.5 l/min (intermittent sinusoidal) or
  95 l/min (continuous)).
  Examples: filter devices with particle filters class P1 or P2 and particle filtering
  half masks; filter devices with full face or half mask and a fan; devices with compressed air-line or assisted fresh air breathing apparatus, in both cases with
  mouthpiece and exhalation valve.
- Class 2: weight of device up to 5 kg
  The resistance to breathing is increased during inhalation and exhalation (above
  5 mbar for a respiratory minute volume of 20×1.5 l/min (intermittent sinusoidal) or 95 l/min (continuous)).
  Examples: filter devices with particle filters P3, with gas filters and combination filters of all classes; regenerating respirators weighing less than 5 kg; assisted fresh air breathing devices; protection devices for sand blasters and protective overalls combined with compressed air line or filter devices.
- Class 3: weight of device over 5 kg
  The resistance to breathing is increased during inhalation and exhalation (up to
  6 mbar for a respiratory minute volume of 20×1.5 l/min (intermittent sinusoidal) or 95 l/min (continuous)).
  Examples: portable self-contained closed-circuit devices such as devices with
  compressed air cylinders; regenerating respirators weighing more than 5 kg;
  protective overalls combined with class 3 devices.

Note: The wearing of protective overalls while using class 3 respirators and regenerating respirators weighing more than 5 kg makes additional demands on the worker. Persons wearing protective overalls are under strain because of the weight they carry, the microclimate, psychic effects (claustrophobia) and the situation (emergency). Regenerating respirators weighing more than 5 kg are a strain because they must be carried for long periods and the inhaled air becomes increasingly warm.

3.2 Functional disorders, symptoms

3.2.1 Acute and subacute effects on health

Acute pulmonary and/or cardiac stress.

3.2.2 Chronic effects on health

not applicable

4 References

Council Directive 89/391/EEC on the introduction of measures to encourage improvements in the safety and health of workers at work

Council Directive 92/85/EEC on the introduction of measures to encourage improvements in the safety and health at work of pregnant workers and workers who have recently given birth or are breastfeeding

G 27   Isocyanates

Committee for occupational medicine, working group "Hazardous substances",
Berufsgenossenschaft der chemischen Industrie, Heidelberg

Preliminary remarks

The present guideline describes a scheme for occupational medical prophylaxis
which aims to prevent or ensure early diagnosis of disorders which can be caused
by isocyanates.

Schedule

G 27

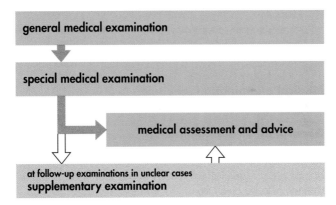

1   Medical examinations

Occupational medical examinations are to be carried out for persons at whose workplaces exposure to isocyanates could endanger health (e.g. the occupational exposure limit value is exceeded) or where direct skin contact can take place.

1.1   Examinations, intervals between examinations

initial examination	before taking up the job
first follow-up examination	after 3–12 months
further follow-up exminations	after 12–24 months and when leaving the job
premature follow-up examination	• after a serious or prolonged illness which could cause concern as to whether the activity should be continued • in individual cases when the physician considers it necessary, e.g. when there is short-term concern about the person's health • when requested by an employee who suspects a causal association between his or her illness and work

1.2   Medical examination schedule

1.2.1   General medical examination

Initial examination

• review of past history (general anamnesis, work anamnesis, symptoms)
Particular attention is to be given to:
• frequent or more serious disorders of the upper and lower airways and the lungs, especially tuberculosis, chronic bronchitis, emphysema, pneumoconiosis
• cardiopulmonary disorders or other disorders causing permanent lung function impairment
• allergic diseases, e.g., hay fever, asthma, tendency to eczema

Follow-up examination

• interim anamnesis (including work anamnesis)
Particular attention is to be given to:
• complaints of shortness of breath, coughing, more expectoration, pronounced breath sounds, especially acute asthmatic attacks, nocturnal dyspnoea, nocturnal coughing
• skin reactions

1.2.2   Special medical examination

Initial examination	Follow-up examination

- spirometry
- large format chest x-ray or use of an x-ray diagnosis which is less than 1 year old (only at initial examinations)

Also helpful:
- full blood count
- erythrocyte sedimentation reaction
- if the anamnesis suggests the presence of the disorders listed in Section 2.1.1, extended lung function tests (whole body plethysmography, examination before and after a work shift with relevant exposure, determination of peak flow, unspecific inhalative provocation in cases where the anamnesis indicates allergic reactions), perhaps blood gas analysis
- ergometry if indicated

If the person is exposed simultaneously to solvents:
- SGPT (ALT) or
- γ-GT

G 27

1.2.3   Supplementary examination

Follow-up examination

In unclear cases:
- determination of specific antibodies against isocyanates (IgE, IgG)
- ergometry with blood gas analysis
- spirometry
- unspecific inhalative provocation
- biomonitoring (see Section 3.1.4)

1.3   Requirements for the medical examinations

- competent doctor or occupational health professional
- laboratory analyses and x-ray examination carried out with appropriate quality control (Good Laboratory Practice)
- necessary equipment:
  - ECG/ergometer
  - equipment for lung function tests

2   Occupational medical assessment and advice

An assessment is only possible when the workplace situation and the exposure of the individual are known. For this purpose a risk assessment as defined in Article 4 Council directive 98/24/EC must have been carried out; it must describe the levels of exposure to isocyanates and specify which technical, organizational and individual protective measures have been applied.

2.1   Assessment criteria

2.1.1   Long-term concern about health

| **Initial examination** | **Follow-up examination** |

Persons with severe disorders such as
- lung disorders with or without impairment of lung function
- chronic obstructive airway disorders
- bronchial asthma
- repeatedly diagnosed bronchial hyperreactivity, symptomatic or in need of treatment
- cardiac disorders
- endogenous eczema

2.1.2   Short-term concern about health

| **Initial examination** |

Persons with the disorders mentioned in Section 2.1.1, provided recovery is to be expected. For a period of 1 to 2 months during convalescence from a disorder of the lungs or pleura which has regressed without sequelae.

| **Follow-up examination** |

As for the initial examination, and persons with acute respiratory tract disorders or those who have just recovered from such.

2.1.3   No concern about health under certain conditions

| Initial examination | Follow-up examination |

If the illnesses or functional disorders mentioned in Section 2.1.1 are less severe, the doctor should establish whether or not it is possible for the person to start work or go on working under certain conditions. The course of the disorder to date and the readiness of the person to co-operate should be taken into account. Such conditions could include
- technical protective measures
- organizational protective measures, e.g., limitation of exposure periods
- transfer to workplaces known to involve lower levels of exposure
- personal protective equipment which takes the individual's state of health into account
- more frequent follow-up examinations

A similar procedure is recommended for persons with atopic disposition (anamnestically detected tendency to develop allergic disorders or detection of increased levels of total IgE) and those with sebostatic eczema (optimal skin protection to be recommended).

G 27

2.1.4   No concern about health

| Initial examination | Follow-up examination |

All other persons, provided there are no restrictions on their employment.

2.2   Medical advice

The advice in an individual case should be commensurate with the workplace situation and the results of the medical examinations. Employees are to be informed about the biomonitoring results and the specific IgE antibody levels.

Employees should be informed about general hygienic measures and personal protective equipment.

Smokers should be told that inhalative smoking also impairs lung function.

If during the course of his work in the company the occupational physician finds indications that the risk assessment should be brought up to date to improve health and safety standards, he is to inform the employer. When this is necessary, the interests of the employee are to be protected (medical confidentiality).

3   Supplementary notes

3.1   External and internal exposure

3.1.1   Occurrence, sources of hazards

Listed below are the kinds of processes, workplaces or activities, including cleaning and repair work, for which exposure to isocyanates must be expected. This must be taken into account during the risk assessment.

- production of isocyanates and their prepolymers
- production of polyurethane plastics (foamed plastics) when volatile isocyanates (e.g. toluene diisocyanate, TDI) are used
- production of rubber-elastic materials (mould making)
- production of paints, glues and bonding agents
- use of isocyanates at high temperatures as glues and coatings or for the production of special plastics (e.g. from naphthalene diisocyanate, NDI)
- dusty processes (e.g. weighing, manual packaging)
- jobs involving exposure to isocyanates as aerosols (spray painting) or as products of the thermal decomposition of polyurethanes (e.g. welding polyurethane-coated objects, removal of coatings), oxygen cutting of metal doors
- in foundries using binder systems containing isocyanates
- sealing of aroma-proof packaging made of plastics containing isocyanates
- use of polyurethane foams, e.g. from spray cans, when this job takes a significant part of the work shift (generally more than half of the shift)
- injection filling jobs
- production and processing of floor coverings for sports halls
- hot wire cutting of polyurethane foam plastics
- handling hot melts containing isocyanates, e.g. lining car roofs, book binding
- use of polyurethanes as slope stabilizers

Occurrence and hazards for specific substances are documented in the information system on hazardous substances (GESTIS) (see Section 4).

3.1.2   Physicochemical properties and classification

It is important to note that isocyanates are available under a wide range of trade names and that the products can contain mixtures of isocyanates.

The substances are mostly liquids (apart from diphenyl methane diisocyanate, MDI) with the general formula

$R-N=C=O$ (R: organic residue).

As isocyanates are mostly taken up by inhalation, the concentration of the substances in the inhaled air is significant (especially also short peak exposures to vapours, aerosols or dust). In addition, intensive skin contact can also lead to pulmonary sensitization. The isocyanate group $(-N=C=O)$ is highly reactive; it reacts primarily

with the "active hydrogen atoms" of a wide range of compounds (e.g. water, alcohols, amines).
In Section 5 some of the toxicologically most important of these compounds are listed. The information system on hazardous substances (GESTIS) provides details of international threshold limit values, classification, evaluation and other substance-specific information (see Section 4).

3.1.3   Uptake
Isocyanates are taken up especially via the airways; intensive skin contact can also lead to dermal uptake.

3.1.4   Biomonitoring
Information about biomonitoring may be found in Appendix 1 "Biomonitoring".

Biological threshold value for occupational exposures from the List of MAK and BAT Values

Substance	Parameter	BLW[1]	Assay material	Sampling time
diphenylmethane-4,4'-diisocyanate (MDI)	4,4'-diaminodiphenylmethane	10 µg/l	urine	end of exposure or end of shift

Threshold values for biological materials reflect the total body burden of a substance taken up by inhalation, through the skin, etc. In persons exposed at work to MDI, the level of 4,4'-diaminodiphenylmethane (MDA) in the urine is a measure of all the absorbed components of a complex MDI mixture because both monomers and oligomers of MDI are metabolized to monomeric MDA, independent of the absorption route.

In contrast, the threshold limit value for MDI in the workplace air takes only the monomeric MDI into account.
The biological threshold value was established by the DFG Commission for the Investigation of Health Hazards of Chemical Compounds in the Work Area (MAK commission) on the basis of correlation with the MAK value for MDI. This correlation is based on the results of several occupational medical workplace studies.
During exposures involving mainly inhalative uptake of MDI for which the relationship between monomers and oligomers or polymers is like that for which the threshold value for the workplace air (MAK value) was derived, the biological threshold value corresponds to the MAK value. In situations where the relationship between

---

[1] Biologischer Leitwert (BLW), see Appendix 1 and List of MAK and BAT Values

monomers and polymers is shifted in favour of more polymer, or when high levels of dermal uptake are involved, the parameter determined in biological material is increased. Thus it is keeping "on the safe side" when the biological threshold value is observed in these cases.

Therefore for persons exposed to unusually high levels of MDI oligomers or polymers and those exposed dermally, observance of the biological threshold value offers more protection than does observance of the threshold limit value for the substance in the workplace air.

Biomonitoring should be carried out with reliable methods and meet quality control requirements (see Appendix 1 "Biomonitoring").

3.2 Functional disorders, symptoms

3.2.1 Mode of action

Isocyanates react in the body with organic substances containing active hydrogen atoms, especially with the hydroxy and amino groups of proteins and lipoproteins. The effects depend on the exposure concentration and time. Inhalation exposure causes gradually increasing effects in the various sections of the respiratory tract.

Low-level exposure causes reversible irritation in the upper airways. Given higher exposure levels, this spreads into the deeper airways.

Direct contact with isocyanates causes superficial brownish skin changes.

Contact of liquid isocyanates with the skin can lead to both irritation and sensitization with urticaria and contact dermatitis. Studies have demonstrated that even a single exposure of a large area of skin to a product containing isocyanates can be sufficient to cause sensitization.

Damage to internal organs has not been shown to be caused by the absorbed substances.

3.2.2 Acute and subacute effects on health

Even low level exposure to isocyanates causes signs of irritation of the eyes (conjunctivitis), nose (rhinitis) and throat (pharyngitis); sometimes the voice is also affected (laryngitis). Such changes are rapidly reversible. Given more intensive exposure and depending on the severity of the damage caused, the symptoms become more pronounced. Severe coughing (tracheitis) and chest pains are associated with dyspnoea (bronchitis, sometimes pneumonia). Attacks of dyspnoea are also observed. After very high-level exposures severe dyspnoea is the main symptom with moist rales and foamy sputum (pulmonary oedema).

Immunologically induced asthma and exogenous allergic alveolitis can also develop after low-level exposures (formation of specific IgE antibodies). However, such reactions are detected in only 20 % to 30 % of persons tested.

Persons with unspecific bronchial hyperreactivity or with acquired specific hypersensitivity to isocyanates can react with bronchospasm (coughing, feeling of tightness in

the chest, shortness of breath, asthma attack) when exposed even to levels below the threshold limit value for the workplace air.
Intensive skin contact can lead to irritation (dermatitis artificialis) and sensitization (urticaria, contact dermatitis).

3.2.3   Chronic effects on health
Specific or unspecific hypersensitivity of the airways can develop which, on re-exposure to very low concentrations of isocyanates, causes coughing, a feeling of tightness in the chest, attacks of dyspnoea, asthma (of immediate type, delayed type or dual type) or alveolitis (with the symptoms of a feverish influenza-like infection). Cases with isolated chronic obstructive bronchitis are rare. In some of the cases with specific respiratory hypersensitivity specific anti-isocyanate antibodies may be detected in blood (sensitization, antibodies detectable with RAST, etc.). Atopic persons have a slightly greater tendency to become sensitized than do normal persons.
Lung function disorders (not including irritation) have not been observed by most authors to result from exposure to low concentrations of isocyanates below the threshold limit value for the workplace air. In very rare cases the hypersensitivity can progress to allergic contact dermatitis of the skin. Evidence of carcinogenic or teratogenic effects of isocyanates has not yet been seen in man.

G 27

4   References
Commission Recommendation 2003/670/EC concerning the European schedule of occupational diseases. Annex I
Council Directive 67/548/EEC on the approximation of the laws, regulations and administrative provisions relating to the classification, packaging and labelling of dangerous substances
Council Directive 98/24/EC on the protection of the health and safety of workers from the risks related to chemical agents at work
Deutsche Forschungsgemeinschaft (German Research Foundation, DFG) (ed) List of MAK and BAT Values 2007. Maximum Concentrations and Biological Tolerance Values at the workplace. Wiley-VCH, Weinheim
Deutsche Forschungsgemeinschaft (German Research Foundation, DFG) (ed) The MAK-Collection for Occupational Health and Safety. Wiley-VCH
    at: www.mrw.interscience.wiley.com/makbat
GESTIS-database on hazardous substances. BGIA
    at: www.dguv.de/bgia/gestis-database
GESTIS-international limit values for chemical agents. BGIA
    at: www.dguv.de/bgia/gestis-limit-values

5   Isocyanates used in industry

The most important of the diisocyanates used in industry are listed below. Threshold limit values and classification of these substance may be found in the information system on hazardous substances (GESTIS) (see Section 4). In the products used at the workplace, however, mixtures of various diisocyanates or polymeric isocyanates may be present.

Aliphatic diisocyanates

HDI = hexamethylene-1,6-diisocyanate

Structural formula $OCN-(CH_2)_6-NCO$
CAS number   822-06-0

Colourless to yellowish liquid with low viscosity and a relatively high vapour pressure.

TMDI = 2,2,4-trimethylhexamethylene-1,6-diisocyanate

Structural formula

$$O=C=N-CH_2-\underset{\underset{CH_3}{|}}{\overset{\overset{CH_3}{|}}{C}}-CH_2-\overset{\overset{CH_3}{|}}{CH}-CH_2-CH_2-N=C=O$$

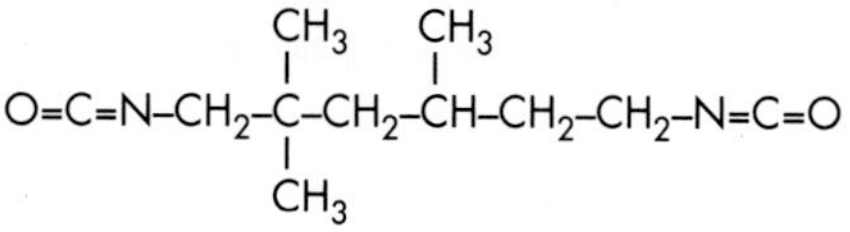

CAS number   16938-22-0

TMDI = 2,4,4-trimethylhexamethylene-1,6-diisocyanate

Structural formula

$$O=C=N-CH_2-\overset{\overset{CH_3}{|}}{CH}-CH_2-\underset{\underset{CH_3}{|}}{\overset{\overset{CH_3}{|}}{C}}-CH_2-CH_2-N=C=O$$

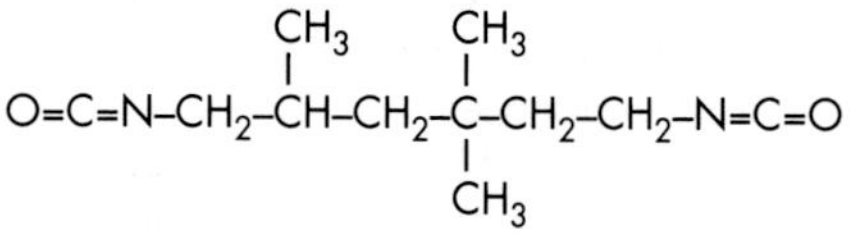

CAS number   15646-96-5

Colourless to yellowish liquid, very poorly inflammable, decomposes in water.

Cycloaliphatic diisocyanates

IPDI = isophorone diisocyanate;
3-isocyanatomethyl-3,5,5-trimethylcyclohexyl-isocyanate

Structural formula

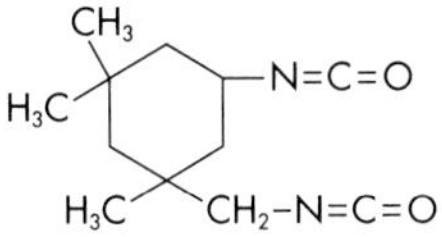

CAS number   4098-71-9

Liquid at normal temperatures, less reactive than the other isocyanates mentioned here.

Aromatic diisocyanates

TDI = toluene diisocyanate

toluene-2,4-diisocyanate
Structural formula

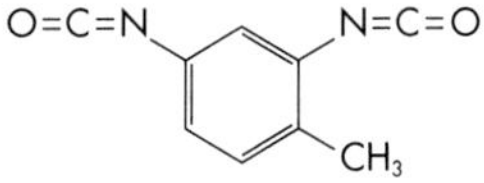

CAS number   584-84-9

toluene-2,6-diisocyanate
Structural formula

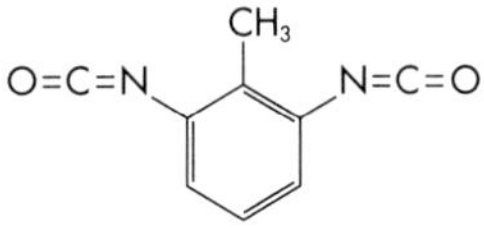

CAS number   91-08-7

toluene diisocyanate (mixture of *2,4-* and *2,6-toluenediisocyanate*)
CAS number   26471-62-5

G 27

NDI = 1,5-naphthylene diisocyanate
Structural formula

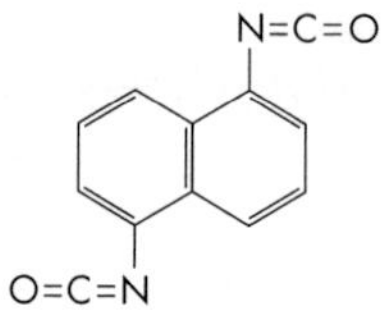

CAS number   3173-72-6

white or yellowish to greyish white flakes

MDI monomer (inhalable fraction) = diphenylmethane-4,4'-diisocyanate
Structural formula

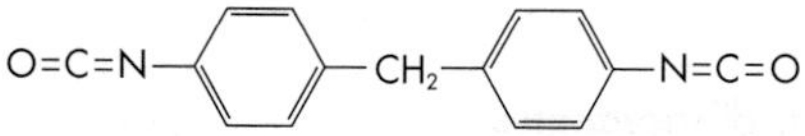

CAS number   101-68-8

MDI monomer (pure): a white to yellowish solid at room temperature, above 40°C a yellowish liquid of low viscosity

MDI polymer* (inhalable fraction)
Structural formula

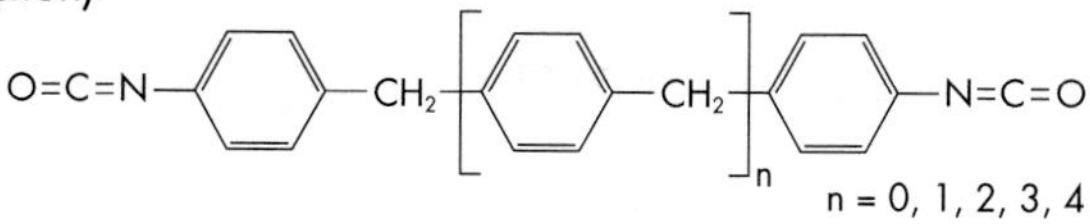

n = 0, 1, 2, 3, 4

CAS number   9016-87-9

As well as the qualities of MDI mentioned above, there are modified formulations which are derived either from monomeric MDI or from polymeric MDI. Their main component is MDI.

---

* MDI polymer = mixture of isomers containing diphenylmethane diisocyanates (diphenyl-
methane-2,2'-diisocyanate, diphenylmethane-2,4-diisocyanate, diphenylmethane-4,4'-diiso-
cyanate) and their prepolymers, 4-methyl-*m*-phenylene diisocyanate, technical MDI
MDI polymer: blackish-brown liquid of medium viscosity

G 29   Benzene homologues (toluene, xylene isomers)

Committee for occupational medicine, working group "Hazardous substances",
Berufsgenossenschaft der chemischen Industrie, Heidelberg

Preliminary remarks

The present guideline describes a scheme for occupational medical prophylaxis
which aims to prevent or ensure early diagnosis of disorders which can be caused
by toluene or xylene. If the toluene or xylene or solvent containing toluene or xylene
contain more than 0.1 % w/w of benzene, then the guideline G 8 Benzene should
be referred to as well.

Schedule

G 29

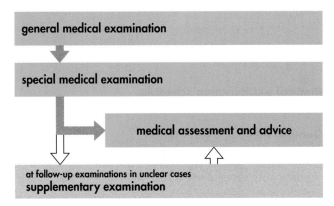

1   Medical examinations

Occupational medical examinations are to be carried out for persons exposed at work to levels of benzene homologues (toluene, xylene isomers) which could have adverse effects on health (e.g. when the occupational exposure limit value is exceeded) or for whom dermal absorption could endanger health.

1.1   Examinations, intervals between examinations

initial examination	before taking up the job
first follow-up examination	after 12–24 months
futher follow-up ecaminations	after 12–24 months and when leaving the job
premature follow-up examination	• after an illness lasting for several weeks or when a physical handicap gives cause for concern about whether the work should be continued • in individual cases when the physician considers it necessary, e.g. when there is short-term concern about the person's health • when requested by an employee who suspects a causal association between his or her illness and work

1.2   Medical examination schedule

1.2.1   General medical examination

Initial examination

• review of past history (general anamnesis, work anamnesis)
• urinalysis (multiple test strips)

Follow-up examination

• interim anamnesis (including work anamnesis)
• particular attention should be paid to: headaches, dizziness, fatigability, nausea, anorexia, weight loss, alcohol intolerance
• urinalysis (multiple test strips)

1.2.2 Special medical examination

Initial examination	Follow-up examination

- full blood count (at two-year intervals in follow-up examinations)
- biomonitoring (see Section 3.1.4) – but not at the initial examination

Also helpful:
- SGPT (ALT), γ-GT
- neurological screening

1.2.3 Supplementary examination

Follow-up examination

In unclear cases further examination by a specialist should be considered.

1.3 Requirements for the medical examinations

- competent doctor or occupational health professional
- laboratory analyses carried out with appropriate quality control (Good Laboratory Practice)

G 29

2 Occupational medical assessment and advice

An assessment is only possible when the workplace situation and the exposure of the individual are known. For this purpose a risk assessment as defined in Article 4 Council directive 98/24/EC must have been carried out; it must specify which technical, organizational and individual protective measures have been applied.

2.1 Assessment criteria

2.1.1 Long-term concern about health

Initial examination	Follow-up examination

Persons with
- marked neurological disorders
- alcohol addiction
- obstructive airway disorders

2.1.2   Short-term concern about health

| Initial examination | Follow-up examination |

Persons with the disorders mentioned in Section 2.1.1, provided recovery is to be expected.

2.1.3   No concern about health under certain conditions

| Initial examination | Follow-up examination |

Persons with
- chronic inflammatory skin disorders
- signs of marked chronic conjunctival irritation

If the illnesses or functional disorders mentioned in Section 2.1.1 are less severe, the doctor should establish whether or not it is possible for the person to start work or go on working under certain conditions. Such conditions could include
- technical protective measures
- organizational protective measures, e.g., limitation of exposure periods
- transfer to workplaces known to involve lower levels of exposure
- personal protective equipment which takes the individual's state of health into account
- more frequent follow-up examinations

2.1.4   No concern about health

| Initial examination | Follow-up examination |

All other persons, provided there are no restrictions on their employment.

2.2   Medical advice

The advice in an individual case should be commensurate with the workplace situation and the results of the medical examinations.

Employees are to be informed about the biomonitoring results.

Employees should be informed about general hygienic measures and personal protective equipment. Because toluene and the xylene isomers readily penetrate the skin, the wearing of protective clothing is of particular significance. Substance-specific protective measures are documented in the information system on hazardous substances (GESTIS) in the section "Handling and usage" (see Section 4).

The employees are to be advised that alcohol consumption potentiates the effects of the substances.

If during the course of his work in the company the occupational physician finds indications that the risk assessment should be brought up to date to improve health and safety standards, he is to inform the employer. When this is necessary, the interests of the employee are to be protected (medical confidentiality).

3   Supplementary notes

3.1   External and internal exposure

3.1.1   Occurrence, sources of hazards

Occurrence and hazards for specific substances are documented in the information system on hazardous substances (GESTIS) (see Section 4).

Health surveillance is necessary for persons working with toluene and xylene isomers, especially for the following kinds of processes, workplaces or activities, including cleaning and repair work:

- use of toluene and xylene together with other solvents in defatting of metals and cleaning of surfaces

Toluene
- recovery from petroleum rich in aromatics and in reforming processes in the petroleum industry; also – currently in unimportant quantities – from the crude benzene of coking plants and from the crude light oil distillation fraction of coal-tar
- processing
- mixing and filling of containers
- cleaning of storage tanks
- use as raw materials in the organic chemicals industry, e.g. in the production of chlorotoluene, nitrotoluene, toluenesulfonic acid, phenol
- use as solvents, cleaners and diluents for printing inks, wood preservatives, resins, paints and glues and processing such formulations

G 29

Xylene isomers
- recovery in reforming processes in the petroleum industry
- mixing and filling of containers
- cleaning of storage tanks
- processing the xylene isomers
- use as solvents, cleaners and diluents for oils, fats, wood preservatives, resins, rubber, paints and lacquers and processing such formulations
- use of xylene in histology laboratories when the workplace is inadequately ventilated

3.1.2   Physicochemical properties and classification

The most important benzene homologues are toluene and the xylene isomers; xylene always occurs as a mixture of *o*-xylene, *m*-xylene and *p*-xylene together with a fourth isomer, ethyl benzene and/or 1,3,5-trimethylbenzene (mesitylene). Mixtures of these benzene homologues are frequently called solvent naphtha. They are mobile, colourless, highly refractive liquids which are very sparingly soluble in water and have a typical benzene-like odour. Toluene is highly volatile. The xylene isomers are much less volatile. The vapour of these substances is heavier than air and can accumulate at floor level.

	Toluene	*Xylene isomers*
Formula	$C_6H_5CH_3$	$C_6H_4(CH_3)_2$
CAS number	108-88-3	1330-20-7
MAK value[1]	50 ml/m^3, 190 mg/m^3	100 ml/m^3, 440 mg/m^3

The information system on hazardous substances (GESTIS) provides details of classification, evaluation and other substance-specific information (see Section 4).

3.1.3   Uptake

The benzene homologues are taken up via the airways and the skin.

3.1.4   Biomonitoring

Information about biomonitoring may be found in Appendix 1 "Biomonitoring". When evaluating the biomonitoring results it should be remembered that in persons exposed to mixtures of solvents the metabolism of the one solvent can be modified by that of the other. Thus it has been reported that in persons exposed to mixtures of *m*-xylene and ethylbenzene the excretion of xylene metabolites is delayed and the concentrations reduced. Co-exposure to *m*-xylene and 2-butanone resulted in an increase in the xylene concentration in blood and a reduction in the amount of methylhippuric (toluric) acid excreted.

---

[1] Maximale Arbeitsplatz-Konzentration = maximum workplace concentration

Biological tolerance value for occupational exposures from the List of MAK and BAT Values

Substance	Parameter	BAT[2]	Assay material	Sampling time
toluene	toluene	1.0 mg/l	whole blood	end of exposure or end of shift
	o-cresol	3.0 mg/l	urine	end of exposure or end of shift; for long-term exposures: after several shifts
xylene (all isomers)	xylene	1.5 mg/l	whole blood	end of exposure or end of shift
	methylhippuric (toluric) acid	2000 mg/l	urine	end of exposure or end of shift

Biomonitoring should be carried out with reliable methods and meet quality control requirements (see Appendix 1 "Biomonitoring").

G 29

3.2   Functional disorders, symptoms

3.2.1   Mode of action

In acute intoxications the narcotic effects are predominant. During acute intoxications, excitation or inebriation, disorders of balance, sensitivity and co-ordination, headaches, tiredness and weakness, feeling dazed and loss of consciousness have been reported.

After long-term exposures, irritation of the mucosa and the eyes can develop. Because the substances defat the skin, they can cause dermatitis. Transient changes in the blood count have been observed. Absorbed toluene and xylene are exhaled (about 20 %) and metabolized (about 80 %). Oxidation takes place mostly on a side chain. The urinary metabolites hippuric acid (toluene) and methylhippuric acid (xylene) are formed via benzoic acid and coupling with aminoacetic acid (glycine).

---

[2] Biologischer Arbeitsstoff-Toleranzwert (BAT) = biological tolerance value for occupational exposures

3.2.2   Acute and subacute effects on health

* prenarcotic symptoms
* excitation stadium mostly with spasms
* narcosis with a risk of central respiratory paralysis

3.2.3   Chronic effects on health

* neurasthenic symptoms
* paraesthesia
* sometimes psychic behavioural disorders
* alcohol intolerance

4   References

Commission Recommendation 2003/670/EC concerning the European schedule of
    occupational diseases. Annex I
Council Directive 98/24/EC on the protection of the health and safety of workers
    from the risks related to chemical agents at work
Deutsche Forschungsgemeinschaft (German Research Foundation, DFG) (ed) List of
    MAK and BAT Values 2007. Maximum Concentrations and Biological Tolerance
    Values at the workplace. Wiley-VCH, Weinheim
Deutsche Forschungsgemeinschaft (German Research Foundation, DFG) (ed) The
    MAK-Collection for Occupational Health and Safety. Wiley-VCH
    at: www.mrw.interscience.wiley.com/makbat
GESTIS-database on hazardous substances. BGIA
    at: www.dguv.de/bgia/gestis-database
GESTIS-international limit values for chemical agents. BGIA
    at: www.dguv.de/bgia/gestis-limit-values

G 30   Hot working conditions

Committee for occupational medicine, Berufsgenossenschaft Nahrungsmittel und Gaststätten, Mannheim

Preliminary remarks

The present guideline describes a scheme for occupational medical prophylaxis which aims to prevent or ensure early diagnosis of disorders which can be caused by working under hot conditions.

Schedule

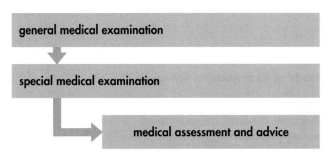

G 30

1   Medical examinations

Occupational medical examinations are to be carried out for persons working under hot conditions.

1.1   Examinations, intervals between examinations

initial examination	before taking up the job
first und further follow-up examinations	• persons up to 50 years old: within 60 months • persons over 50 years old: within 24 months
premature follow-up examination	• after an illness lasting for several weeks or when a physical handicap gives cause for concern about whether the work should be continued • in individual cases when the physician considers it necessary, e.g. when there is short-term concern about the person's health • when requested by an employee who suspects a causal association between his or her illness and work

1.2   Medical examination schedule

1.2.1   General medical examination

Initial examination	Follow-up examination

- review of past history (general anamnesis, work anamnesis, symptoms); particular attention to be paid to: soundness of the cardiopulmonary system, the liver and the upper and lower urinary tract
- urinalysis (multiple test strips)

1.2.2   Special medical examination

Initial examination	Follow-up examination

- ECG with chest lead, at rest and during exercise
- large format posterior-anterior thorax radiograph taken with high kilovolt technique for specific diagnostic purposes, in two planes if indicated
  If a radiograph not more than one year old is available, this should be taken into consideration before deciding on the indicated procedure.

1.3   Requirements for the medical examinations

competent doctor or occupational health professional.

2   Occupational medical assessment and advice

An assessment is only possible when the workplace situation and the exposure of the individual are known. For this purpose a risk assessment as defined in Article 9 Council directive 89/391/EC must have been carried out; it must specify which technical, organizational and individual protective measures have been applied.

2.1   Assessment criteria

2.1.1   Long-term concern about health

Initial examination	Follow-up examination

Persons with
- cardiocirculatory disorders with functional impairment
- disabling pneumoconiosis
- active or extensive latent pulmonary tuberculosis
- chronic obstructive respiratory disease, chronic bronchitis
- bronchial asthma
- seizures – depending on their kind, frequency, prognosis and state of treatment
- incompletely healed skull and brain injuries
- diabetes mellitus
- severe arteriosclerosis
- cataracts (if the exposure is mainly to radiant heat)
- disorders of the kidneys and/or lower urinary tract
- chronic gastrointestinal disorders
- chronic liver disorders
- severe obesity
- chronic recurring and generalized skin disorders
- addiction to alcohol, drugs or medication

G 30

2.1.2   Short-term concern about health

Initial examination	Follow-up examination

Persons with the disorders mentioned in Section 2.1.1, provided recovery is to be expected.

2.1.3   No concern about health under certain conditions

Initial examination	Follow-up examination

If the illnesses or functional disorders mentioned in Section 2.1.1 are less severe, the doctor should establish whether or not it is possible for the person to start work or go on working under certain conditions. Such conditions could include
- improved working conditions
- use of additional personal protective equipment
- more frequent follow-up examinations, etc.

2.1.4   No concern about health

Initial examination	Follow-up examination

All other persons, provided there are no restrictions on their employment.

2.2   Medical advice

The advice in an individual case should be commensurate with the workplace situation and the results of the medical examinations.

The employee should be told about technical and organizational protective measures appropriate for the individual's state of health.

If the results of occupational medical examinations indicate focal cumulation of health risks, the physician, while observing medical confidentiality, is to inform and advise the employer.

3   Supplementary notes

3.1   Heat stress

Climate is defined by the parameters
- air temperature (dry bulb temperature) (°C)
- humidity (expressed as water vapour pressure in hPa or relative humidity in %)
- airflow (wind speed) (m/sec)
- heat flux density (from heat radiation) (W/m^2)

The assessment of heat stress also involves the personal parameters
- work done (energy required) (W or kJ)
- heat transfer through the clothing
- duration of exposure (min)

The heat stress at the workplace is assessed by determining the noon effective temperature for the clothed person, NET (°C), by the method of Yaglou – a measure of climate as felt by a person – and the heat flux density.

The level of work (energy required) is to be determined in a work study and expressed as the mean hourly level.
The determination of the NET is to be carried out at outdoor temperatures which correspond to the average dry bulb temperature of the summer months of June to August and which lie in Germany between 15°C and 18°C.

Example: the dry bulb temperature was found to be 40°C, the relative humidity 33 % (this corresponds to a wet bulb temperature of 26°C), and the wind speed 1 m/sec. According to the nomogram of Yaglou for a clothed person (see Figure) the effective temperature is then NET = 30°C.
The heat stress at the workplace can also be a result of the heat flux density alone or be affected markedly by this. If it cannot be measured directly it can be estimated – admittedly only under constant climatic conditions – with the help of a black globe thermometer.
If the difference between the outdoor temperature and the heat radiation is very large, the effect of the outdoor temperature on the heat stress can be ignored.

3.1.1   Occurrence, sources of hazards

Human thermal comfort is determined essentially by a balance between heat production and heat loss. The same is true for health under conditions of heat stress.

G 30

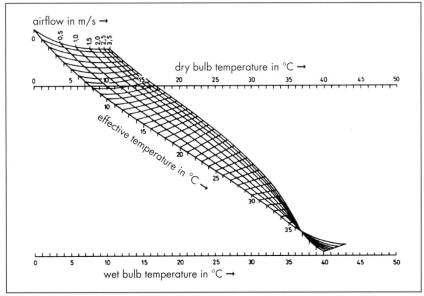

Figure 1: Nomogram for determining the noon effective temperature for a fully clothed person

Heat loss takes place by convection, conduction, radiation and evaporation of sweat. Heat loss may be increased in two main ways:
- by an increase in the peripheral blood supply
- by increased evaporation of sweat

Adverse effects on comfort and health are generally the effect of an imbalance between heat production and heat loss. This imbalance generally arises when the mechanisms for ensuring heat loss are acutely overloaded because of heat stress resulting from a combination of high temperature of the workplace air and heat production from physical work. Thermal imbalance causes an increase in body temperature which can attain or exceed human tolerance limits, above which adverse effects on health may be expected. Depending on the body temperature attained and the rate of the temperature increase, heat stress can result in a variety of disorders.

Occupational medical prophylaxis is necessary even for persons doing only brief or occasional work under hot conditions.

All jobs carried out under hot working conditions involve short-term heat stress if acclimatization of the persons is not to be expected.

Acute illnesses can reduce heat tolerance. Therefore, even when the physician finds nothing serious, during medical examinations in acute cases the sense of well-being of the employee should be taken seriously (willingness, duration of exposure, regulation of breaks).

3.2   Functional disorders, symptoms

- circulatory collapse (heat collapse)
- heat cramp
- heatstroke

4   References

DIN 33 403: Klima am Arbeitsplatz und in der Arbeitsumgebung (Climate at the workplace and its environments); Teil 2: Einwirkung des Klimas auf den Wärmehaushalt des Menschen – (Part 2: Effect of the climate on the heat balance of human beings); Teil 3: Beurteilung des Klimas im Erträglichkeitsbereich (Part 3: Assessment of the climate in the warm and hot working areas based on selected climate indices)

DIN-Fachbericht 128: Klima am Arbeitsplatz und in der Arbeitsumgebung – Grundlagen zur Klimaermittlung. (Climate in the workplace and its environment – Basic principles for the ascertainment of climate).

Directive 89/391/EC on the introduction of measures to encourage improvements in the safety and health of workers at work

EN ISO 7730: Ergonomics of the thermal environment – Analytical determination and interpretation of thermal comfort using calculation of the PMV and PPD indices and local thermal comfort criteria

EN ISO 7933: Ergonomics of the thermal environment – Analytical determination and interpretation of heat stress using calculation of the predicted heat strain

ISO 7726: Ergonomics of the thermal environment – Instruments for measuring physical quantities

Malchaire J, Gebhardt HJ, Piette A (1999) Strategy for evaluation and prevention of risk due to work in thermal environments. Ann occup Hyg 43(5): 367–76

Malchaire J, Kampmann B, Mehnert P, Gebhardt H, Piette A, Havenith G, Holmer I, Parsons K, Alfano G, Griefahn B (2002) Assessment of the risk of heat disorders encountered during work in hot conditions. Int Arch Occup Environ Health 75(3):153–62

Malchaire JB (2006) Occupational heat stress assessment by the Predicted Heat Strain model. Ind Health 44(3): 380–7

Parsons KC (2003) Human Thermal Environments. The effects of hot, moderate and cold environments on human health, comfort and performance. Taylor & Francis, London

G 30

G 31   Hyperbaric pressure

Committee for occupational medicine, working group "Hyperbaric pressure", Arbeitsmedizinischer Dienst der Berufsgenossenschaft der Bauwirtschaft (BG Bau), München

Preliminary remarks
The present guideline describes a scheme for occupational medical prophylaxis which aims to establish whether or not work under conditions of hyperbaric pressure may give rise to concern for the person's health.
The following kinds of work are considered to be work under conditions of hyperbaric pressure:
- work in compressed air at pressures more than 10 kPa (0.1 bar) above atmospheric pressure
- work under water during which the employee is provided with air to breathe via diving equipment.

Schedule

G 31

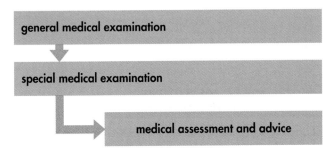

1   Medical examinations

Occupational medical examinations are to be carried out for persons at workplaces where they are exposed to ambient air pressures above atmospheric pressure or when other selection criteria are fulfilled.

1.1   Examinations, intervals between examinations

initial examination	before beginning work at hyperbaric pressure
follow-up examinations	within 12 months
premature follow-up examination	• if the results of a medical examination indicate that shorter intervals between examinations are necessary • after illnesses caused by hyperbaric pressure, after an illness which has lasted longer than 6 weeks or when the person has been ill several times within half a year, it is necessary for the physician to see the employee and decide whether work under hyperbaric pressure is possible again in spite of the illness or whether a premature check-up is necessary; it is also necessary for the person to see the doctor when there is cause for concern about the person's health; this can also be the case after brief illnesses • when requested by an employee who suspects a causal association between his or her illness and work

1.2   Medical examination schedule

1.2.1   General medical examination

Initial examination

• review of past history (general anamnesis, work anamnesis, symptoms)
  Particular attention is to be paid to: results of previous radiological examinations [thorax, joints (date, diagnosis, name of physician)].

Follow-up examination

- interim anamnesis including work anamnesis and for divers inspection of the diving records
  Particular attention is to be paid to:
  - previous work under hyperbaric conditions (duration, pressure levels, symptoms during/after work under hyperbaric conditions, previous pressure chamber treatments)
  - details of first or last follow-up examination (date, results, name of physician)
  - details of radiological examinations carried out since the last examination [thorax, joints (date, diagnosis, name of physician)]

1.2.2   Special medical examination

Initial examination   **Follow-up examination**

- the examination should take into account the workplace situation and the criteria given in Section 2.1 (e.g. inspection of the external auditory canals and the tympanic membranes with Valsalva manoeuvre, Schellong test, dental status)
- urinalysis (multiple test strips: protein, sugar, bile pigments, blood, leukocytes)
- blood count
- haematocrit
- blood sugar
- creatinine in serum
- GGT
- GPT (ALAT)
- blood pressure and pulse rate at rest
- ergometry
- spirometry
- visual acuity in the far range
- air-conduction audiometry (test frequencies 1–6 kHz)
- large or medium format posterior-anterior thorax radiogram (in unclear cases also further planes if the physician considers it necessary) or results of a radiogram taken within the previous 2 years (radiology at follow-up examinations only if strictly indicated, generally not within 5 years)

Also helpful:
- serum urea

Only at the initial examination
- it is helpful to carry out a pressure chamber test up to at least 100 kPa (1 bar) above atmospheric pressure.

G 31

1.3   Requirements for the medical examinations

- competent doctor or occupational health professional
- participation in a recognized specialist training course and regular courses to keep up to date
- equipment required:
  own equipment:
  - ECG with at least 12 leads
  - ergometry equipment for setting physically defined and reproducible work levels (bicycle ergometer)
  - lung function test device, preferably with documentation of the flow-volume curve
  - for eyesight tests an optical instrument or vision testing charts for the far range
  - audiometer
  - otoscope
  own equipment or that of other physicians:
  - laboratory
  - x-ray apparatus for large or medium format radiographs.

2   Occupational medical assessment and advice

An assessment is only possible when the workplace situation and the work of the individual are known. For this purpose a risk assessment as defined in Article 9 Council directive 89/391/EEC must have been carried out; it must specify which technical, organizational and individual protective measures have been applied.

2.1   Assessment criteria

2.1.1   Long-term concern about health

Initial examination	Follow-up examination

Persons with
- general physical weakness, reduced nutritional status, reduced strength
- body weight more than 30% above the normal weight determined by Broca's formula (height in cm minus 100 = normal weight in kg) or by other indices (e.g. BMI > 30)
- disorders of consciousness or balance and seizures of any kind
- disorders or damage of the central or peripheral nervous system with significant functional impairment and their sequelae, functional disorders after head or brain injuries, circulatory disorders in the brain
- emotional or mental disorders, even when these are in the past, if the possibility of recurrence cannot be excluded with sufficient certainty

- abnormal mentality or highly abnormal behaviour
- chronic alcohol misuse, drug-dependence or other addictions
- allergic disorders if these could represent a particular risk for health under the conditions of the job in question
- metabolic disorders, especially diabetes, or other disorders of endocrine glands, especially the thyroid, parathyroid or adrenal glands, if the disorders reduce the person's performance capacity markedly
- pathological disorders of the blood and the haematopoietic organs
- other chronic disorders which cause marked impairment of performance under the specific workplace conditions
- infectious diseases (carriers of dangerous pathogens)
- disorders or alterations of the heart or circulatory system which result in reduced performance or impaired regulation, more severe blood pressure changes, condition after a heart attack
- disorders or alterations of the respiratory organs (especially emphysema, chronic bronchitis, bronchial asthma, pleural fibrosis) which cause marked functional impairment
- active, also latent tuberculosis, extensive inactive tuberculosis and the condition following pleuritis which is perhaps not completely cured
- vital capacity less than 80 % of the calculated normal value and/or forced expiratory volume in one second below the minimum expected value.
- disorders of the gastrointestinal or urogenital systems if they result in sudden symptoms and could cause especially divers to carry out decompression too rapidly
- hernia (also umbilical hernia and incisional hernia)
- disorders of the postural or locomotor system or of the thorax, also rheumatic disorders causing marked functional impairment, with particular attention to the sites most likely to develop decompression-induced aseptic bone necrosis
- malformations or growths which have resulted in functional impairment or which could cause a particular risk for health under the given workplace conditions
- endoprostheses, larger foreign bodies such as screws, nails, etc. in bones or joints
- skin disorders or extensive scars which markedly impair work performance or which can be exacerbated by the work
- bilateral corrected visual acuity <0.7 (<0.63); persons having only one useful eye >0.8 are not automatically excluded from such work
- disorders or alterations of the eyes which markedly impair work performance, e.g. severe myopia with alterations of the fundus oculi, glaucoma, severe nystagmus
- deafness which would endanger reliable communication via the telephone system of the diving equipment or the reliable hearing of warning signals during work under hyperbaric conditions and/or reliable communication via technological communication systems
- perforation of the tympanic membrane and atrophic scars on the tympanic membrane in divers

G 31

- chronic functional disorders of the eustachian tube and chronic disorders of the nasal sinuses
- tendency to develop recurrent or severe disorders caused by hyperbaric pressure
- negative results of multiple pressure chamber tests

2.1.2   Short-term concern about health

Initial examination   **Follow-up examination**

Persons with the disorders mentioned in Section 2.1.1, provided recovery is to be expected.

2.1.3   No concern about health under certain conditions

Initial examination

- not applicable for professional divers
- for persons working under hyperbaric conditions:
  persons with defects or weaknesses of the kind listed in Section 2.1.1 but for whom, in view of the job to be done, no danger is to be expected, either for themselves or for others

Follow-up examination

Persons with defects or weaknesses of the kind listed in Section 2.1 but for whom, in view of the age of the person, the work experience and the job to be done, no danger is to be expected either for themselves or for others.

2.1.4   No concern about health

Initial examination   **Follow-up examination**

All other persons, provided there are no restrictions on their employment.

2.2   Medical advice

Advice for the employee could include suggestions as to behaviour during acute illnesses and after work under hyperbaric pressure.

3   Supplementary notes

3.1   Exposure

3.1.1   Occurrence, sources of hazards

The people to be examined include:
- divers (work under water) whose air supply is provided via compressed air diving equipment
- persons who work at ambient air pressures more than 10 kPa (0.1 bar) above atmospheric pressure

A medical examination is necessary even for single brief jobs or occasional work under hyperbaric conditions.

The following jobs are not considered to involve work under hyperbaric conditions:
- work in rooms in which the air conditioning system produces air pressures which are slightly higher than atmospheric pressure – up to 10 kPa (0.1 bar) above atmospheric pressure
- work with respirators which, in line with DIN 3179, exert pressures up to 20 kPa (0.2 bar) above atmospheric pressure (such persons should be examined according to the Guideline G 26 "Respiratory protective equipment").

3.2   Functional disorders, symptoms

G 31

3.2.1   Mode of action

Persons who work in compressed air and divers are exposed to hyperbaric pressure. The risks involved increase with the pressure level and the duration of exposure. As the pressure increases, the levels of gases from the air which are dissolved in body fluids increase too. The process of dissolution of the gases becomes slower as the concentration of gases in solution increases. Depending on the duration of exposure, first the body fluids become saturated and later, after longer exposure, all the tissues. If the pressure is reduced slowly, the gases which are then released can be eliminated without sequelae via the circulatory system and the lungs. If the pressure is reduced too quickly, gas bubbles are formed in the body fluids and tissues. The consequent gas embolism is the most common cause of damage resulting from work under conditions of hyperbaric pressure. The sequelae can include pain, disorders or functional impairment of the locomotor, nervous or cardiocirculatory systems. Incorrect decompression can set gases free inside cells and cause transient or permanent tissue damage.

3.2.2   Acute and subacute effects on health

Acute disorders caused by increasing pressure (diving, pressure chambers)
A too rapid transition from normal pressure to hyperbaric pressure can cause earache, headaches, balance disorders and toothache.
Problems arise if the pressure equalization with air-filled cavities (e.g. nasal sinuses, tympanic cavity) is prevented. If the eustachian tube is blocked, the tympanic membrane can become perforated.

Acute disorders caused by decreasing pressure (coming up from a dive, pressure chambers)
The transition from hyperbaric to normal pressure can cause more or less severe decompression illness. This can develop during decompression but, in other cases, not until hours later. Most common are joint and muscle pains. Sometimes the persons complain of itching skin: marbling of the skin may develop, especially on the chest, abdomen and thighs. Central nervous symptoms may include dizziness, nystagmus, ringing in the ears, deafness, disorders of vision and speech, difficulties in breathing, paralysis, seizures. More rarely cardiocirculatory or respiratory symptoms may result from an infarction, lung embolism caused by a gas bubble, or pneumothorax. Symptoms like those described above can be caused by air embolism leading to fissures in lung tissue during too rapid decompression.

Therapy of decompression illness
An indispensable therapeutic measure is immediate and sufficient recompression. Delayed and inadequate recompression can put recovery at risk.

3.2.3   Chronic effects on health

Late sequelae are relatively rare. They can develop, however, and then mainly as alterations in the bones or joints, especially in the hip and shoulder regions. They are mainly symptom-free but can cause joint pain. Such symptoms can also develop months after an exposure to hyperbaric pressure.

4   References

Bennett PB, Elliott DH (2003) The Physiology and Medicine of Diving (5th ed). WB Saunders

Bennett, PB, Cronje FJ, Campbell ES (2006) Assessment of Diving Medical Fitness for Scuba Divers and Instructors. Best Publishing Company, U.S.

Bove AA, Davis JC (2003) Diving Medicine (4th ed). WB Saunders

Commission Recommendation 2003/670/EC concerning the European schedule of occupational diseases

Council Directive 89/391/EEC on the introduction of measures to encourage improvements in the safety and health of workers at work

DIN 3179-1 Classification of respiratory equipment – Survey

DIN 13256 Pressure vessels for human occupancy

Edmonds C, Lowry C, Pennefather J, Walker R (2002) Diving and Subaquatic Medicine (4th ed) Arnold, London

Kindwall, EP (2002) Hyperbaric Medicine Practice (2nd ed). Best Publishing Company, U.S.

G 31

G 32   Cadmium and cadmium compounds

Committee for occupational medicine, working group "Hazardous substances",
Berufsgenossenschaft der chemischen Industrie, Heidelberg

Preliminary remarks
The present guideline describes a scheme for occupational medical prophylaxis
which aims to prevent or ensure early diagnosis of disorders which can be caused
by cadmium or cadmium compounds.

Schedule

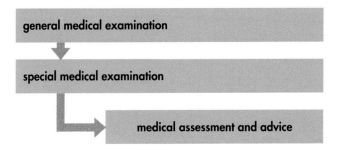

G 32

1   Medical examinations

Occupational medical examinations are to be carried out for persons exposed at work to levels of cadmium or cadmium compounds which could have adverse effects on health (e.g. when the occupational exposure limit value is exceeded) or for whom dermal absorption could endanger health.

1.1   Examinations, intervals between examinations

initial examination	before taking up the job
first follow-up examination	after 12–24 months
further follow-up examinations	after 12–24 months and when leaving the job
premature follow-up examination	• after a serious or prolonged illness which could cause concern as to whether the activity should be continued • in individual cases when the physician considers it necessary, e.g. when there is short-term concern about the person's health • when requested by an employee who suspects a causal association between his or her illness and work

1.2   Medical examination schedule

1.2.1   General medical examination

Initial examination

• Review of past history (general anamnesis, symptoms; particular attention to disorders of the sense of smell)

Particular attention is to be given to:
• disorders of the upper and lower respiratory tract, liver disorders
• kidney damage
• diabetes mellitus
• weight loss
• urinalysis (multiple test strips, sediment)

- interim anamnesis (including work anamnesis)

Particular attention is to be given to:
- disorders of the upper and lower respiratory tract, liver disorders
- functional renal disorders
- disorders of the sense of smell
- urinalysis (multiple test strips, sediment, specific weight)

1.2.2   Special medical examination

Initial examination

- nasal breathing test
- spirometry
- α_1-microglobulin in the urine
- diabetes diagnosis
- N-acetyl-β-D-glucosaminidase in the urine
- erythrocyte sedimentation reaction
- large or medium sized thorax x-ray (not smaller than 10x10 cm) or use of an x-ray diagnosis which is less than 1 year old

Also helpful:
- SGPT (ALT)
- γ-GT

Follow-up examination

- biomonitoring (see Section 3.1.4)
- α_1-microglobulin in the urine
- N-acetyl-β-D-glucosaminidase in the urine

The chest x-ray should be carried out for persons aged 40 years or more, for those who have been exposed for more than 10 years, and when indicated by clinical symptoms, and should be repeated at 12-month intervals.

Also helpful:

see initial examination

G 32

1.3   Requirements for the medical examinations

- competent doctor or occupational health professional
- laboratory analyses and x-ray examination carried out with appropriate quality control (Good Laboratory Practice)
- necessary equipment:
  - spirometer

2   Occupational medical assessment and advice

An assessment is only possible when the workplace situation and the exposure of the individual are known. For this purpose a risk assessment as defined in Article 4 Council directive 98/24/EC must have been carried out; it must describe the levels of exposure to cadmium or cadmium compounds and specify which technical, organizational and individual protective measures have been applied.

2.1   Assessment criteria

2.1.1   Long-term concern about health

Initial examination	Follow-up examination

Persons with severe disorders of
- the upper and lower respiratory tract
- the kidneys (tubulopathy with impaired renal function or diabetic nephropathy; significant impairment of retention)
- the liver

Also persons with
- alcohol addiction and also marked nicotine abuse (danger of inadequate hygiene!)

2.1.2   Short-term concern about health

Initial examination	Follow-up examination

Persons with the disorders mentioned in Section 2.1.1, provided recovery is to be expected.

2.1.3   No concern about health under certain conditions

Initial examination	Follow-up examination

If the illnesses or functional disorders mentioned in Section 2.1.1 are less severe, the doctor should establish whether or not it is possible for the person to start work or go on working under certain conditions. Such conditions could include
- technical protective measures
- organizational protective measures, e.g., limitation of exposure periods
- transfer to workplaces known to involve lower levels of exposure
- personal protective equipment which takes the individual's state of health into account
- more frequent follow-up examinations

2.1.4   No concern about health

Initial examination	Follow-up examination

All other persons, provided there are no restrictions on their employment.

2.2   Medical advice

The advice in an individual case should be commensurate with the workplace situation and the results of the medical examinations.
Employees are to be informed about the biomonitoring results.
The observance of general hygienic measures should be recommended.
The employees should be advised of the potential carcinogenic, germ cell mutagenic and prenatal toxic effects of cadmium and some cadmium compounds and of their toxic effects on reproduction. If during the course of his work in the company the occupational physician finds indications that the risk assessment should be brought up to date to improve health and safety standards, he is to inform the employer. When this is necessary, the interests of the employee are to be protected (medical confidentiality).

3   Supplementary notes

3.1   External and internal exposure

G 32

3.1.1   Occurrence, sources of hazards

Listed below are the kinds of processes, workplaces or activities, including cleaning and repair work, for which exposure to cadmium or cadmium compounds must be expected. This must be taken into account during the risk assessment.

- smelting of lead and zinc ores and production of cadmium or its alloys by thermal processes (roasting, melting, moulding, annealing, quenching, work on post-process dust filters)
- processing of cadmium or cadmium alloys (brazing, welding, annealing, vapour deposition)
- welding and cutting of objects with cadmium coatings
- production of nickel-cadmium accumulators, soluble cadmium compounds (e.g. cadmium sulfate, cadmium nitrate), cadmium pigments and stabilizers containing cadmium
- particular attention require the processing (including recycling) and burning of waste and scrap containing cadmium, removal of coatings containing cadmium (e.g. by burning off) and cutting of metal parts containing cadmium with the welding torch

- smelting of lead and zinc ores and the electrolytic production of cadmium
- demolition jobs on works for production of cadmium or cadmium compounds
- use of pigments containing cadmium to colour plastics and paints
- production and processing of enamel, ceramic colours and glazes containing cadmium
- use of soluble cadmium compounds in the photographic, glass, rubber and jewellery industries
- mechanical processing of materials containing cadmium

In the following activities, heating (brazing, welding, cutting) must be expected to result in the formation of cadmium oxide fumes:

- processing of cadmium-containing plastics, paints, enamel and ceramic colours in the form of pastes
- production and processing of photoelectric cells containing cadmium
- use of cadmium-containing elements and units in television, measuring, controlling and reactor technology and in the motorized vehicle and aircraft industries
- soldering jobs, especially brazing with hard solder containing high levels of cadmium (e.g. production and repair of jewellery)

Occurrence and hazards for specific substances are documented in the information system on hazardous substances (GESTIS) (see Section 4).

3.1.2   Physicochemical properties and classification

Cadmium (Cd) is a silvery white, soft, lustrous metal. Its melting point is 320.9°C, boiling point 767.3°C. In chemical compounds it mostly has a valency of two and also forms complexes with the coordination number four. Cadmium is stable in air; in warm air it forms a skin of the oxide, on heating it burns to form cadmium oxide (CdO). On heating in the presence of halogens, cadmium reacts to form the halides (e.g. cadmium chloride, $CdCl_2$).

Cadmium and cadmium compounds
(bioavailable, in the form of inhalable dusts/aerosols):
Formula (cadmium)   Cd
CAS number (cadmium)   7440-43-9

The information system on hazardous substances (GESTIS) provides details of international threshold limit values, classification, evaluation and other substance-specific information (see Section 4).

Additional information is to be found in the recommendations of the DFG Commission for the Investigation of Health Hazards of Chemical Compounds in the Work Area (List of MAK and BAT Values).

3.1.3   Uptake

The substances are taken up as dust or fumes via the airways and through the gastrointestinal tract.
Cadmium itself and some of its inorganic compounds can also be absorbed into the body through the skin.

3.1.4   Biomonitoring

Information about biomonitoring may be found in Appendix 1 "Biomonitoring".
Cadmium is one of the carcinogenic substances for which correlations ("exposure equivalents for carcinogenic materials", EKA) cannot be evaluated, or only evaluated incompletely, but which are documented in *Biological Exposure Values for Occupational Toxicants and Carcinogens*.
Biomonitoring should be carried out with reliable methods and meet quality control requirements (see Appendix 1 "Biomonitoring").

3.2   Functional disorders, symptoms

3.2.1   Mode of action

A large part of the cadmium absorbed into the body is distributed into the tissues via the liver, where cadmium binds to metallothionein. After long-term exposures, about 50 % to 75 % of the absorbed cadmium is found in the liver and kidney. Most of the cadmium taken up by the body is excreted with the faeces. Absorbed cadmium is excreted very slowly via urine and faeces. The cadmium ion binds, e.g., to sulfhydryl groups in proteins and other molecules. Metallothionein seems to play an important role in the detoxification of cadmium.

G 32

3.2.2   Acute and subacute effects on health

Irritation of the mucous membranes of the nose, throat, larynx and bronchi results from inhalation of cadmium vapour or fumes after a latency period of several hours (to three days):
- coughing, dyspnoea, discomfort on swallowing, chest pains, metal fume fever (fits of perspiration, chills, increased pulse rate), sometimes pulmonary oedema and
- kidney damage

After oral intake (rare at the workplace):
- nausea, vomiting, stomach pains, digestive disorders, diarrhoea, headaches, dizziness, collapse

3.2.3   Chronic effects on health

Chronic intoxication is manifested especially in inflation of the lungs (pulmonary emphysema) and tubular renal damage with proteinuria, in both cases dependent on the intensity of exposure and the individual sensitivity. In addition, anaemia, liver damage and mineralization disorders in the bones can develop. Epidemiological studies provide adequate evidence of a positive correlation between the exposure of humans and the occurrence of lung and kidney cancer.

After exposure for several years, the following symptoms can develop:

- conspicuous tiredness
- chronic rhinitis, atrophy of the nasal mucosa, impairment or loss of the sense of smell
- dyspnoea as a result of obstructive ventilation disorders
- kidney damage
- weight loss
- liver damage
- bronchial or renal carcinoma after high level exposures in certain production processes

4   References

Commission Recommendation 2003/670/EC concerning the European schedule of occupational diseases. Annex I

Council Directive 67/548/EEC on the approximation of the laws, regulations and administrative provisions relating to the classification, packaging and labelling of dangerous substances

Council Directive 98/24/EC on the protection of the health and safety of workers from the risks related to chemical agents at work

Deutsche Forschungsgemeinschaft (German Research Foundation, DFG) (ed) List of MAK and BAT Values 2007. Maximum Concentrations and Biological Tolerance Values at the workplace. Wiley-VCH, Weinheim

Deutsche Forschungsgemeinschaft (German Research Foundation, DFG) (ed) The MAK-Collection for Occupational Health and Safety. Wiley-VCH
at: www.mrw.interscience.wiley.com/makbat

GESTIS-database on hazardous substances. BGIA
at: www.dguv.de/bgia/gestis-database

GESTIS-international limit values for chemical agents. BGIA
at: www.dguv.de/bgia/gestis-limit-values

G 33   Aromatic nitro and amino compounds

Committee for occupational medicine, working group "Hazardous substances",
Berufsgenossenschaft der chemischen Industrie, Heidelberg

Preliminary remarks
The present guideline describes a scheme for occupational medical prophylaxis
which aims to prevent or ensure early diagnosis of disorders which can be caused
by aromatic nitro and amino compounds.

Schedule

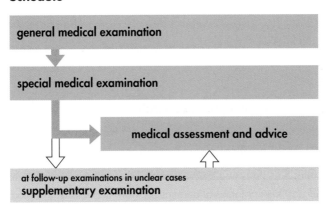

general medical examination

special medical examination

medical assessment and advice

at follow-up examinations in unclear cases
supplementary examination

G 33

1   Medical examinations

Occupational medical examinations are to be carried out for persons exposed at work to levels of aromatic nitro or amino compounds which could have adverse effects on health (e.g. when the occupational exposure limit value is exceeded) or for whom dermal absorption could endanger health.

1.1   Examinations, intervals between examinations

initial examination	before taking up the job
first follow-up examination	after 6–12 months
further follow-up examinations	after 6–12 months and when leaving the job
premature follow-up examination	• after a serious or prolonged illness which could cause concern as to whether the activity should be continued • in individual cases when the physician considers it necessary, e.g. when there is short-term concern about the person's health • when requested by an employee who suspects a causal association between his or her illness and work

1.2   Medical examination schedule

1.2.1   General medical examination

Initial examination

• review of past history (general anamnesis, work anamnesis, symptoms)
• urinalysis (multiple test strips, sediment)

Follow-up examination

• interim anamnesis (including work anamnesis)
• urinalysis (multiple test strips, sediment)

1.2.2   Special medical examination

Initial examination

- full blood count
- SGPT (ALT)
- γ-GT

Also helpful:
- SGOT (AST)
- glucose-6-phosphate dehydrogenase (G6DP) in order to recognize genetically determined enzyme defects which result in increased sensitivity to aromatic nitro and amino compounds
- determination of the acetylator status

The determination of G6DP and the acetylator status may only be carried out if the person gives permission freely; the significance of these tests should be explained. Persons with G6PD deficiency and slow acetylators should be advised not to work with aromatic nitro or amino compounds. If such persons still want to do such work, follow-up examinations should be carried out at shorter intervals.

Follow-up examination

- haemoglobin
- SGPT (ALT)
- γ-GT

Also helpful:
- SGOT (AST)
- differential blood count
- methaemoglobin as an indicator of (acute) exposure

1.2.3   Supplementary examination

G 33

Follow-up examination

- further bladder, kidney and liver diagnosis

In addition, required for persons exposed to carcinogenic aromatic amines:
- urinalysis (multiple test strips, sediment)

Depending on previous findings, every 6–12 months:
- cytological examination of urinary sediment using the Papanicolaou stain (see Section 4). Most suitable for the cytological examination of urinary sediment is so-called mid-stream urine collected early in the morning. An aliquot of at least 20 ml is centrifuged at 2000 rpm and the supernatant decanted to leave a 0.5 ml sample. Depending on the consistency of the sediment, 500 µl (little sediment) or 250 µl (thick sediment) is centrifuged in the Shandon Cytospin II. The sediment which is deposited on the microscope slide in this centrifuge is fixed with a fixation spray. The preparation is then stable for a maximum of 6 days. It is then sent to a pathologist or urologist with experience in assessment of cells; there it must be fixed and stained again. For persons with recurrent micro-

haematuria or for whom pathological cells are detected in the urinary sediment, a urological examination (cytoscopy, ultrasonography) must be carried out.
Optional:
• nuclear matrix protein 22 (NMP22), ELISA test
  This FDA-approved tumour marker has been used for some years now in urological practice both for initial diagnosis and during follow-up care of patients treated for urothelial carcinoma. Prospective studies of symptom-free collectives are not available to date. Use of the NMP22 test in follow-up care has revealed that, if the factors excluding false positives are taken into account, it is as specific as cytology but considerably more sensitive, especially for the common well-differentiated tumours and for early stages. A cut-off value of 10 U/ml has proved useful in interpreting the results; that is, values above 10 require further clarification. False positive results can be obtained when the exclusion criteria (urinary tract infections, urolithiasis, proteinuria, e.g. after heavy physical work) are not taken into account or when the sample is not properly processed (e.g. fixation is not carried out at the proper time). If the urine sample is too dilute, i.e. contains too few cells, both cytology and the NMP22 test can yield false negative results.
A final decision as to whether and when the NMP22 test can replace the cytological examination can be made only when results are available from the occupational medical studies currently being carried out on appropriate risk groups.
Also helpful:
• test for exposure to aromatic amines by their detection in the urine or in their haemoglobin conjugates (see Section 3.1.4)

1.3 Requirements for the medical examinations
• competent doctor or occupational health professional
• laboratory analyses carried out with appropriate quality control (Good Laboratory Practice)

2   Occupational medical assessment and advice

An assessment is only possible when the workplace situation and the exposure of the individual are known. For this purpose a risk assessment as defined in Article 4 Council directive 98/24/EC must have been carried out; it must describe the levels of exposure to aromatic nitro or amino compounds and specify which technical, organizational and individual protective measures have been applied.

2.1   Assessment criteria

2.1.1   Long-term concern about health

Initial examination	**Follow-up examination**

Persons with severe disorders:
- disorders of the blood (e.g. sickle-cell anaemia) and haematopoietic organs
- liver damage
- kidney damage
- chronic disorders of the bladder and the lower urinary tract, especially tumours
- substance-related allergies
- chronic skin disorders with impaired barrier function of the skin
- disorders of the peripheral and central nervous systems
- mental disorders
- addiction to alcohol, drugs or medication

2.1.2   Short-term concern about health

Initial examination

Persons with the disorders mentioned in Section 2.1.1, provided recovery is to be expected.

Follow-up examination

Persons with the disorders mentioned in Section 2.1.1, provided recovery is to be expected. Persons with recurrent microhaematuria until the source of the bleeding has been finally clarified urologically and persons with acute or chronic cystitis until recovery.
After an acute intoxication until the clinical findings and laboratory values have returned to normal.

G 33

2.1.3   No concern about health under certain conditions

Initial examination	Follow-up examination

If the illnesses or functional disorders mentioned in Section 2.1.1 are less severe, the doctor should establish whether or not it is possible for the person to start work or go on working under certain conditions. Such conditions could include

- technical protective measures
- organizational protective measures, e.g., limitation of exposure periods
- transfer to workplaces known to involve lower levels of exposure
- personal protective equipment which takes the individual's state of health into account
- more frequent follow-up examinations

Persons without clinical symptoms whose laboratory values are marginal or lie slightly above or below the normal range. Persons with G6PD deficiency and slow acetylators (see Section 1.2.2).

2.1.4   No concern about health

Initial examination	Follow-up examination

All other persons, provided there are no restrictions on their employment.

2.2   Medical advice

The advice in an individual case should be commensurate with the workplace situation and the results of the medical examinations.

Employees are to be informed about the biomonitoring results.

The observance of general hygienic measures should be recommended.

The employees should be advised of the potentially carcinogenic effects of aromatic nitro and amino compounds.

It should be pointed out that alcohol can increase the toxicity of aromatic nitro and amino compounds enormously.

If during the course of his work in the company the occupational physician finds indications that the risk assessment should be brought up to date to improve health and safety standards, he is to inform the employer. When this is necessary, the interests of the employee are to be protected (medical confidentiality).

3   Supplementary notes

Because of the large number of different aromatic nitro and amino compounds, it must be pointed out that the statements made below apply only for certain members of these groups of substances. Mode of action and clinical symptoms differ from substance to substance or the effects differ in severity.

3.1   External and internal exposure

3.1.1   Occurrence, sources of hazards

Listed below are the kinds of processes, workplaces or activities, including cleaning and repair work, for which exposure to aromatic nitro or amino compounds must be expected. This must be taken into account during the risk assessment.
*   production and processing of colorants, explosives, pesticides and herbicides made from aromatic nitro compounds, and use of the final products when these still contain the free aromatic nitro compound
*   production and processing of synthetic colourants (dyes for leather, paper, fur, hair), insecticides, medicines, and developers in the photographic industry made from aromatic amines, and use of the final products when these still contain the free aromatic amine
*   production and use of aromatic amine reaction accelerators and oxidation inhibitors, e.g. in the rubber industry
*   demolition jobs on production plants for aromatic nitro or amino compounds when previous cleaning and contamination control has not been carried out
Occurrence and hazards for specific substances are documented in the information system on hazardous substances (GESTIS) (see Section 4).

G 33

3.1.2   Physicochemical properties and classification

Because of the large number of different aromatic nitro and amino compounds, it is not possible to give the usual list of the individual substances and their properties here. The reader is referred to the relevant occupational medical and chemical literature.

The information system on hazardous substances (GESTIS) provides details of international threshold limit values, classification, evaluation and other substance-specific information (see Section 4).

Additional information is to be found in the recommendations of the DFG Commission for the Investigation of Health Hazards of Chemical Compounds in the Work Area (List of MAK and BAT Values).

3.1.3   Uptake

The substances are taken up through the airways and the skin. (Contamination of the skin and clothes is a frequent cause of poisoning.)

3.1.4   Biomonitoring

Information about biomonitoring may be found in Appendix 1 "Biomonitoring".
For most of these substances, especially for the carcinogenic aromatic amines, there are no threshold limit values. Nonetheless, the determination of the concentrations in biological material, which is recommended in Section 1.2.3, is very important. The results indicate success or failure of preventive measures.
Biomonitoring should be carried out with reliable methods and meet quality control requirements (see Appendix 1 "Biomonitoring").

3.2   Functional disorders, symptoms

3.2.1   Mode of action

The severity of an intoxication and its effects depend on certain properties of the substance involved and on individual factors. Persons with inherited enzyme defects (e.g. G6DP deficiency) and haemoglobin anomalies are expected to be more than usually sensitive. When the substances are taken up by inhalation, the physical state of the substance (dust particle size, vapour pressure, concentration) is of significance.
Uptake through the skin is determined by the lipoid solubility of the substance. Increased temperature and moistness of the skin increase the absorption rate.
Some of the substances are eliminated, at least in part, via the lungs as the unchanged substance but mostly elimination is via the kidneys, partly as the unchanged substance and partly as the products of oxidative and reductive metabolism, mainly as sulfuric or glucuronic acid conjugates. The aromatic nitro and amino compounds can have the same pathological effects on certain organ systems but they can also differ markedly in their modes of action.
The substances differ in their potency of methaemoglobin formation. In intermediary metabolism, aromatic nitro and amino compounds are converted to the corresponding nitroso compounds and hydroxylamines which are the actual erythrocyte poisons (causing formation of methaemoglobin, verdoglobin and Heinz bodies). These compounds interfere with the enzymatic system of the erythrocytes and cause (reversible) formation of methaemoglobin by oxidation of the bivalent iron of haemoglobin to trivalent iron; that is, in coupled reactions the hydroxylamines are oxidized by oxygen to the corresponding nitroso compounds and haemoglobin is oxidized to methaemoglobin. Because the nitroso compound is reduced back to the hydroxylamine by the enzyme methaemoglobin reductase, the methaemoglobin formation can progress without the person being further exposed to the initial toxin. Methaemoglobin binds oxygen very firmly and causes oxygen deficiency in the organism.

Methaemoglobin formation is reversible. In persons exposed to large amounts of aromatic nitro or amino compounds or exposed for long periods, the haem group of the haemoglobin can be damaged by oxidative cleavage of the porphyrin ring; the result is verdoglobin formation. At the same time, denaturation causes globin damage which can be demonstrated by staining for the so-called Heinz bodies. These changes are not reversible and lead to final breakdown of the haemoglobin and the erythrocytes. Thus, as a result of poisoning with aromatic nitro or amino compounds, Heinz body formation and hypochromic anaemia can develop as well as methaemoglobin and verdoglobin. Extensive erythrocyte breakdown can cause kidney damage. Occasionally changes in the total white count and bone marrow damage have been described.

If the intoxication is very severe, aromatic nitro or amino compounds can cause depression of the central nervous system with inebriation-like symptoms (anilinism), excitation, narcosis or even toxic coma. After exposure to dinitro-o-cresol, hyperthermia is observed. As sequelae of acute and chronic exposure, rare cases of neurological and mental disorders have been described.

Uptake of even small amounts of alcohol increases the toxic effects of aromatic nitro and amino compounds and their metabolites manyfold.

Exposure to aromatic nitro or amino compounds can cause discoloration of the skin and skin appendages. Direct skin contact can cause irritation because of damage to the barrier function of the skin. With certain compounds toxic dermatosis and even blistering are observed. Certain aromatic amino compounds (e.g. *p*-phenylenediamine) can sensitize some individuals and so cause allergic contact dermatitis which recurs when the person is exposed again. Some compounds (e.g. *p*-phenylenediamine) irritate the eyes and airways. Allergic bronchial asthma can be induced in persons with the appropriate disposition.

Poisoning with aromatic nitro or amino compounds is not generally associated with severe liver damage. However, certain compounds (e.g. 4,4'-diaminodiphenylmethane, trinitrobenzene and trinitrotoluene) can cause liver disorders and even toxic hepatitis.

Some aromatic amino compounds can cause acute haemorrhagic cystitis from which the persons generally recover without sequelae. Tumours are not observed in these cases.

Certain diphenylamines and their homologues and 2-naphthylamine form a special group of substances. Some of these are carcinogenic in man and in animals (e.g. 4-aminodiphenyl, benzidine and its salts, 4-chloro-o-toluidine, 2-naphthylamine), others have shown carcinogenic activity to date only in animal studies. In man the tumours develop in the lower urinary tract, especially in the bladder, as broad-based sessile or stalked papillomas. These can become cancerous. Primary transitional cell carcinomas are also observed. These tumours are not different from tumours of other genesis. They can appear long (even decades) after the end of exposure.

G 33

3.2.2   Acute and subacute effects on health

- methaemoglobinaemia with pale grey to blue-grey cyanosis of first the lips, cheeks, ears and nails, later the mucosa
- cardiocirculatory disorders with anxiety, palpitations, fits of perspiration and dyspnoea
- with some compounds irritation of the mucous membranes of the eyes and airways develop
- central nervous disorders such as headaches, weakness, dizziness, nausea, vomiting, torpidity, restlessness
- in severe cases spasms, unconsciousness, coma and death from respiratory paralysis
- a euphoric, inebriated state (anilinism) can be associated with the person's unwillingness to accept that he or she is ill
- haemorrhagic cystitis
- kidney damage and even anuria
- transient blood count changes (including occurrence of Heinz bodies)
- rarely liver damage

3.2.3   Chronic effects on health

- development of Heinz bodies, anaemia
- cystitis
- papillomas and carcinomas of the lower urinary tract, especially the bladder
- damage to the liver parenchyma
- toxic dermatosis and allergic contact dermatitis
- irritation of the eyes and airways

4   References

Commission Recommendation 2003/670/EC concerning the European schedule of
    occupational diseases. Annex I
Council Directive 67/548/EEC on the approximation of the laws, regulations and
    administrative provisions relating to the classification, packaging and labelling of
    dangerous substances
Council Directive 98/24/EC on the protection of the health and safety of workers
    from the risks related to chemical agents at work
Deutsche Forschungsgemeinschaft (German Research Foundation, DFG) (ed) List of
    MAK and BAT Values 2007. Maximum Concentrations and Biological Tolerance
    Values at the workplace. Wiley-VCH, Weinheim
Deutsche Forschungsgemeinschaft (German Research Foundation, DFG) (ed) The
    MAK-Collection for Occupational Health and Safety. Wiley-VCH
    at: www.mrw.interscience.wiley.com/makbat
GESTIS-database on hazardous substances. BGIA
    at: www.dguv.de/bgia/gestis-database
GESTIS-international limit values for chemical agents. BGIA
    at: www.dguv.de/bgia/gestis-limit-values
Papanicolaou GN (1954) Atlas of Exfoliative Cytology. Commonwealth Fund by
    Harvard University Press. Cambridge, Mass.

G 33

G 34   Fluorine and its inorganic compounds

Committee for occupational medicine, working group "Hazardous substances", Berufsgenossenschaft der chemischen Industrie, Heidelberg

Preliminary remarks

The present guideline describes a scheme for occupational medical prophylaxis which aims to prevent or ensure early diagnosis of disorders which can be caused by fluorine or its compounds.

Schedule

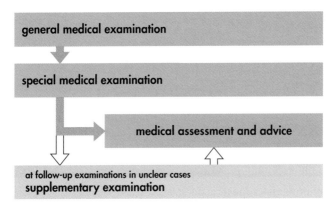

G 34

1 Medical examinations

Occupational medical examinations are to be carried out for persons exposed at work to levels of fluorine or fluorine compounds which could have adverse effects on health (e.g. when the occupational exposure limit value is exceeded) or for whom dermal absorption could endanger health.

1.1 Examinations, intervals between examinations

initial examination	before taking up the job
first follow-up examination	within 12–24 months
further follow-up examinations	within 12–24 months and when leaving the job
premature follow-up examination	• after a serious or prolonged illness which could cause concern as to whether the activity should be continued • in individual cases when the physician considers it necessary, e.g. when there is short-term concern about the person's health • when requested by an employee who suspects a causal association between his or her illness and work

1.2 Medical examination schedule

1.2.1 General medical examination

Initial examination

• review of past history (general anamnesis, work anamnesis, symptoms)
• urinalysis (multiple test strips)

Follow-up examination

• interim anamnesis (including work anamnesis)
  Particular attention is to be given to:
  • complaints of coughing, increased expectoration, harsher breathing noises, shortness of breath when active
  • constipation
  • rheumatic complaints
  • leaden limbs, pain and stiffness in the neck, back pain especially after a shaking
• urinalysis (multiple test strips)

1.2.2   Special medical examination

Initial examination

- large or medium sized thorax x-ray (not smaller than 10x10 cm) or use of an x-ray diagnosis which is less than 1 year old
- spirometry

Also helpful:
- determination of fluoride in urine (initial value)

Follow-up examination

- spirometry
- every 6 months: determination of fluoride in urine (see Section 3.1.4)

1.2.3   Supplementary examination

Follow-up examination

In unclear cases:
- thorax radiograph[1]
- radiograph of the skeletal system with a view to diagnosis of fluorine-induced osteosclerotic changes, formation of bone spurs and trabeculae especially on the pelvis, forearms and lower legs[2]
- if necessary, iliac crest puncture and histological and microanalytical examination of the bone material

1.3   Requirements for the medical examinations

- competent doctor or occupational health professional
- laboratory analyses and x-ray examination carried out with appropriate quality control (Good Laboratory Practice)

G 34

---

[1] Thorax radiographs should be taken when indicated by the clinical picture, and especially after exposure to fluorine, hydrogen fluoride, hydrofluoric acid, or acid fluorides (see Table in Section 3.1.2).

[2] Radiographs of the skeletal system:
AP: the whole pelvis and lumbar spine, dorsolumbar region from the side
AP: both forearms
Differential x-ray diagnosis of other disorders with signs of sclerosis on the bones (e.g. osteoplastic metastasis, osteopetrosis (Albers-Schönberg disease)).

2   Occupational medical assessment and advice

An assessment is only possible when the workplace situation and the exposure of the individual are known. For this purpose a risk assessment as defined in Article 4 Council directive 98/24/EC must have been carried out; it must describe the levels of exposure and specify which technical, organizational and individual protective measures have been applied.

2.1   Assessment criteria

2.1.1   Long-term concern about health

Initial examination	Follow-up examination

Persons with severe disorders such as
- lung disease with significant obstructive and/or restrictive impairment of function
- asthma
- haemodynamic cardiocirculatory disorders
- eczema
- changes in the skeletal system as a result of bone tuberculosis
- chronic rheumatoid arthritis
- Bekhterev syndrome
- stiffness of the spine and the major joints

2.1.2   Short-term concern about health

Initial examination	Follow-up examination

Persons with the disorders mentioned in Section 2.1.1, provided recovery is to be expected.
- for a period of 1 to 2 months during convalescence from a disorder of the lungs or pleura which has regressed without sequelae

2.1.3   No concern about health under certain conditions

Initial examination	Follow-up examination

If the illnesses or functional disorders mentioned in Section 2.1.1 are less severe, the doctor should establish whether or not it is possible for the person to start work or go on working under certain conditions. Such conditions could include
- technical protective measures
- organizational protective measures, e.g., limitation of exposure periods
- transfer to workplaces known to involve lower levels of exposure
- personal protective equipment which takes the individual's state of health into account
- more frequent follow-up examinations

2.1.4   No concern about health

Initial examination	Follow-up examination

All other persons, provided there are no restrictions on their employment.

2.2   Medical advice

The advice in an individual case should be commensurate with the workplace situation and the results of the medical examinations.

Employees are to be informed about the biomonitoring results.

Employees should be informed about general hygienic measures and personal protective equipment.

If during the course of his work in the company the occupational physician finds indications that the risk assessment should be brought up to date to improve health and safety standards, he is to inform the employer. When this is necessary, the interests of the employee are to be protected (medical confidentiality).

G 34

3   Supplementary notes

3.1   External and internal exposure

3.1.1   Occurrence, sources of hazards

Listed below are the kinds of processes, workplaces or activities, including cleaning and repair work, for which exposure to fluorine or its compounds must be expected. This must be taken into account during the risk assessment.

- production, transfer and filling of containers with hydrogen fluoride, hydrofluoric acid, other inorganic acids containing fluorine (e.g. hexafluorosilicic acid, tetrafluoroboric acid), hydrogen fluorides (e.g. ammonium hydrogenfluoride) and other soluble fluorides (e.g. sodium fluoride)
- acid polishing processes in the ceramics and glass industry in which hydrofluoric acid is used and silicon tetrafluoride can be formed
- production of opaque glass
- fused salt electrolysis of substances and formulations containing fluorine
- production and use of wood preservatives containing aqueous solutions of salts of inorganic acids containing fluorine
- surface treatment of metals (e.g. removal of discoloration on stainless steel after welding)
- manual arc welding with alkaline coated electrodes and with special electrodes containing more than 6 % fluorides without appropriate exhaust devices
- inert gas welding and welding without inert gas using filler wire containing more than 6 % fluorides, without appropriate exhaust devices
- working with ceramic cleaners containing hydrofluoric acid
- work with vehicle wheel rim cleaners

Occurrence and hazards for specific substances are documented in the information system on hazardous substances (GESTIS) (see Section 4).

3.1.2   Physicochemical properties and classification

Fluorine is a highly reactive pale yellow gas. Because of its high electron affinity, fluorine reacts with almost all other elements; it forms the electronegative monovalent component of the resulting compound.

Fluorine
Formula   F
CAS number   7782-41-4

Hydrogen fluoride is a colourless gas which, on cooling, becomes a colourless liquid; this is miscible in all proportions with water; the aqueous solutions are called hydrofluoric acid. Fluorides are the salts of hydrofluoric acid (see table).

Hydrogen fluoride
Formula   HF
CAS number   7664-39-3

The information system on hazardous substances (GESTIS) provides details of international threshold limit values, classification, evaluation and other substance-specific information (see Section 4).

Table of substances

Substance	Formula	Acidic reaction of the aqueous solution	Danger of skin damage
hydrogen fluoride (hydrofluoric acid)	HF	+	+
sodium fluoride	NaF	–	(+)
sodium hydrogenfluoride	$NaHF_2$	+	+
potassium fluoride	KF	–	(+)
potassium hydrogenfluoride	KHF_2	+	+
ammonium fluoride	NH_4F	–	(+)
ammonium hydrogenfluoride	NH_4HF_2	+	+
calcium fluoride	CaF_2	–	–
magnesium fluoride	MgF_2	–	–
boron trifluoride	BF_3	(+)	+
tetrafluoroboric acid	HBF_4	+	(–)
sodium tetrafluoroborate	$NaBF_4$	–	–
potassium tetrafluoroborate	KBF_4	–	–
aluminium fluoride	AlF_3	–	(–)
sodium aluminium fluoride (cryolite)	Na_3AlF_6	–	–
silicon tetrafluoride	SiF_4	(+)	+
hexafluorosilicic acid (silico-fluoric acid, fluosilicic acid)	H_2SiF_6	+	(+)
sodium hexafluorosilicate	Na_2SiF_6	–	–
potassium hexafluorosilicate	K_2SiF_6	–	–
magnesium hexafluorosilicate	$MgSiF_6$	–	–
potassium hexafluorotitanate	K_2TiF_6	–	(+)

G 34

3.1.3   Uptake

mainly via the airways;
on direct contact, very ready absorption through the skin, especially of hydrofluoric
acid!

3.1.4   Biomonitoring

Information about biomonitoring may be found in Appendix 1 "Biomonitoring".

Biological tolerance value for occupational exposures

Substance	Parameter	BAT[1]	Assay material	Sampling time
hydrogen fluoride and inorganic fluorine compounds (fluorides)	fluoride	7.0 mg/g creatinine	urine	end of exposure or end of shift
		4.0 mg/g creatinine	urine	at the beginning of the next shift

Biomonitoring should be carried out with reliable methods and meet quality control
requirements (see Appendix 1 "Biomonitoring").

3.2   Functional disorders, symptoms

3.2.1   Mode of action

Hydrogen fluoride, hydrofluoric acid and fluorides (especially hydrogenfluorides)
have local corrosive effects on the mucosa of the eyes and airways and on the skin
(see the table of substances above); low-level exposures cause lacrimation, nasal discharge and irritation of the bronchial mucosa with coughing. Hydrofluoric acid penetrates the skin, destroys deeper tissue layers and, after absorption, can bind chemically to calcium and magnesium ions and so inhibit essential enzymes and cause
acutely dangerous metabolic disorders, e.g., disturbance of the calcium and carbo-
hydrate balance. Inhalation of large amounts in high concentrations can result in immediate death.
Local exposure especially to low concentrations causes local reddening of the skin
and burning pain. It is, however, not unusual for the pain not to begin until hours after the exposure and initially for no skin changes to be evident. Higher concentrations cause typical corrosive burns with severe tissue damage and can also be followed by toxic effects of the absorbed substance.

---

[1] Biologischer Arbeitsstoff-Toleranzwert (BAT) = biological tolerance value for occupational
exposures

Prolonged (years of) uptake of high levels of fluorine can cause mineralization disorders which result in severe bone damage, mostly of the osteosclerotic kind (bone fluorosis).

3.2.2   Acute and subacute effects on health

Local exposure to high concentrations of fluorine compounds as gas, fumes or dust causes local irritation, lacrimation, sneezing, coughing and dyspnoea. Inhalation of large doses can cause pulmonary oedema, in rare cases also immediate death.
On contact with the skin, hydrofluoric acid penetrates the epidermis rapidly, damages the subepidermal tissue and causes necrosis. The absorbed substance can cause systemic toxicity.
Oral intake of fluorine compounds causes – depending on the dose and concentration – irritation and corrosion of the oral cavity, oesophagus and stomach and can cause spasms and acute heart, liver and kidney damage.

3.2.3   Chronic effects on health

Long-term exposure to high concentrations of fluorine or fluorides causes rheumatic disorders considered to be the result of osteosclerosis, mainly of spongy bone such as the pelvis, spinal column and ribs.
x-ray examination can differentiate:
- stadium I: increased sclerosis of the bones; coarse, indistinct trabeculae on the vertebrae, ribs and pelvis
- stadium II: increasingly homogeneous bone density in radiographs, osteophyte development on the spinal column, narrowing of the medullary cavity of long tubular bones
- stadium III: eburnation of the spinal column (bamboo-like appearance); extensive calcification of tendons, joint capsules, membranes; multiple periosteum reactions, exostosis, ankylosis of the sacroiliac articulation

The skull, intervertebral joints, hands and feet remain free of pathological changes for a long period.
Dental fluorosis is only possible if fluorides are taken up while the ameloblasts are still active. Once these cells have stopped functioning (after age 14 years), fluoride intake is no longer associated with a serious risk for the teeth.

G 34

4   References

Commission Recommendation 2003/670/EC concerning the European schedule of occupational diseases. Annex I

Council Directive 67/548/EEC on the approximation of the laws, regulations and administrative provisions relating to the classification, packaging and labelling of dangerous substances

Council Directive 98/24/EC on the protection of the health and safety of workers from the risks related to chemical agents at work

Deutsche Forschungsgemeinschaft (German Research Foundation, DFG) (ed) List of MAK and BAT Values 2007. Maximum Concentrations and Biological Tolerance Values at the workplace. Wiley-VCH, Weinheim

Deutsche Forschungsgemeinschaft (German Research Foundation, DFG) (ed) The MAK-Collection for Occupational Health and Safety. Wiley-VCH
    at: www.mrw.interscience.wiley.com/makbat

GESTIS-database on hazardous substances. BGIA
    at: www.dguv.de/bgia/gestis-database

GESTIS-international limit values for chemical agents. BGIA
    at: www.dguv.de/bgia/gestis-limit-values

G 35   Work abroad under exceptional climatic conditions and with other health risks

Committee for occupational medicine, working group "Work abroad", Berufsgenossenschaft der chemischen Industrie, BV Köln

Preliminary remarks

The present guideline describes a scheme for occupational medical prophylaxis of persons working abroad under exceptional climatic conditions and exposed to other health risks. Consultation with a medical specialist before beginning the work abroad is intended to provide the employee with information about any exceptional climatic conditions and health risks and about the medical care available in the foreign country. Medical examinations should help to establish whether there is any medical cause for concern about the person's working in these regions or under which conditions this concern may be put aside. The follow-up examination, especially that carried out on the person's return, is intended to ensure early diagnosis of diseases which can develop in these regions.

Schedule

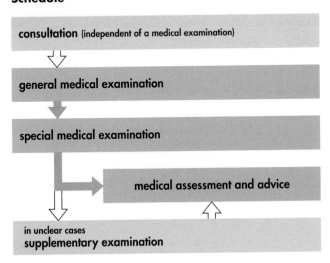

G 35

1 Medical consultation and examination before beginning work abroad

1.1 Medical consultation/examinations, intervals between examinations

consultation	Consultation with a medical specialist before beginning work abroad is intended to provide the employee with information about any exceptional climatic conditions and health risks and about the medical care available in the foreign country. The consultation is to be documented.
	Independent of the duration of the work abroad, if the conditions to be expected at the new workplace or in the new job are exceptional (e.g. if the medical care available is particularly poor, if the workplace changes continually, if the risk of infection is very high, or if the work involves unusual stress) the consultation is to be followed by a medical examination.
initial examination	For all persons intending to work abroad for a total of more than 3 months per year, a medical examination must be carried out before the first trip abroad.
	Before the person goes abroad to work again, an initial examination is not necessary provided that the follow-up examination on return from the previous trip was carried out during the previous 1 year. Nonetheless, medical consultation is necessary in this case too.
first and further follow-up examinations	after 24–36 months
premature follow-up examination	• follow-up examination within 8 weeks of the return from a job abroad which lasted longer than 1 year
	• after an illness lasting several weeks or a physical impairment which could give rise to concern about health
	• in individual cases when the physician considers it necessary, e.g. when there is short-term concern about the person's health
	• when the person is moving to a country with very different climatic conditions or health risks
	• when requested by an employee who suspects a causal association between his or her illness and work

1.2   Medical examination schedule

1.2.1   General medical examination

Initial examination

- review of past history (general anamnesis, work anamnesis taking special account of earlier periods working abroad)
- detailed physical examination taking into account the region where the person is to work and job to be done

Particular attention is to be given to:
- regions where the person is to work
- accommodation and working conditions
- medical care abroad

Follow-up examination

- interim anamnesis (including work anamnesis)
- otherwise as for the initial examination

1.2.2   Special medical examination

Initial examination

- urinalysis (multiple test strips, sediment)
- erythrocyte sedimentation rate
- blood count
- γ-GT, GPT
- total cholesterol
- blood sugar
- creatinine
- resting ECG

Follow-up examination

(also when the person returns from working abroad)
- interim anamnesis (including work anamnesis)
- medical examination: see initial examination

In addition:
- stool examination (parasitology, perhaps bacteriology)
- the employee should be advised as to the possibility of late-developing symptoms (latency)

G 35

1.2.3   Supplementary examination

Initial examination

Further tests may be indicated, e.g.
- test for anti-HIV antibodies (the employee should be advised that the test is sensible but requires his or her consent; the explanation should be documented)
- for women: gynaecological examination
- tests for anti-HBc, anti-HAV, anti-HCV antibodies
- for persons more than 45 years old: Hemoccult test, ergometry

If the tests carried out so far make it seem necessary, further tests including a dental examination may be carried out or arranged.

Follow-up examination

- medical examination: see initial examination
- in unclear cases, especially if it is suspected that the person has a tropical disease or another disorder with
- unexplained raised temperature
- persistent diarrhoea
- marked weight loss
- generalized swelling of the lymph nodes
- raised eosinophil counts
- urticarial, puriform, ulcerative skin changes
  or
- if it is not possible to answer the question as to whether a continuation of work abroad is medically advisable, further tests by an institution or specialist for tropical diseases should be arranged

1.3   Requirements for the medical examinations

The consultations and examinations may be carried out by a competent doctor or occupational health professional who
- has sufficient experience in examining persons working abroad and
- can demonstrate knowledge of tropical workplaces. It is sufficient proof if the physician can show that he has worked in the tropics as a doctor for a period of at least 14 days.

Physicians who have specialized in tropical medicine are qualified to carry out G 35 consultations and examinations.

2   Occupational medical assessment and advice

An assessment is only possible when the workplace situation and the exposure of the individual in the foreign country are known. For this purpose a risk assessment as defined in Article 9 Council directive 89/391/EEC must have been carried out; it must specify which general and personal protective measures have been applied.

Whether or not adequate medical care is available in the foreign workplace should be taken into account.

2.1   Assessment criteria

2.1.1   Long-term concern about health

Initial examination	Follow-up examination

Persons who require constant medical attention and whose illness must be expected to get worse under the conditions of working abroad

The assessment must take into account especially the severity of the disorder, functional deficits and the possibilities for treatment in the foreign country.

2.1.2   Short-term concern about health

Initial examination	Follow-up examination

Persons with temporary health problems provided that
* recovery is expected
* a necessary supplementary examination has not yet been carried out

2.1.3   No concern about health under certain conditions

Initial examination	Follow-up examination

Persons with disorders which can be given appropriate medical care or medicinal treatment in the foreign country and for whom the risk of deterioration under the conditions abroad is small

G 35

2.1.4   No concern about health

Initial examination	Follow-up examination

All other persons.

2.2   Medical advice

The consultation which follows the examination should take into account the workplace situation and the results of the medical examinations. At the follow-up examination carried out when the employee returns from abroad, the possibility of late-developing symptoms arising during a period of one year after the end of the period abroad should be pointed out.

3   Supplementary notes

3.1   Exceptional geographic and climatic conditions

Exceptional conditions for health and hygiene are not restricted to the tropics or subtropics. Also for individuals working in areas outside this zone, depending on the working conditions and the results of a health risk assessment, a medical consultation should take place and perhaps even medical examinations as given in this guideline. The "warm countries" lie between the latitudes 30° north and 30° south. Heat, humidity and sunshine produce a climate to which the individual must become acclimatized. This applies particularly for the tropics (between the latitudes 23°27' north and south). Living at high altitudes there requires additional adaptation processes. The physically and mentally healthy person can generally cope with the climatic stress and can adjust (acclimatization). Persons who are not completely healthy can also travel to warm countries and work there provided that they have been given appropriate medical advice and have access to medical care in the foreign country. Acute illnesses and certain chronic complaints involve health risks during short visits or longer periods in foreign countries.

3.2   Exceptional hygienic conditions

Particularly in warm countries, the climate favours the occurrence and reproduction of insects which can communicate diseases and serve as interim hosts for parasitic infections. Many animals – including pets – serve as pathogen reservoirs. Poor sanitary standards favour worm infections. Water from the public water supply can generally not be considered to be hygienically fit to drink.

3.3   Diseases in warm countries

Many of the diseases which are nowadays called tropical diseases occur most frequently in these countries but are not necessarily restricted to the region. Only very few tropical diseases occur only in the tropics (African and South American trypanosomiasis, filariasis, yaws and yellow fever). Most of the diseases which affect people in the warm countries of the world today used to be prevalent in temperate climates as well. Cholera, plague and smallpox, for example, are under control or have been eradicated. Other infectious diseases (malaria, tuberculosis, schistosomiasis, whipworm, hookworm and ascaris infections, leprosy, amoebiasis and other intestinal infections, virus hepatitis and generalized mycoses) are very widely distributed.

Some tropical diseases which can be acquired even during a brief stay can result in death or severe health defects if they are not recognized and treated (e.g. malaria, amoebiasis, schistosomiasis). Other infections require long-term exposure (e.g. filariasis). It is possible to protect oneself against most tropical diseases – also long term: vaccination, prophylactic medication, hygiene and a healthy life style, all based on information which everyone should and can have before going abroad to work.

Recently some tropical diseases have developed new momentum. Malaria, for example, is becoming increasingly common all over the world. The disease is spreading into regions which were still free of malaria not long ago. In addition, the mosquitoes which transmit the disease have developed insecticide resistance, and this makes economical control more difficult. In many parts of the world the dangerous malaria tropica pathogen has become resistant to a number of medications. The construction of irrigation and drainage systems has led to the dissemination of schistosomiasis. In a number of tropical countries HIV-infection is very widely distributed. Thus in such places there is an increased risk of infection, e.g. via injections or blood transfusions. Therefore special measures, especially with respect to personal hygiene and behaviour, are required.

Health defects or diseases can be diagnosed and, in most cases, successfully treated. From a medical point of view, a consultation and/or examination as given in the guideline G 35 is also necessary for partners and children who travel abroad with the employee.

4   References

Ashford RW et al (2001) Encyclopedia of Arthropod-transmitted Infections of Man and Domesticated Animals. CABI Publishing, Wallingford

Chiodini PL (2002) Atlas of Travel Medicine and Health. BC Decker, Hamilton

Chiodini PL et al (2001) Atlas of Medical Helminthology and Protozoology. Churchill, Livingstone

Cohen J, Powderly WG (2004) Infectious Diseases. Mosby, London

Commission Recommendation 2003/670/EC concerning the European schedule of occupational diseases

Cook GC, Zumla A (eds) (2002) Manson's Tropical Diseases. WB Saunders, London

Dawoo R (2002) Travellers' Health. How to stay healthy abroad. Oxford University Press

Directive 89/391/EEC on the introduction of measures to encourage improvements in the safety and health of workers at work

Eddleston M, Pierini S (1999) Oxford Handbook of Tropical Medicine. Oxford University Press

Ericsson CD et al (2003) Travelers' Diarrhea. BC Decker, Hamilton

G 35

European Centre for Disease Prevention and Control (ECDC) at: www.ecdc.eu.int/
Fields BN et al (2001) Virology. Lippincott Williams & Wilkins, Philadelphia
Gillespie SH, Pearson RD (2001) Principles and Practice of Clinical Parasitology. John Wiley & Sons, Chichester
Guerrant RL et al (1999) Tropical Infectious Diseases. Principles, Pathogens, & Practice. Churchill, Livingstone, Philadelphia
Jong EC, McMullen R (2003) The Travel and Tropical Medicine Manual. WB Saunders, Philadelphia
Keystone JS et al (2003) Travel Medicine. Mosby, Edinburgh
Long SS et al (2003) Principles and Practice of Pediatric Infectious Diseases. Churchill Livingstone, New York
Mandell GL et al (2000) Principles and Practice of Infectious Diseases. Churchill Livingstone, New York
Mehlhorn H (2001) Encyclopedic Reference of Parasitology: Biology, Structure, Function. Diseases, Treatment, Therapy. Spinger, Berlin
Palmer PES, Reeder MM (2001) The Imaging of Tropical Diseases. Springer, Berlin
Peters W, Pasvol G (2002) Tropical Medicine and Parasitology. Mosby, London
Plotkin SA, Orenstein WA (2004) Vaccines. WB Saunders, Philadelphia
Shakir RA et al (ed) (1996) Tropical Neurology. WB Saunders, London
Steffen R et al (2003) Manual of Travel Medicine and Health. BC Decker, Hamilton
Strickland GT (2000) Hunter's Tropical Medicine and Emerging Infectious Diseases. WB Saunders, Philadelphia

G 36   Vinyl chloride

Committee for occupational medicine, working group "Hazardous substances", Berufsgenossenschaft der chemischen Industrie, Heidelberg

Preliminary remarks

The present guideline describes a scheme for occupational medical prophylaxis which aims to prevent or ensure early diagnosis of disorders which can be caused by vinyl chloride.

Schedule

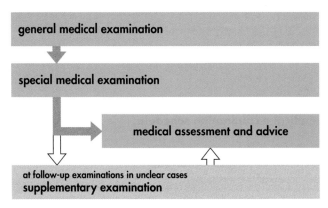

1   Medical examinations

Occupational medical examinations are to be carried out for persons exposed at work to levels of vinyl chloride which could have adverse effects on health (e.g. when the occupational exposure limit value is exceeded) or for whom dermal absorption could endanger health.

1.1   Examinations, intervals between examinations

initial examination	before taking up the job
first follow-up examination	after 12–24 months
further follow-up examinations	after 12–24 months and when leaving the job
premature follow-up examination	• after a serious or prolonged illness which could cause concern as to whether the activity should be continued • in individual cases when the physician considers it necessary, e.g. when there is short-term concern about the person's health • when requested by an employee who suspects a causal association between his or her illness and work

1.2   Medical examination schedule

1.2.1   General medical examination

Initial examination

• review of past history (general anamnesis, work anamnesis, symptoms)
• urinalysis (multiple test strips, sediment)

Follow-up examination

• interim anamnesis (including work anamnesis)
• urinalysis (multiple test strips, sediment)
Particular attention is to be given to:
• upper abdominal symptoms, anorexia (aversion to fat), paraesthesia in the fingers, dizziness

1.2.2   Special medical examination

Initial examination   **Follow-up examination**

- full blood count with thrombocytes
- SGPT (ALT)
- γ-GT
- alkaline phosphatase

Also helpful:
- further liver parameters
- sonography of the epigastric region paying particular attention to the liver

1.2.3   Supplementary examination

Follow-up examination

In unclear cases:
biomonitoring (see Section 3.1.4)

1.3   Requirements for the medical examinations

- competent doctor or occupational health professional
- laboratory analyses carried out with appropriate quality control (Good Laboratory Practice)

2   Occupational medical assessment and advice

An assessment is only possible when the workplace situation and the exposure of the individual are known. For this purpose a risk assessment as defined in Article 4 Council directive 98/24/EC must have been carried out; it must describe the levels of exposure and specify which technical, organizational and individual protective measures have been applied.

G 36

2.1 Assessment criteria

2.1.1 Long-term concern about health

Initial examination	Follow-up examination

Persons with severe disorders:
- systemic blood diseases
- scleroderma-like skin disorders
- acro-osteolysis
- disorders of the central and peripheral nervous systems
- vascular changes (especially Raynaud's disease)
- markedly impaired respiratory function
- liver disease, current or during the previous 2 years
- diabetes mellitus (insulin-dependent)
- alcohol, medicament or drug abuse or addiction

2.1.2 Short-term concern about health

Initial examination	Follow-up examination

Persons with the disorders mentioned in Section 2.1.1, provided recovery is to be expected

2.1.3 No concern about health under certain conditions

Initial examination	Follow-up examination

If the illnesses or functional disorders mentioned in Section 2.1.1 are less severe, the doctor should establish whether or not it is possible for the person to start work or go on working under certain conditions. Such conditions could include
- technical protective measures
- organizational protective measures, e.g., limitation of exposure periods
- transfer to workplaces known to involve lower levels of exposure
- personal protective equipment which takes the individual's state of health into account
- more frequent follow-up examinations

2.1.4 No concern about health

Initial examination	Follow-up examination

All other persons, provided there are no restrictions on their employment.

2.2   Medical advice

The advice in an individual case should be commensurate with the workplace situation and the results of the medical examinations.
Employees are to be informed about the biomonitoring results.
Employees should be informed about general hygienic measures and personal protective equipment.
Employees should be advised as to the carcinogenic effects of vinyl chloride.
If during the course of his work in the company the occupational physician finds indications that the risk assessment should be brought up to date to improve health and safety standards, he is to inform the employer. When this is necessary, the interests of the employee are to be protected (medical confidentiality).

3   Supplementary notes

3.1   External and internal exposure

3.1.1   Occurrence, sources of hazards

Exposure is possible in works which produce vinyl chloride, polymerize it to PVC, store, transport or process vinyl chloride. Higher level exposures can occur occasionally during plant breakdowns (e.g. leaks) and during cleaning, servicing and repair jobs.
This must be taken into account during the risk assessment.

3.1.2   Physicochemical properties and classification

Under normal conditions, vinyl chloride is a colourless, readily inflammable gas which smells slightly sweet. At 101.3 kPa (760 Torr) and −14°C it condenses to a colourless mobile liquid. Vinyl chloride is readily soluble in almost all organic solvents. In water vinyl chloride is poorly soluble but if it is stirred with suspending agents, stabilizers or emulsifiers, a fine suspension in water can be formed. In the absence of air and light, pure dry vinyl chloride liquid and gas are stable and not corrosive. Chemical reactions of vinyl chloride are almost entirely restricted to reactions of the double bond. The chlorine atom, the second functional group, may be replaced only with difficulty. The most important property of vinyl chloride is its ability to polymerize.

G 36

Vinyl chloride
Formula C_2H_3Cl
CAS number   75-01-4

The information system on hazardous substances (GESTIS) provides details of international threshold limit values, classification, evaluation and other substance-specific information (see Section 4).
Additional information is to be found in the recommendations of the DFG Commission for the Investigation of Health Hazards of Chemical Compounds in the Work Area (List of MAK and BAT Values).

3.1.3   Uptake
The substance is taken up mainly via the airways and also via the skin.

3.1.4   Biomonitoring
Information about biomonitoring may be found in Appendix 1 "Biomonitoring".
Exposure equivalents for carcinogenic substances (EKA: see the current List of MAK and BAT Values) give the relationships between the concentration of a substance in the workplace air and that of the substance or its metabolites in biological material. From these relationships, the body burden which results from uptake of the substance exclusively by inhalation may be determined. They are intended to provide the physician with a tool to help in the assessment of the analytical results. The EKA are not threshold values but data from occupational medical examinations.

Exposure equivalents for carcinogenic materials (EKA[1]) from the List of MAK an BAT Values

Vinyl chloride		
air vinyl chloride		Sampling time: after several shifts urine
(ml/m^3)	(mg/m^3)	thiodiglycolic acid (mg/24 h)
1	2.6	1.8
2	5.2	2.4
4	10	4.5
8	21	8.2
16	41	10.6

Biomonitoring should be carried out with reliable methods and meet quality control requirements (see Appendix 1 "Biomonitoring").

---

[2] Expositionsäquivalente für Krebserzeugende Arbeitsstoffe = exposure equivalents for carcinogenic materials

3.2   Functional disorders, symptoms

3.2.1   Mode of action
Vinyl chloride is metabolized via intermediates to yield mainly thiodiglycolic acid. The carcinogenic effects of vinyl chloride are ascribed to DNA alkylation by reactive metabolites.
Vinyl chloride and its metabolites have their main effects in the liver (carcinogenic effects), blood, skin, vascular and skeletal systems.

3.2.2   Acute and subacute effects on health
Exposure to very high doses of vinyl chloride results in tiredness, dizziness, a prenarcotic syndrome, and narcosis leading occasionally to death.

3.2.3   Chronic effects on health
Liver damage including malignant growths, varices in the oesophagus and fundus of the stomach, enlargement of the spleen, thrombocytopenia, circulatory disorders (especially Raynaud's disease), acro-osteolysis, morphological changes in the phalanges of the fingers, scleroderma-like skin changes.

4   References

Council Directive 67/548/EEC on the approximation of the laws, regulations and administrative provisions relating to the classification, packaging and labelling of dangerous substances

Council Directive 98/24/EC on the protection of the health and safety of workers from the risks related to chemical agents at work

Deutsche Forschungsgemeinschaft (German Research Foundation, DFG) (ed) List of MAK and BAT Values 2007. Maximum Concentrations and Biological Tolerance Values at the workplace. Wiley-VCH, Weinheim

Deutsche Forschungsgemeinschaft (German Research Foundation, DFG) (ed) The MAK-Collection for Occupational Health and Safety. Wiley-VCH
    at: www.mrw.interscience.wiley.com/makbat

GESTIS-database on hazardous substances. BGIA
    at: www.dguv.de/bgia/gestis-database

GESTIS-international limit values for chemical agents. BGIA
    at: www.dguv.de/bgia/gestis-limit-values

G 36

G 37   VDU (visual display unit) workplaces

Committee for occupational medicine, working group "VDU workplaces", Verwaltungs-Berufsgenossenschaft, Hamburg

Preliminary remarks

The present guideline describes a scheme for occupational medical prophylaxis which aims to prevent or ensure early diagnosis of adverse effects on health which can be caused by work with visual display units.

Schedule

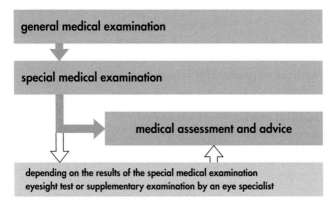

general medical examination

special medical examination

medical assessment and advice

depending on the results of the special medical examination
eyesight test or supplementary examination by an eye specialist

1   Medical examinations

1.1   Examinations, intervals between examinations

initial examination	before starting work at a VDU workplace
first follow-up examination and all later follow-up examinations	while employed at a VDU workplace • persons up to 40 years old: within 60 months • persons over 40 years old: within 36 months
premature follow-up examination	• after illnesses which cause concern as to whether this kind of work should be continued • when requested by an employee who suspects a causal association between his or her symptoms or illness and work, independent of any results of previous medical examinations • in individual cases when the physician considers it necessary, e.g. when there is cause for concern about the person's health in the short term

1.2   Medical examination schedule

1.2.1   General medical examination

Initial examination	Follow-up examination

- Review of past history
- General anamnesis, symptoms:
  for example
  - symptoms and disorders of the eyes
  - symptoms and disorders of the musculoskeletal system
  - neurological disorders
  - metabolic disorders
  - high blood pressure
  - long-term medication
- Work anamnesis:
  for example
  - workplace
  - job
  - training
  - working hours

G 37

If the findings and symptoms suggest that it is necessary, specific examinations focussed on work at the VDU workplace may be carried out.

1.2.2   Special medical examination

| Initial examination | Follow-up examination |

- visual acuity in the far range (with corrective appliances if the person wears them)
- visual acuity in the near range relevant for the workplace (with corrective appliances if the person wears them)
- stereopsis (three-dimensional sight)
- phoria (alignment of the eyes)
- central visual field (for persons 50 years old or more or given appropriate indications)
- colour vision[1]

The minimum requirements for the parameters tested in the special examination are shown in Table 1, a review of procedures in Table 2.

Table 1: Minimum values for the parameters tested in the special medical examination

Parameter	Minimum values
visual acuity in the far range	0.8/0.8
visual acuity in the near range relevant for the workplace	0.8/0.8
central visual field	normal
colour vision[1]	normal

Table 2: Review of the procedures to be used in the special medical examination

Parameter	Equipment or procedure
visual acuity in the far range	test procedure: EN ISO 8596 and 8597
visual acuity in the near range	test procedure: EN ISO 8596 and 8597
phoria	optical instruments
stereopsis	optical instruments
central visual field	standard charts
colour vision[1]	colour charts (e.g. Ishihara) or optical instruments

When selecting appropriate instruments – in line with EN ISO 8598 – the recommendations of the ophthalmologic societies should be taken into consideration.

---

[1] only when the ability to distinguish colours is required

Assessment scheme 1: "Special medical examination"

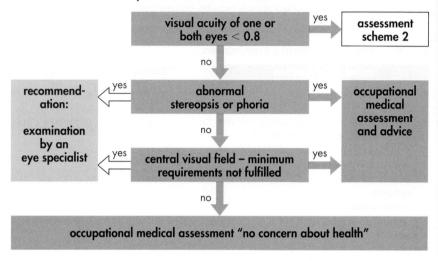

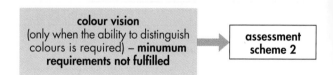

Results and assessment
a) minimum requirements for visual acuity fulfilled
   visual acuity of both eyes ≥ 0.8 (in the far and near ranges)[2]
b) minimum requirements for visual acuity not fulfilled for the
   - visual acuity of one eye < 0.8 (in the near and far ranges): recommendation that measures to improve visual acuity be sought and, e.g., the person be sent to see an eye specialist of his or her choice[3]
   - visual acuity of both eyes < 0.8 (in the near and far ranges): recommendation that measures to improve visual acuity be sought and e.g. the person be sent to see an eye specialist of his or her choice[3]; the visual acuity test may then be repeated:

---

[2] For persons with visual acuity < 1.0 an ophthalmologic examination is to be recommended, but this is not part of the present occupational medical examination.

[3] Costs which result from the recommendation that the person sees an ophthalmologist of his or her choice are not considered to be part of this occupational medical examination.

- minimum requirements fulfilled
- minimum requirements not fulfilled: supplementary examination by an eye specialist

c) minimum requirements for central visual field and colour vision fulfilled
d) disorders of stereopsis and/or phoria, minimum requirements for central visual field not fulfilled: recommendation that the person sees an eye specialist of his or her choice to clarify the findings. The test for visual acuity is not repeated.
e) disorders of colour vision in persons whose work requires them to distinguish colours, e.g. at CAD workplaces: supplementary examination by an eye specialist.

Assessment scheme 2: "Abnormalities in the special medical examination"

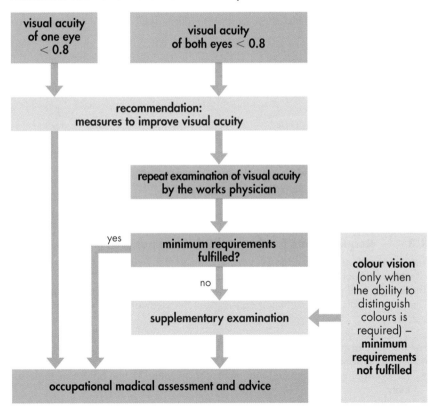

1.2.3   Supplementary examination

| Initial examination | Follow-up examination |

A supplementary medical examination by an eye specialist is indicated when
- abnormal findings or symptoms persist and clarification is necessary
- the minimum values are still not attained and clarification is necessary
- effects on the continuing work at a VDU workplace are conceivable.

The supplementary medical examination is oriented on the results of the special examination as described in Section 1.2.2.

The eye specialist reports to the occupational physician the results of the supplementary examination, his ophthalmologic assessment and suggestions for further measures. The occupational physician has to make out the medical certificate, taking the ophthalmologic assessment into account.

The supplementary ophthalmologic examination includes:

1. *General examination:*
   - anamnesis
   - general examination of the eyes

2. *Special examination:*
   - refractometry
   - quantitative determination of the visual field with a perimeter
   - examination of colour vision with the anomaloscope, determination of anomaly ratio

3. *Ophthalmologic assessment*
   Further ophthalmologic examinations may be carried out if justified.

1.3   Requirements for the medical examinations

The examinations described in Sections 1.2.1 and 1.2.2 are to be carried out by a competent doctor or occupational health professional.

Those described in Section 1.2.3 are to be carried out by an eye specialist.

The requirements to be met when carrying out the medical examinations are listed below:

For the special medical examination (only for competent doctors or occupational health professionals)
- for eyesight tests an optical instrument recommended by the ophthalmologic society
- facilities for determining visual acuity in the near and far ranges, phoria (alignment of the eyes), stereopsis (three-dimensional vision) and colour vision
- optical instrument with which the visual acuity in the near range can be determined for the distance relevant at the workplace
- standard chart for determining the visual field

For the supplementary examination (only for doctors qualified as eye specialists)

- fully equipped ophthalmologic practice
- facilities for carrying out standard ophthalmologic examinations
- facilities for determining visual acuity according to EN ISO 8596
- anomaloscope to determine the anomaly ratio
- facilities for quantitative determination of the visual field with the perimeter

For doctors qualified as eye specialists who carry out the examinations specified in sections 1.2.1 and 1.2.2 as well as the supplementary examinations, the following requirements apply:
- access to the firms
- the possibility of carrying out an examination of the workplace situation to assess ergonomics and, e.g., orthopaedic questions associated with having to work in awkward positions.

2   Occupational medical assessment and advice

An assessment is only possible when the workplace situation and the work of the individual are known. For this purpose a risk assessment as defined in Article 9 Council directive 89/391/EEC must have been carried out; it must specify which technical, organizational and individual protective measures have been applied.

2.1   Assessment criteria

2.1.1   Long-term concern about health

Initial examination	Follow-up examination

Persons with serious health defects, e.g., disorders of the musculoskeletal system, if they *cannot* be compensated by
- technical or organizational measures
- medical therapy

2.1.2   Short-term concern about health

Initial examination	Follow-up examination

Persons with serious disorders which are expected to be cured.

2.1.3   No concern about health under certain conditions

Initial examination	Follow-up examination

Persons with serious health defects which *can* be compensated by
- technical or organizational measures
- medical therapy

Shorter intervals between follow-up examinations may be necessary.
For persons with severe visual defects or blindness the assessment is carried out in co-operation with a rehabilitation centre for blind and partially sighted persons or a similar institution.

2.1.4   No concern about health

Initial examination	Follow-up examination

All other persons
Note: having only one eye does not rule out work with a visual display unit.

2.2   Medical advice

The medical advisor requires personal knowledge of the particular workplace situation. The advice in an individual case should be commensurate with the workplace situation and the results of the medical examinations. Of particular relevance are
- that ergonomic data be taken into account
- organizational measures in work planning
- the wearing of corrective appliances for eyesight at the VDU workplace

If the results of occupational medical examinations indicate focal cumulation of health risks, the physician, while observing medical confidentiality, is to inform and advise the employer.

3   Supplementary notes

3.1   Definitions

A visual display unit is a display screen for alphanumeric or graphic display, regardless of the display process employed.
A VDU workplace is a workplace with a visual display unit that can be equipped with
1. input devices,
2. software available to the employee to perform tasks

3. additional accessories and elements that pertain to the operation and use of the visual display unit or
4. other work equipment and the immediate work environment

Employees are employees who habitually use visual display units as a significant part of their normal work.

3.2   Adverse effects on health

Depending on the intensity and duration of work with a visual display unit, persons with inadequate eyesight or working in ergonomically ill-designed VDU workplaces can develop asthenopic symptoms such as headaches, burning and watering of the eyes, flickering vision or symptoms caused by poor working positions.

3.3   Corrective appliances designed for the workplace

If special corrective appliances for the eyes are required at the workplace, these must be designed to take into account the distances and angles of vision obtaining at the workplace.

4   References

Directive 89/391/EEC on the introduction of measures to encourage improvements in the safety and health of workers at work

Directive 90/270/EEC on the minimum safety and health requirements for work with display screen equipment

EN ISO 8596 Visual acuity test types. Specification for Landolt ring optotype for non-clinical purposes

EN ISO 8597 Visual acuity test types. Method for correlating optotypes used for non-clinical purposes

EN ISO 8598 Optics and optical instruments. Focimeters

5   Forms

Protocol sheet "VDU workplaces"

G 37 VDU workplaces

Surname	First name
Address: street	
Postcode, town	
Employer	
Address: street	
Postcode, town	
Place of work	
Kind of job	

Date ___.___._____   ☐ Initial examination   ☐ Follow-up examination

1   General anamnesis

1.1 Sight problems
(e.g. blurred vision, lacrimation, seeing double, pain, feeling of pressure, burning sensation, pain on moving the eyes, itching)   ☐ yes   ☐ no

    at work   ☐ yes   ☐ no

    when reading   ☐ yes   ☐ no

1.2 Glasses or contact lenses for

    the far range   ☐ yes   ☐ no

    the near range   ☐ yes   ☐ no

    the near and far ranges   ☐ yes   ☐ no

    ☐ bifocals   ☐ trifocals   ☐ varifocals   ☐ contact lenses

    Date of the last prescription for glasses   ___.___._____

1.3 Eye disorders (e.g. injuries, operations, allergies)   ☐ yes   ☐ no

    Which?

    Special aids for persons with visual disabilities   ☐ yes   ☐ no

1.4 Symptoms of the postural and locomotor system   ☐ yes   ☐ no

    Which and since when?

1.5 Disorders or symptoms of the nervous system
(e.g. migraine, headaches, dizziness)   ☐ yes   ☐ no

1.6 Metabolic disorders
(e.g. diabetes, thyroid function)   ☐ yes   ☐ no

1.7 High blood pressure   ☐ yes   ☐ no

1.8 Long-term medication   ☐ yes   ☐ no

    Which?

G 37

2	**Work anamnesis**		
2.1	Instruction in working at a visual display unit (VDU)	☐ yes	☐ no
2.2	Working time at a VDU	__ __ hours/day	

First Special medical examination

visual acuity with optimal correction

far range	VDU distance	near range		normal	
R [ ] L	R [ ] L	R [ ] L	visual field	☐ yes	☐ no
			colour vision	☐ yes	☐ no
			phoria	☐ yes	☐ no
Second Special medical examination			stereopsis	☐ yes	☐ no
far range	VDU distance	near range	phoria	☐ yes	☐ no
R [ ] L	R [ ] L	R [ ] L	stereopsis	☐ yes	☐ no

Comments

Results

no concern about health	☐
no concern about health under certain conditions*	☐
concern about health*	☐
Supplementary examination required	☐
Next examination	____ _____ month/year

* Recommendations

Date, stamp, signature of the physician

G 38   Nickel and nickel compounds

Committee for occupational medicine, working group "Hazardous substances", Berufsgenossenschaft der chemischen Industrie, Heidelberg

Preliminary remarks

The present guideline describes a scheme for occupational medical prophylaxis which aims to prevent or ensure early diagnosis of disorders which can be caused by nickel or nickel compounds.

Schedule

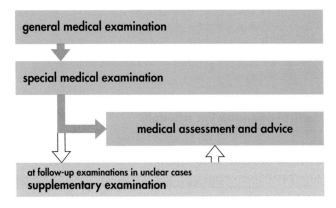

1   Medical examinations

Occupational medical examinations are to be carried out for persons exposed at work to levels of nickel or nickel compounds which could have adverse effects on health (e.g. when the occupational exposure limit value is exceeded) or for whom dermal absorption of nickel carbonyl could endanger health.

1.1   Examinations, intervals between examinations

initial examination	before taking up the job
first follow-up examination	after 24–60 months
further follow-up examinations	after 24–60 months and when leaving the job
premature follow-up examination	• after a serious or prolonged illness which could cause concern as to whether the activity should be continued • in individual cases when the physician considers it necessary, e.g. when there is short-term concern about the person's health • when requested by an employee who suspects a causal association between his or her illness and work

1.2   Medical examination schedule

1.2.1   General medical examination

Initial examination

• review of past history (general anamnesis, smoking anamnesis, work anamnesis – also with respect to previous exposures to carcinogenic substances – symptoms, allergic disposition, respiratory diseases)
• urinalysis (multiple test strips)
particular attention to be paid to eczema and skin allergies

Follow-up examination

• interim anamnesis (including work anamnesis and smoking anamnesis)
• urinalysis (multiple test strips)
particular attention to be paid to eczema and skin allergies

1.2.2   Special medical examination

Initial examination

- examination of the nose with the speculum
- large or medium sized thorax x-ray (not smaller than 10x10 cm) or use of an x-ray diagnosis which is less than 1 year old
- spirometry

For persons exposed to nickel carbonyl or during electrolytic isolation of nickel also:
- erythrocyte sedimentation reaction

Follow-up examination

- examination of the nose with the speculum
- chest x-ray for persons aged 40 years or more and for persons who have been exposed for more than 10 years
- spirometry

For persons exposed to nickel carbonyl or during electrolytic isolation of nickel also:
- erythrocyte sedimentation reaction

Also helpful: biomonitoring (see Section 3.1.4)

1.2.3   Supplementary examination

Follow-up examination

In unclear cases:
- x-ray examination of the nasal sinuses
- for persons with unexplained allergic skin diseases – examination by a skin specialist

1.3   Requirements for the medical examinations

- competent doctor or occupational health professional
- laboratory analyses and x-ray examination carried out with appropriate quality control (Good Laboratory Practice)
- necessary equipment:
  - spirometer
  - nasal speculum

2   Occupational medical assessment and advice

An assessment is only possible when the workplace situation and the exposure of the individual are known. For this purpose a risk assessment as defined in Article 4 Council directive 98/24/EC must have been carried out; it must describe the levels of exposure and specify which technical, organizational and individual protective measures have been applied.

2.1   Assessment criteria

2.1.1   Long-term concern about health

Initial examination	Follow-up examination

Persons with severe disorders:
- respiratory diseases (e.g. severe airway obstruction) or chronic bronchitis, bronchiectasis, pleural fibrosis
- skin disorders (eczema and skin allergies)

2.1.2   Short-term concern about health

Initial examination	Follow-up examination

Persons with the disorders mentioned in Section 2.1.1, provided recovery is to be expected.

2.1.3   No concern about health under certain conditions

Initial examination	Follow-up examination

If the illnesses or functional disorders mentioned in Section 2.1.1 are less severe, the doctor should establish whether or not it is possible for the person to return to work or go on working under certain conditions. Such conditions could include
- technical protective measures
- organizational protective measures, e.g., limitation of exposure periods
- transfer to workplaces known to involve lower levels of exposure
- personal protective equipment which takes the individual's state of health into account
- more frequent follow-up examinations

2.1.4   No concern about health

Initial examination	Follow-up examination

All other persons, provided there are no restrictions on their employment.

2.2   Medical advice

The advice in an individual case should be commensurate with the workplace situation and the results of the medical examinations.

Employees are to be informed about the biomonitoring results.

Employees should be informed about general hygienic measures and personal protective equipment. They should be told about the sensitizing and carcinogenic effects of metallic nickel and some nickel compounds. The pathogenic effects of cigarette smoking should be mentioned.

If during the course of his work in the company the occupational physician finds indications that the risk assessment should be brought up to date to improve health and safety standards, he is to inform the employer. When this is necessary, the interests of the employee are to be protected (medical confidentiality).

3   Supplementary notes

3.1   External and internal exposure

3.1.1   Occurrence, sources of hazards

Listed below are the kinds of processes, workplaces or activities, including cleaning and repair work, for which exposure to nickel or nickel compounds must be expected; this must be taken into account during the risk assessment.

- preparation and processing of nickel ores to obtain nickel or nickel compounds (including work on post-process dust filters)
- electrolytic deposition of nickel using non-consumable anodes
- production and processing of nickel or nickel compounds in powder form
- use of finely divided nickel as large-scale process catalyst in organic chemistry
- production of accumulators, magnets and loops containing nickel
- inert gas welding of metals and manual arc welding with high alloy materials (containing 5 % w/w or more nickel) and arc welding with materials containing more than 5 % w/w nickel in small spaces especially, e.g., small cellars, tunnels, pipes, wells, tanks, vats and other containers, coffer-dams and cells between double walls in ships or in inadequately ventilated spaces without local exhaust systems
- plasma arc and laser cutting of materials containing 5 % w/w or more nickel

- thermal spraying (flame, arc and plasma arc spraying) with spray materials containing more than 5 % w/w nickel
- grinding and polishing of nickel and alloys containing more than 5 % w/w nickel (e.g. magnets)
- demolition jobs on works for production of nickel or nickel compounds
- in electroplating, manually controlled, open, air-operated nickel baths at temperatures above 65°C
- foundries and steel manufacture when adding nickel to molten iron in alloy production
- in the preparation of special steels containing nickel

Nickel carbonyl is produced during nickel production by the carbonyl process in which a mixture of sulfides is reacted with carbon monoxide. However, the unintentional production of nickel carbonyl must also be expected whenever carbon monoxide comes into contact with nickel in a reactive form. The threshold limit value for the workplace is considered to have been exceeded if skin contact with nickel carbonyl occurs.

Occurrence and hazards for specific substances are documented in the information system on hazardous substances (GESTIS) (see Section 4).

3.1.2   Physicochemical properties and classification

Nickel is a silvery metal which melts at 1453°C. Finely divided nickel reacts with air and can ignite spontaneously.

Inorganic nickel compounds are solids, some of which are very readily soluble in water (e.g. nickel sulfate, nickel acetate, nickel nitrate), others practically insoluble (nickel carbonate, nickel hydroxide, nickel oxide, nickel sulfide).

Nickel
Formula   Ni
CAS number   7440-02-0

Nickel carbonyl is a readily inflammable, colourless, odourless liquid. It boils at 43°C; the vapour forms an explosive mixture with air.

Nickel carbonyl
Formula $Ni(CO)_4$
CAS number   13463-39-3

The information system on hazardous substances (GESTIS) provides details of international threshold limit values, classification, evaluation and other substance-specific information (see Section 4).

Additional information is to be found in the recommendations of the DFG Commission for the Investigation of Health Hazards of Chemical Compounds in the Work Area (List of MAK and BAT Values).

3.1.3   Uptake

Nickel and nickel compounds are taken up mainly via the airways in the form of dust, fumes or aerosols (sprayed droplets), through the skin (only nickel carbonyl) and through the gastrointestinal tract.

3.1.4   Biomonitoring

Information about biomonitoring may be found in Appendix 1 "Biomonitoring". Exposure equivalents for carcinogenic substances (EKA: see the current List of MAK and BAT Values) give the relationships between the concentration of a substance in the workplace air and that of the substance or its metabolites in biological material. From these relationships, the body burden which results from uptake of the substance exclusively by inhalation may be determined. They are intended to provide the physician with a tool to help in the assessment of the analytical results. The EKA are not threshold values but data from occupational medical examinations.

Exposure equivalents for carcinogenic materials (EKA[1]) from the List of MAK and BAT Values

Nickel (nickel metal, oxide, carbonate, sulfide, sulfidic ores)	
air nickel (mg/m^3)	Sampling time: after several shifts urine nickel (µg/l)
0.10 0.30 0.50	15 30 45

Nickel (readily soluble nickel compounds such as nickel acetate and similar soluble salts, nickel chloride, nickel hydroxide, nickel sulfate)	
air nickel (mg/m^3)	Sampling time: after several shifts urine nickel (µg/l)
0.025 0.050 0.100	25 40 70

---

[1] Expositionsäquivalente für Krebserzeugende Arbeitsstoffe = exposure equivalents for carcinogenic materials

Biomonitoring should be carried out with reliable methods and meet quality control requirements (see Appendix 1 "Biomonitoring").

3.2   Functional disorders, symptoms

3.2.1   Mode of action
- local carcinogenic effects in the airways and nasal mucosa after inhalation
- sensitization on skin contact

3.2.2   Acute and subacute effects on health
Toxic concentrations of nickel carbonyl cause damage especially in the airways and lungs (interstitial pneumonia), sometimes pulmonary oedema. In contrast, the oral and inhalative toxicity of nickel or other nickel compounds is not high enough to cause poisoning of persons exposed at the workplace.

3.2.3   Chronic effects on health
Inhalation of especially inorganic nickel compounds such as trinickel disulfide (nickel subsulfide Ni_3S_2) and nickel oxide (NiO) can lead in rare cases to cancer of the nasal passages, nasal sinuses and lungs.
For the various nickel compounds there is probably no relationship between the carcinogenic potential and how readily the substance is absorbed – and thus no relationship with the levels of nickel excreted in the urine.
Skin contact can lead to allergic dermatitis, occasionally associated with allergic bronchial asthma.

4   References

Commission Recommendation 2003/670/EC concerning the European schedule of occupational diseases. Annex I

Council Directive 67/548/EEC on the approximation of the laws, regulations and administrative provisions relating to the classification, packaging and labelling of dangerous substances

Council Directive 98/24/EC on the protection of the health and safety of workers from the risks related to chemical agents at work

Deutsche Forschungsgemeinschaft (German Research Foundation, DFG) (ed) List of MAK and BAT Values 2007. Maximum Concentrations and Biological Tolerance Values at the workplace. Wiley-VCH, Weinheim

Deutsche Forschungsgemeinschaft (German Research Foundation, DFG) (ed) The MAK-Collection for Occupational Health and Safety. Wiley-VCH
      at: www.mrw.interscience.wiley.com/makbat

GESTIS-database on hazardous substances. BGIA
      at: www.dguv.de/bgia/gestis-database

GESTIS-international limit values for chemical agents. BGIA
      at: www.dguv.de/bgia/gestis-limit-values

G 38

4   References

Commission Recommendation 2003/670/EC concerning the European schedule of occupational diseases, Annex I.)

Council Directive 67/548/EEC on the approximation of the laws, regulations and administrative provisions relating to the classification, packaging and labelling of dangerous substances

Council Directive 98/24/EC on the protection of the health and safety of workers from the risks related to chemical agents at work

Deutsche Forschungsgemeinschaft (German Research Foundation) (Ed.) (2011): List of MAK and BAT Values 2011, Maximum Concentrations and Biological Tolerance Values at the workplace, Wiley-VCH, Weinheim

European Risk Assessment Report, Chemical Agents Evaluation Institution, DRAR ref. The ULLMANN sheet on The Chemical and Health and Safety, Wiley VCH http://www.mrw.interscience.wiley.com/ullmann

GESTIS-Database on hazardous substances, BGIA
of www.hvbg.de/d/bia/fac/stoffdb/index.html

DNEL-Informationsdatenbank, Data values for chemical agents, DGUV, Germany IFA
of www.dguv.de/bgia/gestis-dnel-werte

G 39   Welding fumes

Committee for occupational medicine, working group "Welding fumes", Maschinen-bau- und Metall-BG, Düsseldorf

Preliminary remarks

The present guideline describes a scheme for occupational medical prophylaxis which aims to prevent or ensure early diagnosis of adverse effects on health which can be caused by exposure to welding fumes.

If the exposures are to respirable and inhalable dust in general or to substances with germ cell mutagenic, carcinogenic, fibrogenic or other toxic effects, the relevant Guidelines for Occupational Medical Examinations should be consulted.

In addition, the present guideline also contains suggestions for examination of persons exposed to welding fumes containing aluminium oxide which aim to prevent or ensure early diagnosis of adverse effects on health which can be caused by exposure to welding fumes containing aluminium.

Schedule

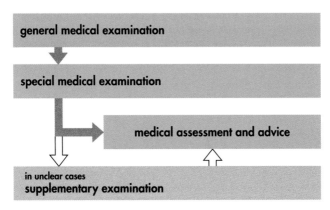

1   Medical examinations

Occupational medical examinations are to be carried out for persons at whose workplaces during welding and separating of metal parts exposure to welding fumes could endanger health (e.g. the occupational threshold limit value[1] is exceeded).

1.1   Examinations, intervals between examinations

initial examination	before taking up the job
first follow-up examination	after 36 months
further follow-up examinations	after 36 months and when leaving the job
premature follow-up examination	• after an illness lasting for several weeks or when a physical handicap gives cause for concern about whether the work should be continued (especially symptoms suggesting a bronchial or pulmonary disorder) • in individual cases when the physician considers it necessary, e.g. when there is short-term concern about the person's health • when requested by an employee who suspects a causal association between his or her illness and work • for persons exposed to aluminium welding fumes in addition and within at most 3 months if the BAT value of 200 μg aluminium/l urine has been exceeded and if unfavourable exposure conditions (e.g. welding in confined spaces) make a rapid increase in aluminium levels conceivable

---

[1] In Germany the statutory limit value for welding fumes is a concentration of 3 mg/m^3 (shift mean value) measured as respirable dust.

1.2   Medical examination schedule

1.2.1   General medical examination

| Initial examination | Follow-up examination |

general anamnesis, differentiated work anamnesis, detailed smoking anamnesis[2]
* non-smokers, smokers, ex-smokers
* cigarettes, cigars, pipes (number per day)
* year of starting and, if applicable, ending tobacco consumption (number of cigarette pack years)

1.2.2   Special medical examination

| Initial examination |

* physical examination
* spirometry
* large format posterior-anterior thorax radiograph taken with high kilovolt technique unless results are available from such an x-ray examination which has been carried out within the previous year; if digital techniques are used, the current radiography regulations must be observed.
* determination of the aluminium concentration in urine if the anamnesis suggests previous exposure to aluminium (see Appendix 1)

| Follow-up examination |

As for the initial examination.
* posterior-anterior thorax radiograph after 6 years, earlier if specifically indicated

1.2.3   Supplementary examination

| Initial examination |

Depending on the posterior-anterior radiogram and any previous x-ray results, an additional lateral radiogram may be necessary.
Where indicated, more extensive lung function tests (e.g. whole body plethysmography, inhalation test for unspecific bronchial hyperreactivity).

---

[2] For details of recording tobacco consumption see protocol sheet for anamnesis "Mineral dust" (G 1.1, G 1.2, G 1.3) in the guideline G 1.1.

As for the initial examination.

For persons exposed to aluminium welding fumes it should be remembered that nowadays early diagnosis of aluminosis is possible by means of high resolution computed tomography (HRCT). This can be indicated occasionally, especially for persons in whom the BAT value for aluminium is exceeded over long periods.

1.3 Requirements for the medical examinations
• competent doctor or occupational health professional

2 Occupational medical assessment and advice

An assessment is only possible when the workplace situation and the exposure of the individual are known. For this purpose a risk assessment as defined in Article 9 Council directive 89/391/EEC must have been carried out; it must specify which technical, organizational and individual protective measures have been applied.

2.1 Assessment criteria

2.1.1 Long-term concern about health

Initial examination	Follow-up examination

Persons with
• manifest obstructive or restrictive airway disorders, particularly bronchial asthma, chronic bronchitis especially with obstructive components and/or emphysema
• clinically manifest, irreversible bronchial hyperreactivity (for longer than 6 months)
• dust lung demonstrated radiographically (conventionally or with HRCT), silicosis (1/1 or greater), asbestosis (1/0 to 1/1 and greater), asbestos-induced pleural changes and also other fibrotic or granulomatous changes in the lungs including thorax deformities affecting lung function, pleural thickening (e.g. of tuberculous origin)
• existing cardiac insufficiency or diseases which often cause cardiac insufficiency
• where there is exposure to aluminium welding fumes, also persons with aluminosis

2.1.2   Short-term concern about health

Initial examination	Follow-up examination

Persons with
- the disorders mentioned in Section 2.1.1 provided recovery is to be expected
- acute respiratory disorders (e.g. acute bronchitis, tuberculosis, pneumonia),
- and also for persons exposed to aluminium welding fumes when the BAT value of 200 μg aluminium/l urine is exceeded. In these cases frequent determination of the aluminium concentration in urine is necessary.

2.1.3   No concern about health under certain conditions

Initial examination	Follow-up examination

If the illnesses or functional disorders mentioned in Section 2.1.1 are less severe, the doctor should establish whether or not it is possible for the person to start work or go on working under certain conditions.

In such cases the level and duration of exposure at the workplace should be established and taken into account in the assessment.

In addition, for persons exposed to aluminium welding fumes for whom the BAT value of 200 μg aluminium/l urine is exceeded, frequent determination of the aluminium concentration in urine is necessary.

2.1.4   No concern about health

Initial examination	Follow-up examination

All other persons, provided there are no restrictions on their employment.

2.2   Medical advice

The advice in an individual case should be commensurate with the workplace situation and the results of the medical examinations.

Cigarette smoking is the main cause of lung cancer and of the development of chronic obstructive airway diseases. Stopping inhalative tobacco consumption has been shown to result in an improvement of lung function and in a reduction of the overall risk of developing cancer, especially lung cancer. The physician is to inform the smoker of these facts and that treatment can be successful in helping him or her to stop smoking.

3   Supplementary notes

3.1   Exposure

3.1.1   Production of welding fumes

Welding fumes are dispersions of very finely divided solid matter in air; they are produced during thermal welding processes.

The emission of welding fumes affected by numerous parameters. These include

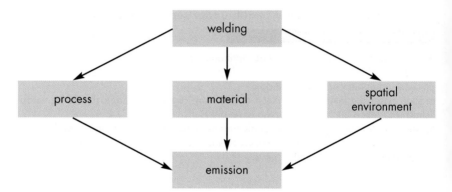

Type of welding process as a factor affecting the emission of welding fumes:

Of the fusion welding processes,
*   arc welding processes such as
    *   arc welding with a hand welding unit
    *   inert gas welding
    *   metal active gas welding (MAG)
    *   metal inert gas welding (MIG)
    *   tungsten inert gas welding (TIG)
    *   powder welding processes
*   beam welding processes such as
    *   plasma welding processes
    *   laser beam welding processes
are of considerable industrial importance.

Of the *forge welding processes* especially the resistance welding processes
*   spot welding and
*   projection welding
are of considerable industrial importance.

Also of importance for the emission of welding fumes are the **process parameters** such as
- amount of welding current
- alternating or direct current
- angle of the electrode

Type of material being welded as a factor affecting the emission of welding fumes: Basic materials of considerable importance in industry include
- steels
  - unalloyed construction steel
  - low alloy steels (containing < 5 % Cr, Ni, Mo, Mn, etc.)
  - high alloy steels (containing > 5 % Cr, Ni, Mo, Mn, etc.)
- aluminium and aluminium alloys
Accessory materials in the form of
- wire (as rods or on spools with or without coatings/fillings)
- powder
- solder
The accessory materials affect the composition of the welding fumes markedly.

Other factors affecting the emission of welding fumes include
- state of the surfaces (contamination, coatings)
- additives (inert gas, flux)

Spatial environment as a factor affecting the emission of welding fumes
Because of the spatial circumstances and the construction of the work pieces being welded:
- position of the welder's head and body caused by the position of the joint to be welded
- welding work in confined spaces (containers, silos, double walls, etc.)
- ventilation measures (e.g. exhaust systems near the point of emission)
In addition to the particulate components of the welding fumes, gaseous substances can be produced and these too should be taken into account in the risk assessment.

3.1.2   Occurrence, sources of hazards

The text below gives examples of welding processes during which the threshold limit value of 3 mg/m^3 is readily exceeded:
- manual arc welding with coated electrodes, unless adequate ventilation is ensured
- MIG and MAG welding, especially with filler wire and self-shielded flux-cored wire, unless adequate ventilation is ensured
- plasma cutting without an exhaust system or not under water
- mechanical oxygen cutting without an exhaust system
- flame, arc and plasma arc spraying in incompletely closed systems

- laser beam welding with and without accessory materials without an exhaust system
- laser beam cutting without an exhaust system
- flame gouging
- compressed air arc gouging
- flash butt welding

aluminium welding
- MIG welding of aluminium work pieces, unless adequate ventilation is ensured
- plasma cutting of aluminium work pieces without an exhaust system or not under water
- flame, arc and plasma arc spraying in incompletely closed systems.

According to the results of scientific studies and workplace analyses, in the processes listed below there is a possibility of exposure to chromates and nickel (see Section 3.2.1.4) if the work is carried out without ventilation or if the ventilation is inadequate.

There is a risk of exposure to higher levels of Cr(VI) compounds during work with chromium-nickel materials during the following welding processes:
- manual arc welding with coated electrodes
- MAG welding with filler wire
- plasma cutting
- laser beam cutting
- thermal spraying.

Plasma cutting, laser beam cutting and thermal spraying can result in simultaneous exposure to high levels of nickel oxides.

During work with nickel and nickel-based materials there is a risk of exposure to high levels of nickel oxides during the following welding processes:
- MAG welding with solid wire
- MIG welding
- plasma cutting
- laser beam cutting
- thermal spraying

3.1.3   Welding jobs

Welding jobs can be classified into three groups:
- full time welder
  Employees whose main job is welding: the welding jobs take more than 85 % of the working day. In the remaining working time, minor extra jobs are carried out.
- welder with more other jobs
  Employees who carry out welding jobs and other jobs associated with welding: 20 % to 85 % of the working day is spent doing welding jobs. Normally the remaining working time is spent doing other more or less time-consuming jobs such as
  - setting up the workplace at the construction site
  - preparing welding joints, correcting and filling the weld joint

- grinding the weld joint
- tack welding the work pieces
- mounting the work pieces in the positioning fixtures
- transport of the work pieces
- occasional welder
  Employees who carry out occasional welding jobs at work but generally do other jobs closely associated with welding work. On average not more of 20 % of the working day (about 1.5 hours per shift) is spent doing welding jobs. Typical professions include: fitters, fitters on building sites, welders doing repair jobs, panel-beaters, smiths, etc.

Table 1: Arc time/welding time

welding process	manual arc welding	MIG/MAG	TIG
full time welder	max. 50%	max. 70%	max. 60%
welder with more other jobs	12%–50%	20%–70 %	12%–60 %
occasional welder	max. 12%	max. 20%	max. 12%

3.1.4   Uptake

The fumes are taken up via the airways.

3.2   Functional disorders, symptoms

3.2.1   Mode of action

3.2.1.1   Irritative toxic effects

Welding fumes do not generally have chemically irritating or toxic effects on mucous membranes, the bronchial system or the lungs, given appropriate occupational hygiene and ventilation.

However, welding fumes emitted by certain work pieces and accessory materials can have chemically irritating effects on the bronchial system, for example when the fumes contain chromates (especially during manual arc welding with high alloy coated electrodes containing >5 % chromium), oxides of some other alloy metals and fluorides (during manual arc welding with basic coated electrodes).

Also some gases released during certain processes – such as nitrogen oxides (especially during autogenous welding), ozone (especially during MIG and TIG welding of aluminium work pieces) and pyrolysis products (e.g. of plastic, paint or mineral oil coatings) – are potentially irritative or toxic for the respiratory passages.

3.2.1.2 Sensitization and metal fume fever

Certain metals (e.g. copper, zinc) and their oxides in welding fumes can cause metal fume fever in predisposed persons (for symptoms see Section 3.2.2). The pathogenicity of this syndrome is still not completely understood.

A few individual cases of allergic sensitization (immediate type) of the bronchial system to certain metals (cobalt, chromium, nickel) have been described.

There is no evidence that welding fumes containing aluminium can cause metal fume fever or have sensitizing effects of immediate type on the bronchial system.

3.2.1.3 Pneumoconiosis

Welding fumes and welding gases are complex mixtures of hazardous substances. The iron oxide contained in welding fumes can be deposited in the pulmonary interstitial tissues in the form of dust depots which can be detected radiologically. The changes detected in the radiogram, so-called siderosis, can be reversible after the end of exposure to welding fumes. These changes are generally not associated with adverse effects on health nor with a clinically relevant impairment of lung function.

In rare individual cases after high level exposures, reactive fibrotic changes in the sense of a clinically manifest pulmonary fibrosis (siderofibrosis) can develop in the areas close to the deposits of welding fume particles (see also Section 3.2.2).

After sufficient exposure to aluminium, aluminosis can develop. Aluminosis, also called aluminium dust lung, is characterized by diffuse interstitial pulmonary fibrosis which is manifested most markedly in the upper and middle fields of the lung. In the advanced stages it is characterized by subpleural emphysema which is associated with an increased risk of spontaneous pneumothorax.

The risk of developing aluminosis depends primarily on the level, nature and duration of exposure. In addition, currently available information suggests that the individual disposition also plays a role. The risk seems to be particularly high for persons exposed to uncoated or lightly oiled stamped aluminium powder at stamping machines in the aluminium powder producing industry. Recent results also indicate that lung diseases can also develop in aluminium welders.

Radiological diagnosis of the early stages of aluminosis was, until recently, very difficult. Recent studies have shown that high resolution computed tomography (HRCT) provides more sensitivity and specificity in cases of aluminosis than do conventional radiographs. With HRCT it is also possible to detect early stages of aluminosis. The radiograph shows small, flat, round and irregular opacities which are manifested mainly in the upper fields of the lung. Sometimes the appearance of the radiograph is like that seen in cases of alveolitis with the characteristic "ground-glass pattern". In advanced stages the effects become spread over the whole lung and the incidence of linear opacities increases, a sign of progressive fibrosis.

3.2.1.4   Mutagenicity and carcinogenicity

The vast majority of welding fumes contain no particulate or gaseous substances which are known to have mutagenic or carcinogenic potency. However, the fumes from accessory substances containing chromium and/or nickel which are used in welding have been shown to have mutagenic effects and, under certain conditions, carcinogenic effects. This applies especially for fumes from high alloy coated electrodes. In welders who have worked with these kinds of high alloy accessory substances or who have cut high alloy work pieces using thermal processes, mostly for many years under unfavourable conditions of occupational hygiene, bronchial carcinoma has been diagnosed and recognized as an occupational disease.

In the year 1990, the International Agency for Research on Cancer (IARC) classified welding fumes as possibly carcinogenic to humans (Group 2 B). To some extent this is a result of the fact that welders can be exposed to a wide variety of substances, depending on the welding process being used, and that it is difficult to record the exposures in epidemiological studies. In addition to the components of actual welding fumes, welders can also be exposed to asbestos, aromatic amines (from azo colourants and tar paints), products of the pyrolysis of organic material (burning, sanding, removal of coatings containing tar and of oils and fats) and chromates in paints.

Especially in cohort studies the risk of developing tumours of the respiratory tract has been shown to be increased, but only rarely was the increase significant. Case-control studies more often show clear evidence of pulmonary carcinogenicity. In an extensive meta-analysis, Stern (1987) came to the conclusion that welding in general led to an increased risk of developing lung cancer. More recent meta-analyses have been published by Danielsen (2000) and Ambroise et al. (2006).

Essentially, an analytical assessment of causality requires differentiation of the welding processes and especially of the levels of exposure to the carcinogenic chromium(IV) compounds and nickel oxides. To be considered toxicologically relevant in the sense of having potential carcinogenic effects in the respiratory tract are, in particular, exposures during several years to very high levels of chromates and/or nickel oxides (see Section 3.1.2). The average latency period for tumours induced by welding fumes is about 20 years. In persons exposed to excessive amounts of chromates and/or nickel oxides, shorter latency periods are also conceivable.

3.2.2   Acute and subacute effects on health

Exposure to welding fumes does not generally cause acute or subacute illness. Type I allergic reactions (immediate type) are generally not induced in the airways.

In persons with the appropriate disposition, some metals and their oxides can cause metal fume fever. This is a syndrome which develops after a latency period of only a few or up to 10 hours and is manifested in respiratory distress and general symptoms of raised temperature, chills and exhaustion. The symptoms generally regress completely within hours or days. Persistent symptoms have not yet been observed. Acclimatization is known; in such cases, the respiratory symptoms may be expected to appear again when the person is re-exposed after long periods away from work.

In individual cases after exposure to toxicologically relevant levels of chemically irritative components of welding fumes or gases, acute irritation of the eyes or upper airways, coughing, expectoration and/or airway obstruction may develop. The symptoms generally increase in severity gradually during the work shift or after work. They are usually reversible after an exposure-free period. After exposure for long periods, however, persistent airway obstruction can develop.

In persons with existing unspecific bronchial hyperreactivity, chronic bronchitis or manifest obstructive airway disease, exposure to welding fumes can cause acute airway obstruction or persistent exacerbation of the bronchial symptoms.

Ozone and nitrogen oxides in higher concentrations are also potentially toxic for mucous membranes. Toxic pulmonary oedema has been observed in persons exposed to nitrogen oxides (e.g. as a result of working with the large flame in inadequately ventilated confined spaces). It should be taken into account that toxic effects on the bronchioli and alveoli and even, in individual cases, life-threatening toxic pulmonary oedema can develop after longer latency periods of 1 to 2 days after the end of exposure to such substances. The syndrome is generally reversible; however, in individual cases persistent impairment of lung function is possible.

Exposure to welding fumes containing aluminium does not generally cause acute or subacute illness.

3.2.3   Chronic effects on health

The normal exposure to welding fumes does not generally cause chronic disorders. In epidemiological studies to date, a significant excess of obstructive airway diseases could not be demonstrated in welders. Independent of these results, in individual cases there can be a risk especially for persons working with the processes mentioned in Section 3.1.2.

After long-term exposure to chemical irritants in welding fumes or to welding fumes with toxic components or after acute intoxications resulting from accidents, persistent alterations in lung function have been described in individual cases.

There are just a few reports of interstitial siderofibrosis of the lung in persons exposed intensely for many years to welding fumes under unfavourable conditions of occupational hygiene. The radiograph reveals mostly small irregular opacities of the forms s and t. In the early stages, the symptoms of gas exchange and diffusion disorders depend on the level of physical activity. Reduction in vital capacity as a sign of a restrictive ventilation disorder does not appear until the disease reaches the advanced stages. Use of electron microscopy and energy dispersive x-ray microanalysis reveals the dust particles deposited in the fibrotic lung areas to have the same elementary composition as the welding fumes at the workplace.

Morphological examination with the light microscope reveals that the interstitial fibrosis in the lung tissue is generally topographically close to the dust deposits.

The early symptoms of aluminosis are, like those of all pneumoconioses, uncharacteristic with chronic coughing and expectoration and/or dyspnoea during physical activity. In the advanced stages the patients complain of dyspnoea even at rest. As the disease progresses further, chronic cor pulmonale can develop. As a consequence of the pulmonary emphysema in patients with aluminosis, pneumothorax, also bilateral, develops frequently. The disease is also seen to progress after the end of exposure. Lung function tests in patients with advanced aluminosis reveal mainly restrictive ventilation disorders and perhaps disorders of gas exchange.

3.3   Comments

To avoid multiple medical examinations, the necessity for the application of other guidelines should be checked. To be considered are especially the guidelines G 1.1, G 1.4, G 15, G 26 and G 38.

G 39

4   References

Ambroise D, Wild P and Moulin J-J (2006) Update of a meta-analysis on lung cancer and welding. Scand J Work Environ Health 32: 22

Antonini JM et al (2003) Pulmonary effects of welding fumes: review of worker and experimental animal studies. Am J Ind Med 43: 350–360

Becker N (1999) Cancer mortality among arc welders exposed to fumes containing chromium and nickel. Results of a third follow up: 1989–1995. J Occup Envivon Med 41: 294–303

Commission recommendation 2003/670/EC concerning the European schedule of occupational diseases

Council Directive 89/391/EEC on the introduction of measures to encourage improvements in the safety and health of workers at work

Council Directive 92/85/EEC on the introduction of measures to encourage improvements in the safety and health at work of pregnant workers and workers who have recently given birth or are breastfeeding

Council Directive 98/24/EC on the protection of the health and safety of workers from the risks related to chemical agents at work

DIN EN 481: Workplaces atmospheres; size fraction definitions for measurement of airborne particles

Danielsen TE, Langard S, Andersen A (2000) Incidence of cancer among welders and other shipyard workers with information on previous work history. J Occup Environ Med 42: 101–109

Deutsche Forschungsgemeinschaft (German Research Foundation, DFG) (ed) List of MAK and BAT Values 2007. Maximum Concentrations and Biological Tolerance Values at the workplace. Wiley-VCH, Weinheim

Jöckel KH, Ahrens W, Pohlabeln H et al. (1998) Lung cancer risk and welding: results from a case-control study in Germany. Am J Ind Med 33: 313–320

Mur JM, Pham QT, Teculescu D et al. (1989) Arc welders respiratory health evolution over five years. Int Arch Occup Environ Health 61: 321–327

Rösler J, Woitowitz HJ (1998) Pulmonary fibrosis after heavy exposure to welding fumes. Eur J Oncol 3: 391–394

Stern RM (1987) Cancer incidence among welders: possible effects of exposure to extremely low frequency electromagnetic radiation (ELF) and to welding fumes. Environ Health Perspect 76: 221–229

Simonato L, Fletcher AC, Andersen A et al. (1991) A historical prospective study of European stainless steel, mild steel, and shipyard welders. Br J Ind Med 48: 145–154

Vogelmeier C, König G, Bencze K, Fruhmann G (1987) Pulmonary involvement in zinc fume fever. Chest 92: 946–948

G 41   Work involving a danger of falling

Committee for occupational medicine, working group "Work involving a danger of falling", Arbeitsmedizinischer Dienst der Berufsgenossenschaft der Bauwirtschaft, Zentrum Köln

Preliminary remarks

The present guideline describes a scheme for occupational medical prophylaxis which aims to ensure early diagnosis of disorders which could result in an increased risk of falling (see Section 2.1.1)

Schedule

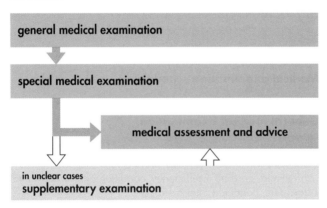

1   Medical examinations

1.1   Examinations, intervals between examinations

initial examination	before beginning a job which involves a danger of falling	
first and further follow-up examinations	until age 25 years	after 36 months
	from age 25 years to 49 years	after 24–36 months
	from age 50 years	after 12–18 months
premature follow-up examination	• after an illness lasting for several weeks or when a physical handicap gives cause for concern about whether the work should be continued	
	• in individual cases when the physician considers it necessary, e.g. when there is short-term concern about the person's health	
	• when requested by an employee who feels that continuing to work in the job involving a risk of falling is dangerous for health reasons	
	• if there are other indications which cause concern as to whether this kind of work should be continued	

1.2   Medical examination schedule

1.2.1   General medical examination

Initial examination	Follow-up examination

review of past history (general anamnesis, work anamnesis)
- cardiac arrhythmia, cardiac insufficiency, condition after a heart attack
- vascular disorders, condition after a stroke
- injuries to the skull and brain or cervical spine
- renal disorders
- diabetes mellitus or other endocrine disorders
- neurological or neuro-otological disorders
- psychiatric disorders
- intake of medicines or drugs: sedatives or drugs with sedative side effects, diuretics, aminoglycosidic antibiotics, antivertiginous drugs, alcoholic beverages, addictive drugs
- visus disorders: blurred vision, double vision, moving images, visual field defects
- symptoms of balance disorders: feeling as if the floor is moving, feeling of being in a lift, feeling of spinning around, tendency to fall, feeling faint, unsteadiness
- vegetative symptoms: sweating, nausea, retching, vomiting, collapse

- ear disorders: tinnitus, hearing loss, deafness, condition after an ear operation
- symptoms of other disorders of the brain nerves (disorders of taste and smell)
- trigeminus symptoms
- facial paralysis: peripheral, central

1.2.2   Special medical examination

Initial examination	Follow-up examination

Particular attention should be given to disorders of balance or consciousness and to locomotor disorders.
- tests of the head and body balance functions including the Romberg test for standing posture and the Unterberger-Fukuda stepping test (in each case for 1 minute), if possible with objective, quantitative documentation of the results (e.g. craniocorpography)
- tests of visual acuity and colour vision
- perimetry at every second examination
- hearing tests
- ECG
- ergometry for persons who are 40 years old or more, for those doing heavy physical work and/or in unclear cases
- urinalysis (multiple test strips)
- blood sugar, gamma-GT, blood count, creatinine

1.2.3   Supplementary examination

Initial examination	Follow-up examination

- in unclear cases further laboratory tests (blood/urine)
If the findings are unclear, further examinations by appropriate specialists (e.g. ENT specialist with experience in neuro-otology, neurologist, etc.) may be indicated.

1.3   Requirements for the medical examinations

- competent doctor or occupational health professional
- laboratory analyses carried out with appropriate quality control (Good Laboratory Practice)
- Equipment required:
  Own equipment:
  - electrocardiograph with 12 leads (extremities and thorax) for resting ECG
  - ergometry unit
  - device or chart for vision testing
  - colour charts or device for testing colour vision
  - perimeter

Own equipment or that of other physicians:
* laboratory
* craniocorpograph

2 Occupational medical assessment and advice

An assessment is only possible when the workplace situation and the exposure of the individual are known. For this purpose a risk assessment as defined in Article 9 Council directive 89/391/EEC must have been carried out; it must specify which technical, organizational and individual protective measures have been applied.

2.1 Assessment criteria

2.1.1 Long-term concern about health

Initial examination	Follow-up examination

Persons
* swaying sideways in the stepping test by more than 20 cm or by more than 80° to the right or 70° to the left
* swaying to and fro in the standing test by 12 cm or more and/or swaying sideways in the standing test by 10 cm or more
* with chronic attacks of dizziness with severe vestibular or retinal disorders affecting eye movement which can be detected electronystagmographically
* seeing moving images, persons with blurred vision
* with severe restriction of mobility, strength or sensitivity of a limb which is important for the job
* with disorders or alterations of the heart or circulatory system which result in reduced performance or impaired regulation, more severe blood pressure changes, condition after a heart attack or stroke
* who are overweight with BMI above 30 or comparable indices in a similar range
* who suffer from seizures – depending on their kind, frequency, prognosis and state of treatment
* with metabolic disorders, especially medically treated diabetes mellitus with a tendency to hypoglycaemia, disorders of the thyroid, parathyroid or the adrenal glands
* with corrected visual acuity of less than 0.7/0.7 or less than 0.8 in the far range for both eyes
* with colour vision disorders if a good colour vision is relevant for safety
* with restriction of the normal field of vision in the 30° central area
* with hearing acuity less than 3 m normal speech for both ears

- with emotional or mental disorders, even when these are in the past, if the possibility of recurrence cannot be excluded with sufficient certainly, abnormal mentality or highly abnormal behaviour
- with addiction to alcohol, drugs or medicines

2.1.2   Short-term concern about health

Initial examination	Follow-up examination

Persons with the diseases or functional disorders mentioned in Section 2.1.1 provided recovery or sufficient improvement is to be expected (see Section 3.1, second paragraph).

2.1.3   No concern about health under certain conditions

Initial examination	Follow-up examination

Persons with the diseases or functional disorders listed in Section 2.1.1 if under certain conditions (e.g. shorter intervals between follow-up examinations, specific working conditions) it need not be feared that the persons are a danger to themselves or others.

2.1.4   No concern about health

Initial examination	Follow-up examination

All other persons, provided there are no restrictions on their employment.

2.2   Medical advice

The advice in an individual case should be commensurate with the workplace situation and the results of the medical examinations. The employee should be told that premature follow-up examinations are to be carried out after illnesses of long duration and especially after acute disorders of the balance organ.

The employer should be advised as to any necessary technical, organizational and personal working conditions, provided that medical confidentiality can be observed.

3   Supplementary notes

3.1   Human balance

Human postural balance is achieved by spatial orientation of the body according to the force of gravity as detected by the vestibular receptors in the inner ear, via spatial hearing, via the eyes and visual information about the environment and finally by the postural regulation of the body via proprioceptive sensors. The cooperation of these four senses may be called the balance tetrad. The vestibular system is optimally adjusted horizontally and vertically when the head and gaze are directed forward and bent downwards by 30°. The visual stabilization point then lies about 3 metres in front of a normal adult on level ground.

The particular characteristics of the human balance system make it possible to compensate disorders. In certain kinds of cases, therefore, a repeat examination after one year can be indicated. After four years an improvement is generally no longer to be expected.

3.1.1   Occurrence, sources of hazards

An increased risk of falling may be assumed for work at the processes, workplaces or activities listed below and for similar situations:
- overhead cables and contact lines
- aerials
- bridges, masts, towers, chimneys
- floodlighting systems
- assembly and dismantling of self-supporting constructions (e.g. steel-girder constructions, constructions of prefabricated reinforced concrete parts, wooden constructions)
- shafts in mines
- work on scaffolding, roofs and facades of buildings

In these jobs employees are sometimes not secured against falling. For employees who suffer from the diseases or functional disorders listed in Section 2.1.1, the danger of falling is then increased.

An increased danger of falling at such workplaces is not to be assumed if the employees are always secured against falling by technical measures (railings, side panels, walls, etc.) or personal protective equipment.

4   References

Claussen C-F, Claussen E (2000) Cranio-corpo-graphy (CCG) – 30 years of equilibriometric measurement of spatial head, neck and trunk movements. Excerpt Medical, International Congress Series, 1201, Elsevier Publishers, Amsterdam, Lausanne, New York, Oxford, Shannon, Tokyo, 245–260

Claussen C-F, Haralanov S (2002) Cranio-Corpo-Graphy for objective monitoring of alcohol withdrawal syndrome. Neurootology Newsletter 8: 60–61

Directive 89/391/EEC on the introduction of measures to encourage improvements in the safety and health of workers at work

G 42   Activities with a risk of infection

Committee for occupational medicine, working group "Risk of infection"; Berufsgenossenschaft für Gesundheitsdienst und Wohlfahrtspflege, Hamburg

G 42

Preliminary remarks

The present guideline describes a scheme for occupational medical prophylaxis for
persons exposed at work to pathogens which can cause infectious diseases.
The prophylaxis aims to prevent adverse effects on health which can be caused by
infectious pathogens, or to recognize them at an early stage.

This guideline consists of 2 main sections:
The first section *"Basics"* describes the basic examinations and criteria for occupational medical assessment and advice on protection from infectious diseases which
apply for all activities involving a risk of infection including work in the biotechnol-
ogy sector.
The second section *"Specific infections"* contains pathogen-specific information and,
where relevant, also details of sensitizing or toxic effects.

Schedule

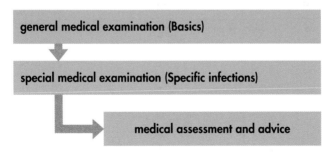

Basics

1   Medical examinations

Occupational medical examinations are to be carried out for persons at workplaces involving a risk of infection.

1.1   Examinations, intervals between examinations

intial examination	before taking up the job
first follow-up examination	• within 12 months • after vaccination depending on the period of immunity
further follow-up examinations*	• within 36 months • after vaccination depending on the period of immunity
premature follow-up examination	• after an infection or a serious or prolonged illness which could cause concern as to whether the activity should be continued • after injuries which could enable the pathogens to enter the organism • in individual cases when the physician considers it necessary, e.g. when there is short-term concern about the person's health • when requested by an employee who suspects a causal association between his or her illness and work • after accidents or incidents
final follow-up examination	after the end of an activity with a risk of infection

---

* For persons with life-long immunity (natural or acquired by vaccination) follow-up examinations are unnecessary.

1.2   Medical examination schedule

1.2.1   General medical examination

Initial examination

- review of past history (general anamnesis, work anamnesis, symptoms); vaccination anamnesis, past or present infections or infectious diseases. Particular attention is to be paid to disorders of the immune system or to disorders and therapeutic measures which affect the immune system.
- general physical examination, urinalysis (multiple strip tests, sediment if indicated), erythrocyte sedimentation rate, blood count (haemoglobin, erythrocytes, leukocytes), γ-GT, SGPT, blood sugar

G 42

When necessary, or when indicated by the anamnesis and/or the results of the medical examination:

- immunoelectrophoresis
- spirometry
- x-ray examination of the thorax or reference to an x-ray diagnosis which is not more than 12 months old

When necessary, effective vaccines should be made available for those workers who are not already immune to the biological agents.

Follow-up examination

- interim anamnesis (including work anamnesis)
- medical examination: see initial examination

For persons who have been vaccinated against the vaccinable biological agents at the workplace, follow-up examinations are not necessary as long as adequate immunity persists.

Final follow-up examination: advice as to conceivable manifestations of disease after the end of the incubation period.

1.2.2   Special medical examination

Initial examination   **Follow-up examination**

For pathogen-specific information, see "Specific infections".

1.3   Requirements for the medical examinations

- competent doctor or occupational health professional
- laboratory tests to be carried out in compliance with national regulations (medical councils, etc.) for quality control of quantitative medical laboratory analyses

2   Occupational medical assessment and advice

An assessment is only possible when the workplace situation and the exposure of the individual are known. For this purpose a risk assessment as defined in Article 9 Council directive 89/391/EEC and Article 3 Council Directive 2000/54/EC must have been carried out; it must specify which technical, organizational and individual protective measures have been applied.

2.1   Assessment criteria

2.1.1   Long-term concern about health

Initial examination	Follow-up examination

Persons with permanently impaired immune defence, e.g., with
- chronic (inherited or acquired) diseases which permanently weaken the defensive mechanisms of the body
- immune system altered by therapy with immunosuppressants, cytostatic agents, ionizing radiation, etc.
- long-term systemic treatment with corticosteroids or antibiotics which permanently weaken the defensive mechanisms of the body
- chronic, therapy-resistant eczema on the hands which impairs the protective function of the skin against infectious pathogens
- defective cellular and humoral immune response
- in persons whose spleen has been removed and who handle Streptococcus pneumoniae (except in persons who were immunized against pneumococci before the spleen was removed)

2.1.2   Short-term concern about health

Initial examination	Follow-up examination

Persons with temporarily impaired immune defence systems, e.g., with
- infectious diseases
- decompensated diabetes mellitus
- systemic medication with corticosteroids
- acute eczema on the hands which impairs the protective function of the skin against infectious pathogens or makes skin decontamination more difficult

2.1.3   No concern about health under certain conditions

| Initial examination | Follow-up examination |

In cases of less serious disorders (in the sense of impairment of immune defence) the doctor is to establish whether under certain conditions (improved workplace conditions, use of special individual protective equipment, reduced intervals between follow-up examinations, etc) it is possible for the person to start work or return to work.

2.1.4   No concern about health

G 42

| Initial examination | Follow-up examination |

All other persons, provided there are no restrictions on their employment (see Section 4).

2.2   Advice on protection from infections/infectious diseases

- information as to direct and indirect transmission routes (contact, droplet and indirect infection)
- hygienic measures
- personal protective equipment (in addition to working clothes):
  - skin protection
  - gloves
  - (waterproof) aprons
  - overalls
  - goggles
  - masks
  - respirator
  - particle filter masks
- vaccination (active, passive, contraindications, vaccination calendar, right to claim in the case of vaccination damage)
- immediate measures for accidents

3   Supplementary notes

3.1   Exposure

3.1.1   Occurrence, sources of hazards

see "Specific infections", "Occurrence".

3.1.2   Uptake

see "Specific infections", "Transmission route, immunity".

3.1.3   Mode of action

see "Specific infections", "Symptoms".

3.2   Functional disorders, symptoms

see "Specific infections", "Symptoms".

4   References

Commission recommendation 2003/670/EC concerning the European schedule of
    occupational diseases
Directive 89/391/EEC on the introduction of measures to encourage improvements
    in the safety and health of workers at work
Directive 92/85/EEC on the introduction of measures to encourage improvements in
    the safety and health at work of pregnant workers and workers who have re-
    cently given birth or are breastfeeding
Directive 2000/54/EC on the protection of workers from risks related to exposure to
    biological agents at work

Specific infections

Contents

G 42

Note: in Part 2 of the German version of G42 there are also details of the following pathogens:

Ancylostoma duodenale	Hepatitis E virus (HEV)
Ascarias lumbricoides	Hepatitis G virus (HGV)
Balantidium coli	Herpes simplex virus
Bartonella spp.	*Histoplasma capsulatum*
Coxiella burnetii	*Orthopoxvirus vaccinia*
Cryptococcus neoformans	*Orthopoxvirus bovis, O. simiae*
Cryptosporidium spp.	*Parapoxvirus bovis,*
Echinococcosus spp.	other animal poxviruses
Entamoeba histolytica	*Plasmodium* spp.
Erysipelothrix rhusiopathiae	*Pneumocystis carinii*
Francisella tularensis	Semliki Forest Virus (SFV)
Fusarium spp.	*Trichinella spiralis*
Giardia lamblia	*Tropheryma whipplei*

Adenovirus (HAd, VI – 47)

1   Infectious agent

Adenovirus (human adenovirus, species VI with 47 serotypes), DNA virus without an envelope, 240 hexon capsomers (group-specific antigen); 12 penton capsomers (serotype-specific antigen), also as model virus (molecular biology/gene therapy), environmentally stable (remains infectious for weeks); family Adenoviridae; classification in group 2 as defined in the Directive 2000/54/EC.

G 42

2   Occurrence

General
Adenoviruses are distributed ubiquitously all over the world (man/animals), sporadic, endemic, epidemic; 7 % to 17 % of all intestinal infections, 5 % to 10 % of respiratory infections, epidemic keratoconjunctivitis, locally frequent, outbreaks, miniepidemics, in Germany 138 adenovirus infections (2005), probably a considerable number of unreported cases.

Occupational
The health service (hospitals, outpatient clinics, ophthalmological practices, communal institutions), research establishments, consulting laboratories, social work, metalworking industry ("shipyard eye").

3   Transmission route, immunity

Source of infection: acutely infected persons (saliva, stool, urine, blood), persons with inapparent infections (fluctuating levels in saliva); airways (*droplet infection*), faecal-oral (*indirect infection*), sexual (*contact infection*), perhaps nosocomial, iatrogenic; conjunctiva (*indirect infection*); persistent serotype-specific *immunity*, re-infection possible with other serotypes, immunosuppressive therapy reactivates inapparent infections: virus persistence especially in lymphoid tissue, perhaps in the kidneys.

4   Symptoms

Mostly localized; in persons with severe immunosuppression life-threatening multiorgan involvement; the course of the infection is subclinical with 2/3 of the human pathogenic serotypes (at present 51 types), otherwise with raised temperature and with or without organ manifestations; primary infection in the first years of life is frequent; *incubation period* 2–12 days; *contagious* from person to person as long as the virus is detectable in secretions and excretions: in the throat 2–5 days, in the eye up to 2 weeks, in the airways 3–6 weeks, in cases of gastroenteritis up to 10 days or more, infections of the urinary tract can persist for months to years, in immunodeficient or immunosuppressed persons 2–12 months; contagiousness particularly high in cases of keratoconjunctivitis, gastroenteritis, pneumonia.

Acute febrile pharyngitis (serotypes 1–3, 5–7)
5 % of all acute respiratory tract infections; coughing, rhinitis, pharyngitis, exudative tonsillitis, cervical/preauricular lymphadenopathy with concomitant general symptoms; mostly sporadic in babies, infants, immunodeficient and immunosuppressed persons.

Acute respiratory syndrome (serotypes 1–3, 4, 6, 7, 14, 21)
Febrile uncharacteristic infections: rhinitis, tonsillitis, laryngitis (serotypes 1–3, 5–7), tracheobronchitis, cervical/preauricular lymphadenopathy; as complications pneumonia (serotypes 1–4, 7), acute otitis media; outbreaks among babies, infants, adolescents, life-threatening in immunodeficient and immunosuppressed persons.

Pharyngoconjunctival fever (serotypes 3, 7, 14)
Duration of illness 3–5 days, painful, mostly mild unilateral follicular conjunctivitis (serotypes 3, 4, 7) with cervical lymphadenopathy (swimming pool conjunctivitis), photophobia, lacrimation, inflammation of the plica semilunaris and caruncula lacrimalis, later roundish subepithelial corneal infiltrations; heals mostly without sequelae (often after a period of several months), transiently impaired visus; in severe cases pneumonia (types 1–4, 7); outbreaks among pre-school children, sporadic in adults.

Epidemic keratoconjunctivitis (serotypes 8, 19, 37)
All age groups, highly contagious nosocomial infections especially in ophthalmological clinics (outpatient and in the wards); favoured by epithelial injury, lacrimal probe, caustic vapours; virus excretion generally in the first two (or three) weeks of illness; mostly unilateral sudden onset, painful follicular conjunctivitis, itching, feeling of a foreign body in the eye, lacrimation, photophobia, inflammation of the plica semilunaris and caruncula lacrimalis, eyelid oedema with ptosis, cervical lymphadenopathy; sometimes after 1 week (20 %–90 % of cases) corneal involvement with whitish subepithelial infiltrations of roundish keratitic foci; symptoms regress after 2–4 weeks, cloudy cornea, mostly heals completely, occasionally impaired visus, haemorrhagic conjunctivitis.

Follicular conjunctivitis (serotypes 3, 4, 7)
Mild bilateral conjunctivitis (swimming pool conjunctivitis), photophobia, lacrimation, inflammation of the plica semilunaris and caruncula lacrimalis, later roundish subepithelial corneal infiltrates; accompanied by cervical lymphadenopathy, mostly heals without sequelae (not uncommonly after a period of several months), transient impaired visus; sporadic occurrence or outbreaks (summer).

Gastroenteritis (serotypes 31, 40, 41)
Second commonest form of viral enteritis in man (after rotavirus enteritis); cardinal symptom diarrhoea (up to 10 days); rarely with raised temperature, vomiting, dehydration; occasional respiratory symptoms; *with mesenteric lymphadenopathy* (serotypes 1, 2, 5, 6) simulates appendicitis, rare ileac intussusception.

Acute haemorrhagic cystitis (serotypes 11, 21)
Microhaematuria, dysuria, temperature not raised, high blood pressure, normal renal function, only male babies and infants, self-limiting syndrome.

5   Special medical examination

Detection of infectious agent
Electron microscopy: especially for viruses which cannot be cultivated; *culture:* virus isolation in cell cultures from blood, liquor, stool, urine, swabs, secretions (days 3–7), perhaps long-term culture (tissue/biopsy specimens) with latency period up to 3 weeks; *molecular biology:* PCR; restriction analysis, DNA hybridization with group-specific DNA probes.

Detection of antigens
Immunocytology (swab material) with the direct immunofluorescence test, enzyme immunoassay. Note: under some conditions false positive results for antigen in stool, check positive results perhaps with complement fixation reaction; serotype identification with the neutralization test, haemagglutination inhibition test;

Detection of antibodies
From week 2 of the illness, confirmation of the diagnosis by taking 2 blood samples 14 days apart: group specific antigens with complement fixation reaction, type-specificity with haemagglutination inhibition test, IgM/IgG enzyme immunoassay.

6   Specific medical advice

Before exposure
Exposure prophylaxis: personal protective equipment, general hygienic and disinfection measures, if possible equipment that operates without contact (e.g. tonometer).
Disposition prophylaxis (vaccination): use of vaccine not permitted in Germany; in the USA live vaccine against serotypes 3, 4, 7, 21 (acute respiratory syndrome).

After exposure
Medicinal therapy: specific therapy not available (antiviral substances are being tested); otherwise treatment according to symptoms.

7   Additional notes

Any national notification regulations and restrictions on activities and employment are to be observed.

G 42

Aspergillus fumigatus

1   Infectious agent

Aspergillus (A.) *fumigatus,* facultative pathogen (opportunist); mycotoxin producer (aflatoxin); thermotolerant (up to 50°C); form-class Deuteromycetes, class Hyphomycetes, most common agent (90%) causing invasive Aspergillus mycosis; of less relevance for human medicine: *A. flavus, A. nidulans, A. niger, A. ochraceus, A. repens, A. terreus, A. versicolor;*
classification in group 2, A: potential allergenic effects, as defined in the Directive 2000/54/EC.

2   Occurrence

General
Worldwide, sporadic in man, epidemic in horses, cattle, sheep, poultry, birds (feathers, droppings, nests); damp organic material, e.g. foodstuffs (over-ripe fruit); concentrated feedstuffs, feather grass, hay, jute, hemp, cereals, wood (sawdust), paper (records), rubbish (especially organic rubbish); building dust (stonework, cellulose-based insulation material); damp parts of air-conditioning systems, especially if not serviced properly; private living areas (room insulation); contaminated soil, e.g. of pot plants; invades (allochthonous) healthy human bodies without causing symptoms, e.g. paranasal sinuses, skin, intestinal tract, e.g. from mouldy foodstuffs.

Occupational
Production and use of fungal cultures (moulds) (special laboratories), reference centres, consulting laboratories, handling animals, plants or other biological products which are colonized, infected or contaminated; regular contact with infected samples or samples suspected of being infected or with contaminated pathogen-containing objects or materials, or materials which release fungal elements: e.g. veterinary medicine, laundries, textile production, pest control, breeding of birds, poultry; archives, depots, stockrooms and restoration workshops for books; industrial production of citric acid, kojic acid (*A. niger*), cereal silos, recycling industry with waste and recycling areas, e.g. disposal of organic waste (collection, transport, storage), composting of garden waste, sorting and processing of recyclable materials, mould-infested areas in farming, forestry, timber industry, building, gardening; sewage treatment; purification of drinking water, humidifier water in ventilation and air-conditioning systems.

3   Transmission route, immunity

Aerogenic infection with colonization of the airways including the paranasal sinuses, especially via so-called bioaerosols, that is, airborne reproductive fungal material (spores) or vegetative mycelium; indirect infection via surgical body openings, urinary catheters, transplantations, infection facilitated by immunodeficiency and by viral infections (e.g. Epstein-Barr virus, cytomegaly virus); contact infection via injured skin or burns, on contact with ornamental and pet birds; endogenous infection (controversial) in persons with persistent immunodeficiency and concomitant pathological colonization (rare) by allochthonous fungal material; other factors predisposing to infection: incompetent immune system, diabetes mellitus, long-term wide-spectrum antibiotic therapy, mucoviscidosis, lack of immunity.

4   Symptoms

Invasive pulmonary aspergillosis

G 42

Incubation period cannot be determined; *contagiousness* persists as long as infectious fungal spores can reach persons (generally immunodeficient) directly or indirectly, e.g. from macrocultures (special laboratories), samples for examination or other organic material; untreated high proportion of fatalities (90 %); in about ¼ of autopsies of tumour patients aspergillosis can be demonstrated, up to 55 % of pulmonary mycoses are caused by *Aspergillus* spp.; acute/chronic course with pneumonia-like symptoms: radiology reveals diffuse shadows or recurring, sometimes moving, solitary infiltrates with air trapped around round foci, sometimes pleural effusion, Wegner's triad (pulmonary infarction, haemorrhagic diathesis, thrombocytopenia), haemoptysis (cardinal symptom), necrotic erosion, rupture possible (lung bleeding).

Other organ involvement

After initial colonization of the lungs, haematogenic dissemination or dissemination *per continuitatem* in predisposed persons: encephalon/meninges: colonization after advanced dissemination or via the nasopharynx, paranasal sinuses, eye sockets, ears; encephalitis (base of brain), meningoencephalitis; paranasal sinuses: maxillary sinusitis; eyes: especially postoperatively in the form of endophthalmitis, chorioretinitis; keratoconjunctivitis (wearers of contact lenses) with involvement of the tear ducts, colonization of the eye socket from the paranasal sinus with destruction of adjacent bony structures; ears: otomycosis as secondary infection of the external auditory canal, more frequently with *A. niger*, in cases of chronic otitis media; skin: 2 %–5 % of cases, multiple maculopapular efflorescences, liver/kidneys: necrosis; bones: osteomyelitis, heart: endocarditis, pericarditis; sepsis: e.g. if the diagnosis and therapy come too late, mostly fatal.

Allergic bronchopulmonary aspergillosis (ABPA)

Organic dust toxic syndrome (ODTS); in immunocompetent persons after inhalation of spores (colonization) and the resulting sensitization of the airways with transient dual allergies: IgE-mediated immediate type (type I) with influenza-like symptoms (rhinitis, conjunctivitis), bronchial asthma, IgE-independent immune complex (type III) in the form of exogenous allergic alveolitis (EAA) or toxic as organic dust toxic syndrome (ODTS): raised temperature, coughing with expectoration (grey-brownish, purulent mucous), retrosternal pain, exertional dyspnoea, eosinophilia (blood, sputum); recurrent infiltrates, sacciform central bronchiectasis (rare).

Aspergilloma
Secondary infection of already damaged lung or bronchial tissue with coughing, raised temperature (rare), recurring haemoptysis (60 %), e.g. in cases of pneumoconiosis, tuberculosis, sarcoidosis, chronic bronchitis, but also in persons without apparent predisposition; localized ball-shaped, sometimes calcified fungal masses in abscess cavities, bronchiectasis dilations, bullae, fistulae, caverna, cysts; in the radiograph irregular limited roundish shadows or (more marked) with a sickle-shaped mass of air over a large ball of fungus, reactive thickening of the pleura.

5   Special medical examination

Detection of infectious agent
Microscopic: in special laboratories direct preparations from sputum, broncho-alveolar lavage, pus, tissue, skin material; macroculture (smoky green with *A. fumigatus*), *culture:* micromorphological culture preparation with aerial mycelium (thallus) which can be used for identification; positive culture result on its own without diagnostic significance; blood cultures and liquor almost always free of pathogen; histological detection in ventilated lung sections (open lung biopsy) without species-specific relevance.

Detection of antibodies
If clinically indicated antibody detection by RAST, immunoelectrophoresis, ELISA, double radial immunodiffusion (Ouchterlony); complement fixation reaction; DNA detection: PCR (early recognition of the invasive pulmonary form); antibody detection in blood does not automatically indicate infection/allergic disorder.

6   Specific medical advice

Before exposure
Exposure prophylaxis: personal protective equipment: in risk areas respiratory protection with particle filtering FFP2/FFP3 half mask; workplace dust-reducing measures; general hygienic and disinfection measures; air-conditioning units to be serviced regularly, persons with permanently impaired immune function should not be employed in moving or processing contaminated soil or building rubble, in demolition work, at workplaces in the recycling industry, in areas with paper dust (printers, archives).
Disposition prophylaxis (vaccination) not available.

After exposure
In infected persons, operate on localized processes; for the allergic bronchopulmonary form glucocorticoids, anti-asthmatics, mucolytics; for the invasive bronchopulmonary form and dissemination standard parenteral systemic antimycotic therapy.

7   Additional notes

Any national notification regulations are to be observed.

Bacillus anthracis

1   Infectious agent

Bacillus (B.) *anthracis*, Gram-positive sporulating aerobic bacillus, high resistance to environmental factors (spores); family Bacillaceae; classification in group 3 as defined in the Directive 2000/54/EC.
Has been placed in category A on the list of potential bioterrorism agents by the US Center for Disease Control and Prevention (CDC).

2   Occurrence

General
Worldwide in man and animals; in Germany and other industrial countries (Central and Northern Europe, North America) practically eradicated, the last case of cutaneous anthrax in Germany was registered in 1994 (sporadic appearance); soil as pathogen reservoir, spores viable for decades; primary infection of herbivorous animals, e.g. grazing farm animals, wild animals; infections via imported feed and animal products (hair, skins, fur).

Occupational
Research institutes, laboratories (regular work and contact with infected animals/ samples, samples and animals suspected of being infected, other contaminated objects or materials containing the infectious agent, given a practicable route of transmission), veterinary medicine, farming, forestry, hunting, firms and industries processing animal material including transport, work in areas where the disease is endemic.

3   Transmission route, immunity

Contact and indirect infection, most frequent route of entry through skin lesions by inoculation of the pathogen or spores from infected animals: blood, body fluids, organs, raw animal products; infections via the mucosa of mouth and eyes possible, also via insects; more rarely by inhalation (droplet, dust infection) of aerosols containing spores, e.g. when spreading contaminated fertilizer; when eating food which has not been cooked thoroughly (meat, milk); transmission from person to person practically impossible; humoral immunity to cutaneous anthrax of unknown duration.

4   Symptoms

All forms of anthrax can become systemic infections: as sepsis (lethal within a few hours) and/or haemorrhagic meningitis (convulsions/loss of consciousness); typical autopsy findings: enlarged and blackish red discoloured (necrotizing) spleen; the forms are distinguished by the ports of entry:

Cutaneous anthrax (pustula maligna): most frequent form (95 %); *incubation period* 2–10 days; itching papular efflorescences, development of blisters (malignant carbuncles), later usually painless erythematous ulcers (pustules) with a bluish black necrotic centre; in benign cases remains local without raised temperatures until the scab is sloughed off (10–15 days); in some cases released toxins induce high temperatures, dizziness and arrhythmia, untreated is fatal in 5 %–20 % of cases.

Inhalation anthrax: *incubation period* up to 5 days (depending on the infection dose), initially symptoms of an acute airway infection; then (within 2–4 days) fulminant syndrome: sepsis and/or meningitis, atypical bronchopneumonia with pulmonary necrosis; haemorrhagic thoracic lymphadenitis/mediastinitis; shock symptoms; untreated fatal within 3–5 days.

Intestinal anthrax: *incubation period* a few days, raised temperature, dramatic haemorrhagic gastroenteritis with haematemesis, bloody serous diarrhoea, peritonitis (ascites); prognosis unfavourable.

5   Special medical examination

Detection of infectious agent
Microscopic staining method, e.g. Gram stain, direct immunofluorescence test (capsule) and/or isolation of the pathogen from swab material, sputum, stool, blood.

Detection of antibodies
Antibody determination (capsule and toxin) possible, in diagnosing acute cases of less importance; nucleic acid amplification technique (PCR) possible in specialized laboratories; recently developed test systems (Light Cycler technology) provide identification within a few hours.

6   Specific medical advice

Before exposure
Exposure prophylaxis by monitoring imported animal products; if necessary decontamination of animal material; technical safety requirements to be met in specialized laboratories; personal protective equipment: in risk areas respiratory protection with a particle filtering half mask FFP3;
Disposition prophylaxis (vaccination) not currently available in Germany; killed vaccine in the USA.

After exposure
Isolation of exposed/infected persons generally not necessary; antibiotic therapy in cases of local cutaneous anthrax: ciprofloxacin and penicillin V (7 days); surgical

procedures contraindicated; in all forms of systemic infections also doxycycline (60 days); when applied in the early phase: fatalities approach 0 % (cutaneous anthrax), 50 % (inhalation anthrax, intestinal anthrax); if the pathogen has been disseminated intentionally, e.g. bioterrorist attack, modified therapies could be necessary, e.g. combination of several antibiotics; medicinal prophylaxis only after exposure: ciprofloxacin, doxycycline or amoxicillin.

7   Additional notes
Any national notification regulations are to be observed.

G 42

Bordetella pertussis

1   Infectious agent
Bordetella (B.) *pertussis*, coccoid Gram-negative bacterium, also *B. parapertussis* (5–20 % of cases); classification in group 2 as defined in the Directive 2000/54/EC.

2   Occurrence
General
Worldwide, man is the only natural host; highest incidence (Central Europe) in autumn/winter; prevalence dependent on vaccination, about 46 % of the pre-school age group is completely vaccinated against whooping cough, vaccination behaviour has moved infections to the youth and adult age range; eradication currently not possible.

Occupational
Facilities for medical examination, treatment and nursing of children and for care of preschool children, care of pregnant women, obstetrics, research institutes, consulting laboratories.

3   Transmission route, immunity
Droplet infection; indirect infection cannot be ruled out; asymptomatic, ill or contact persons can have transient carrier status, increasingly also vaccinated persons; natural infection produces immunity of limited duration (15–20 years), after complete vaccination about 10 years; it is possible in principle to suffer from the disease a second time as an adult.

4   Symptoms

Incubation period 7–20 days; contagious for 3 weeks, beginning at the end of the incubation period, ending in the early paroxysmal stage; infection without predisposing factors, particularly severe course in babies and infants.

Catarrhal stage
Duration 1–2 weeks, prodromal influenza-like symptoms with subfebrile temperatures.

Paroxysmal stage
Duration 4–8 (20) weeks, staccato coughing (max. 40–50 attacks/day) productive of viscous mucous; inspiratory stridor with vomiting, ends in expiratory apnoea attacks; more frequent and more severe at night; often induced by physical exertion, eating, mental factors; fatal in 0.6 % of cases, affects especially very young babies (acute attacks); in adults frequently takes the form of persistent coughing without paroxysms.

Stadium decrementi
Duration 6–10 weeks, gradual decrease in coughing attacks; intercurrent respiratory infections can cause a recurrence of clinical symptoms.

Complications
Mainly in the first year of life; about 25 % bacterial aspiration pneumonia, responsible for half of the deaths, secondary infections *(H. influenzae, Str. pneumoniae et pyogenes, S. aureus)*, convulsions (2 % of treated children), occasional encephalopathy with residual defects.

5   Special medical examination

Diagnosis primarily clinical (classical symptoms), 80 %–85 % success rate; laboratory tests (alternatives):

Detection of infectious agent
Isolation of pathogen from swabs of the posterior nasopharynx (special transport medium!) offer the best chance of success in the early paroxysmal stage; direct immunofluorescence test for screening; PCR in all stages;

Detection of antibodies
ELISA; circulating antibodies first appear 15–25 days after the start of the illness.

6   Specific medical advice

Before exposure
Exposure prophylaxis: if necessary particle-filtering half mask FFP2; general hygienic and disinfection measures (prophylaxis);

Disposition prophylaxis (vaccination): one vaccination dose at each of ages 2, 3, 4 and 11 to 14 months; boosters at age 5 to 6 years and 9 to 17 years with polyvalent combination vaccines (monovalent vaccines are not available); booster for adults generally after 10 years, a single vaccination with a combination vaccine (Tdap, TdapIPV) if possible not sooner than 5 years after the last dose of the other antigen in the vaccine (Td); vaccination is recommended for unvaccinated adults caring for children, for paediatrics personnel, persons caring for pregnant women, persons working in obstetrics, in hospitals for infectious diseases and in centres for preschool children and children's homes if possible four weeks before the birth of a child; *medicinal prophylaxis:* e.g. with erythromycin for not immune persons in close contact and members of the same household, as a precaution also vaccinated persons if they are in contact with persons at risk such as babies and children with cardiac or pulmonary disorders.

G 42

After exposure
Unvaccinated persons in close contact in families, communal centres for pre-school children and children's homes; antibiotic therapy makes sense only during catarrhal stage, without affecting the attacks of coughing it has anti-epidemic effects, reduces mortality/fatalities, recommended for carriers; macrolides, e.g. erythromycin (drug of choice), alternatively azithromycin, clarithromycin, roxithromycin, co-trimoxazole (in each case for 10 days); supported by mucolytics, sedation, plenty of liquids.

7   Additional notes

Any national notification regulations and rules for avoiding infection are to be observed.

Borrelia burgdorferi, Borrelia burgdorferi sensu lato

1   Infectious agent

Flexible Gram-negative spirochaete, sensitive to environmental factors; complex of human pathogens in Europe includes the species *Borrelia* (B.) *burgdorferi sensu lato* (Bbsl), *B. garinii, B. afzelii,* 10 species in all; classification in group 2 as defined in the Directive 2000/54/EC.

2   Occurrence
General
Global distribution, correlates closely with the vector hard tick/sheep tick (*Ixodes ricinus* in Europe), northern hemisphere: North America, Europe, Asia, case reports from Australia; risk of infection may be assumed for all parts of Germany, endemic

infection levels vary regionally 7 %–10 %; annual incidence (Germany) 100–200 cases/100000 inhabitants, mostly sporadic infections; pathogen reservoir rodents, birds, wild animals as hosts for the vector; biotope low vegetation, undergrowth, bushes, high grass; seasonally most frequent March–October with peak June–July; after a bite 3 %–6 % of persons infected (seroconversion), 0.3 %–1.4 % develop manifest illness.

Occupational
Farming, forestry and timber industry, gardening, kindergartens in the woods, research institutes, reference centres, regular work in low vegetation and in woods.

3   Transmission route, immunity
Vectorial via the bite of a female tick; infection dependent on period the tick remains on the person's skin: <12 hours unlikely, 24–48 hours about 5 %, 48–72 hours about 50 %, >72 hours 100 %; delayed humoral and rapid cellular immune responses, no reliable immunity; previous infection/increased antibody titre (serum) generally does not protect against re-infection; transplacental transmission possible.

4   Symptoms
Incubation period variable, depending on stadium: days to weeks (I), weeks to months (II), months to years (III); not *contagious* from person to person; any stadium can be omitted, all clinical manifestations can appear in isolation or in various combinations, spontaneous recovery without sequelae is possible in any stadium.
Stadium I: typical erythema (chronicum) migrans, in 40 %–60 % of infected persons; initial papules, then sharply delimited, painless erythema with a pale centre and centrifugal spread, sometimes associated with general influenza-like symptoms (arthralgia, swollen lymph nodes, sometimes a stiff neck); lymphadenosis *cutis benigna* Bäfverstedt (*Borrelia* lymphocytoma): circumscribed soft, livid reddish tumour covered by thinned skin, sometimes ulcerous and disintegrating (lobes of the ears, mamilla, scrotum).
Stadium II (disseminated infection): acute lymphocytic meningopolyneuritis (neuroborreliosis), is the most frequent clinical manifestation, cardinal symptom: initial painful radiculitis (generally at night); in 90 % of cases asymmetrical limp paralysis; mainly unilateral acute peripheral facial paralysis; loss of sensibility in more than two thirds of cases; episcleritis, keratitis, chorioretinitis; sometimes deafness; moving, sometimes severe joint and muscle pain; rarely meningitis, encephalitis, myocarditis, pericarditis, pancarditis.
Stadium III (late manifestations): Lyme arthritis after one in two untreated erythema migrans, intermittent/chronic monoarticular or oligoarticular arthritis (most often in the knee, also ankle, elbow, finger, toe, wrist and mandibular joints); persistent in 10 % of cases; sometimes myositis, bursitis, tenosynovitis; acrodermatitis *chronica atrophicans* Herxheimer, initially infiltrating livid atrophy of the skin of the extensor sides of the extremities; later arthropathy, peripheral polyneuropathy; chronic

encephalomyelitis affecting concentration, memory and behaviour, paraparesis, tetraparesis.

5   Special medical examination

Detection of infectious agent
Microscopic: directly from biopsy material (skin), joint aspirate, liquor with the direct immunofluorescence test; culture: *culture* on special medium (Kelly medium); both procedures possible in principle but little used in routine diagnosis.

G 42

Detection of antibodies
Detection of specific antibodies (serum, liquor); step-wise diagnosis: ELISA (or indirect immunofluorescence test), if result positive, immunoblot (confirmation test); differentiation by direct immunofluorescence test (skin biopsy, liquor), perhaps PCR (joint aspirate, synovial fluid). Note: one in two cases with erythema migrans is seronegative; reliable IgM antibody detection; IgG antibodies persist for years after infection (70 %–100 %), also after inapparent infection (10 % of the general population), serological tests should nonetheless be carried out; persistence also after successful therapy; false positive reactions, e.g. from persons with autoimmune disorders, herpesvirus infections, syphilis

6   Specific medical advice

Before exposure
Exposure prophylaxis with repellents; clothing that covers the body, e.g. long trousers, long-sleeved shirts, socks, closed shoes;
Disposition prophylaxis (vaccination): vaccine currently not available (Europe), in USA recombinant vaccine on the basis of an external membrane protein.

After exposure
After spending time in a tick-infested area, carefully search the body for ticks; remove ticks; disinfect wounds; after a tick bite recommended medicinal therapy with tetracycline (e.g. doxycycline) for five days; therapy most successful in the early phase; duration 2 weeks (3–4 weeks for late manifestations); tetracycline (drug of choice), e.g. doxycycline; for pregnant women and children penicillin G, amoxycycline; for carditis, neuroborreliosis: cephalosporins; isolation of infected persons not necessary, no measures necessary for contact persons.

7   Additional notes

Any national notification regulations are to be observed.

Brucella melitensis

1 Infectious agent

Brucella (B.) abortus (abortus fever), B. melitensis (Malta fever), B. suis (swine brucellosis), Gram-negative rod-shaped coccobacilli; classification in group 3 as defined in the Directive 2000/54/EC.
Has been placed in category B on the list of potential bioterrorism agents by the US Center for Disease Control and Prevention (CDC).

2 Occurrence

General
Worldwide and closely associated with the occurrence of brucellosis in animals, particularly common in certain Western European and Mediterranean countries (B. abortus especially in Central and Northern Europe).

Occupational
Research institutes, laboratories, meat processing, knackers' yards, farming, veterinary medicine, animal-keeping, hunting, artificial insemination, work in areas where the disease is endemic.

3 Transmission route, immunity

Infection by contact with secretions or excretions from infected animals via wounded skin or mucous membranes, by consumption of contaminated, non-pasteurized milk products, aerogenic infection possible; immunity for years to decades.

4 Symptoms

Incubation period 1–3 weeks (B. melitensis), 2 weeks to several months (B. abortus, B. suis); no contagion from person to person; up to 90 % of infections sub-clinical; early symptoms include headaches, joint and muscle pain, gastrointestinal disorders, moderately high temperature; at the beginning of the generalization stage high temperature with maximum about 40°C (undulant or continuous), recurrent in 5 % of cases within two years of the start of the illness; chronic course over >2 years with hepatosplenomegaly, lymphadenitis, occasionally hepatitis with icterus, haemorrhage, orchitis, chronic bronchopneumonia, endocarditis, meningoencephalitis (neurobrucellosis).

5 Special medical examination

Detection of infectious agent
Blood (from febrile persons), sternum or joint aspirates, biopsy material (lymph gland, liver, spleen); culture in liquid medium (tryptose or brain-heart infusion broth)

followed by solid medium (liver broth agar as described by Stafseth), identification with anti-Brucella antisera, biochemical performance tests.

Detection of antibodies
To establish the susceptibility to infection, disease anamnesis is not sufficient; detection of specific antibodies with heat-killed *Brucella* (slow agglutination in a suspension test), positive for 7–10 days *post infectionem*, proof is a 4-fold titre increase (after an interval of 10–14 days); complement fixation reaction (from week 4 of the illness) positive, ELISA detects recent infections (IgM antibodies, chronic infections IgG antibodies).

G 42

6   Specific medical advice

Before exposure
Exposure prophylaxis: personal protective equipment when brucellosis is present or suspected, general hygienic and disinfection measures;
Disposition prophylaxis (vaccination): vaccine is being tested (USA, France).

After exposure
In case of an infection, medicinal therapy (antibiogram): doxycycline combined with streptomycin or rifampicin; alternatively co-trimoxazole with rifampicin.

7   Additional notes

Any national notification regulations are to be observed.

Burkholderia pseudomallei (Pseudomonas pseudomallei)

1   Infectious agent

Burkholderia (B.) *pseudomallei*, pleomorphic, Gram-negative rod, motile, obligate pathogen, causes the potentially life-threatening infectious disease melioidosis; other human pathogens *B. cepacia* (bacterial rot of onions/mucoviscidosis), *B. mallei* (glanders); classification in group 3 as defined in the Directive 2000/54/EC.
Has been placed in category B on the list of potential bioterrorism agents by the US Center for Disease Control and Prevention (CDC).

2   Occurrence

General
Endemic between latitudes 20° north and 20° south, in Europe only imported cases (rare), also associated with natural disasters; in contaminated surface water (rivers,

ocean), damp soil (*B. pseudomallei* can survive for years), rice paddies; prevalence in areas where the pathogen is not endemic is probably underestimated.

Occupational
Research institutes, laboratories, the health service, veterinary medicine (veterinary practices), farming, zoological gardens, work in areas where the pathogen is endemic.

3   Transmission route, immunity

Pathogen reservoir: fundamentally all animal species can carry the pathogen; especially small mammals, pets; aerogenic (*dust infection*); percutaneous/transcutaneous (*indirect infection*); rarely oral via contaminated surface water/soil; contaminated foodstuffs, meat, milk from infected animals (*alimentary infection*); handling infected/diseased pets (*contact infection*); no immunity, not even after recurrent infections.

4   Symptoms

Pathogenesis (melioidosis) largely unclear; granulomas characteristic; diabetes mellitus, chronic lung diseases, renal insufficiency, alcohol abuse predispose to infection; uncharacteristic course with multiple granulomatous or abscess-like lesions of internal organs, the skin, skeletal muscles, bones; immune status has a significant effect on clinical severity and prognosis.
Incubation period depends on the pathogen level: 2–21 days after skin injury, decades after inapparent infections; *contagious* as long as the pathogen is excreted, transmission from person to person possible (rare); *pulmonary form:* acute course (75 %) with raised temperature, pneumonia, sometimes lung abscesses, pleural empyema; *localized form:* multiple abscesses/ulcers with lymphadenitis; *chronic form:* multiple abscess formation in visceral organs, skin, skeletal muscles, bones; *sepsis:* fatal in about 50 % of cases, pulmonary form may develop concomitantly.

5   Special medical examination

Detection of infectious agent
From sputum, tracheal secretion, swab material, blood culture, urine; *microscopic colour test:* Gram stain, methylene blue, Wright stain; bipolar staining; *culture:* pathogen not difficult to culture, aerobic culture on routine or selective media, blood culture media; biochemical differentiation not reliable; serological identification with monoclonal antibodies, e.g. (latex) agglutination tests, direct immunofluorescence test, enzyme immunoassay (capture ELISA).

Detection of antibodies
IgM ELISA, IgM immunofluorescence test, indirect haemagglutination test; results are difficult to interpret because of high infection levels and cross reactions; detection by molecular biological methods (PCR) only possible in special laboratories.

6   Specific medical advice

Before exposure
Exposure prophylaxis: in areas where the pathogen is endemic, close contact with surface water should be avoided, especially by persons with skin injuries;
Disposition prophylaxis (vaccination) not available.

After exposure
If clinically indicated for persons who have spent time in areas where the pathogen is endemic, even decades later (travel anamnesis!), laboratory tests necessary; persons who have had the illness must be observed medically life-long (early detection of relapses);

G 42

Medicinal therapy: after visiting areas where the pathogen is endemic and given clinical indications initial parenteral therapy, oral maintenance therapy for several weeks; fatal in 20 % of cases in spite of therapy.
B. pseudomallei is a potential *bioterrorism agent;* the infection dose is small (aerosols), intentional dissemination by bioterrorists would probably not result in an epidemic, transmission from person to person is rare; has been placed in category B on the list of potential bioterrorism agents by the US Center for Disease Control and Prevention (CDC).

7   Additional notes

Any national notification regulations are to be observed.

Candida albicans, C. tropicalis

1   Infectious agent

Candida (*C.*) *albicans,* yeast (Deuteromycetes, class Blastomycetes), *C. tropicalis* second most common yeast in man, facultative pathogen (opportunists); 15 other species relevant in human medicine including *C. glabrata, C. guilliermondii, C. krusei, C. lusitaniae, C. parapsilosis,* classification in group 2 (A: potential allergenic effects), as defined in the Directive 2000/54/EC.

2   Occurrence

General
Worldwide, ubiquitous, transient on skin (rare), mucous membranes (gastrointestinal tract is a natural reservoir) of man and animals (birds, pets, wild animals), plants; colonizes about 30 % to 50 % of healthy persons. *Candida* may be isolated in 79 % of cases of nosocomial mycethaemia; *C. tropicalis:* man is not a reservoir, ubiquitous in soil (damp milieu); 30 % of persons are colonized orally/gastrointestinally with

Candida sp., duration of colonization (of persons in hospital) increases with the time spent in the ward.

Occupational
The health and social services, hydrotherapy, balneotherapy, microbiological laboratories, reference centres, veterinary medicine, animal breeding, soil disinfection, sewage works, recycling industry.

3   Transmission route, immunity

Endogenous (increasingly also exogenous) infection given predisposing factors: marked immune deficiency of the host is necessary; entry when barrier functions disturbed (injury, dermatosis, chronic maceration, tissue damage caused by bacterial or viral infections); no immunity.

4   Symptoms

Incubation period unknown; *contagious* as long as the pathogen is excreted, e.g. from ulcers or secretions (sputum, tracheal secretion, bronchial lavage, pus) or excretions (urine, faeces) and makes contact with immunodeficient persons.

Surface candidiasis (most common form)
Oral mucosa "thrush": focal whitish removable deposits on reddened tissue, stomatitis, candida leukoplakia, glossitis, angular cheilitis;
Body flexurae: favoured by hyperhidrosis, obesity, diabetes mellitus, weeping itching foci (intertrigo), skin between toes and fingers with macerations, whitish scales;
Skin appendages: inflammation of the nail folds (paronychia), brittle discoloured nail plates (onychomycosis).

Local invasive candidiasis (mostly in the form of ulcers)
Respiratory tract: tracheitis, bronchitis, pneumonia (rare), systemic spread possible;
Urogenital tract: vulvovaginitis, itching, discharge; urethritis, balanitis, balanoposthitis;
Gastrointestinal tract: oesophagitis (AIDS-defining condition); colonization without symptoms (half of all clinically healthy persons) or uncharacteristic symptoms (stomach, duodenum), haematemesis, risk of progression to generalized candidiasis.

Generalized candidiasis
Haematogenic dissemination from the intestines, in the form of sepsis (fatal in >50 % of cases), establishment in the heart (endocardium), eye (endophthalmitis), CNS, lymphatic tissue, kidneys, peritoneum, thyroid gland, liver, testes (rare); skin (candida granuloma).

Chronic mucocutaneous candidiasis
Caused by hereditary immune defect with autosomal recessive inheritance: persistent foci and granulomas (mouth, skin, nails, airways), largely resistant to treatment.

Systemic invasive candidiasis
Haematogenic dissemination (candidemia) in the form of sepsis (lethal in $> 50\ \%$ of cases); intraparenchymatous colonization, heart (endocardium), eye (endophthalmitis), CNS (meningitis), lymph nodes, spleen, kidneys, peritoneum, thyroid gland, liver, testes (rare), *C. tropicalis* disseminates more frequently than *C. albicans* especially in persons with haematological disorders (neutropenia), infection of liver and spleen is a late complication, in immunosuppressed persons and those with damage to the gastrointestinal mucosal barrier; *C. tropicalis* accounts for 25 % of cases of candida sepsis, nosocomial, pneumonia (tuberculosis-like symptoms).

G 42

5   Special medical examination

Only when the clinical symptoms are associated with the job and/or when infection, e.g. nosocomial infection, is suspected

Detection of infectious agent
Tracheal secretion, bronchial lavage, stool, mid-stream urine, swabs; for systemic infection: blood culture (positive in 25 % to 60 % of cases), liquor, tissue samples, aspirates; *microscopic detection:* native preparation or stained (e.g. Gram-stain); *culture:* macroculture on special media, germ tube test as rapid test *(C. albicans)*, staining with methylene blue, lactophenol blue; species determination by biochemical performance tests, in cases of nosocomial infection strain determined by pulsed field gel electrophoresis, DNA probe method; clinical intestinal manifestation: pathogen count (colon) $>10^6$/g stool characteristic, 10^4–10^6 requires checking, $<10^4$/g clinically insignificant (commensal mycoflora).

Detection of antibodies
Indirect haemagglutination test, ELISA, indirect immunofluorescence test, radioimmunoassay; tests cannot distinguish absolutely between colonization and infection; clinical intestinal (colon) manifestations should be verified quantitatively: pathogen count $>10^6$/g stool characteristic, 10^4–10^6/g require checking, $<10^4$/g clinically insignificant (commensal mycoflora).

6   Specific medical advice

Before exposure
Exposure prophylaxis: e.g. avoidance of occlusive clothing and damp milieu; *Disposition prophylaxis* (vaccination) not available.

After exposure
In case of illness polyene anti-mycotics (e.g. amphotericin, nystatin, natamycin), imidazole derivatives (e.g. miconazole).

7   Additional notes
Any national notification regulations are to be observed.

Central European encephalitis (CEE) virus

1   Infectious agent
Central European (tick-borne) encephalitis (CEE) virus, RNA virus, family Flaviviridae; classification in group 3(**) as defined in the Directive 2000/54/EC.

2   Occurrence
General
Endemic natural sources of infection (high risk areas) in temperate climatic zones; main risk areas in Germany: Bavaria (most frequent), Baden-Württemberg, Hessen, Rheinland-Palatinate, Thuringia; sporadic local sources of infection in Saarland, Saxony, Brandenburg; other European countries, e.g. Austria, Switzerland, Alsace, some Eastern European, Scandinavian and Balkan countries; natural habitats (ticks) along the edges of woods, wooded river valleys; seasonal from April until November; worldwide about 10000 cases annually, in Germany 255 reported cases (in the year 2001); pathogen reservoir in animals living in the wild (squirrel, lizard, yellow-necked mouse *(Apodemus flavicollis)*, bat, fox, hare, mouse, hedgehog, mole, roe-deer, red deer, wild pig, birds); domesticated animals (dog, horse, sheep, goat); in animals the disease is very rarely clinically manifest.

Occupational
In areas in which the organism is endemic: farming, forestry, timber industry, gardening, animal dealing, hunting, research institutes, reference centres, laboratories, consulting laboratories, regular work in low vegetation and in woods, work involving frequent direct contact with wild animals.

3   Transmission route, immunity
Virus not directly transmissible from person to person; heterogeneous chains of infection involving bites by blood-sucking hard ticks (*Ixodes ricinus*/sheep tick) infected with the virus (1 %–5 % of the tick population) with life-long persistence of the virus within the population, ticks drop from bushes and high grass, also found in dust; no

ticks found at high altitudes above 1000 m; almost one in two persons does not remember the tick bite; alimentary (rare in Germany) via unpasteurized milk from infected cows, sheep or goats, or products made from these; rare (aerogenic) laboratory infections; life-long immunity, also after inapparent infections; cellular immunity
probable.

4   Symptoms

Incubation period 3–14 (40) days; not contagious; virus multiplication at the site of
entry (e.g. in macrophages, granulocytes, endothelial cells); only 10 %–30 % of infections are manifest and show the two-phase course of the disease.

Primary phase (first viraemic phase), typically with peak illness after 3–14 days (in
90 % of all persons with the illness); influenza-like symptoms (4–6 days), associated
with uncharacteristic, catarrhal, sometimes gastrointestinal symptoms, temperature
generally not above 38°C, mostly followed by a symptom-free interval (6–20 days);
Secondary phase (second viraemic phase), severe illness, temperature up to 40°C,
organ manifestations: CNS-symptoms (in 10 % of those affected); isolated cases of
(acute lymphocytic) meningitis, mainly in children, occasional vertigo, fixation nystagmus, abducens paralysis, in general recovery without sequelae; meningoencephalitis is the most common form in adults, occasional disorders of consciousness,
concentration or memory, ataxia, hemiparesis, epileptic seizures; involvement of
cerebral nerves (loss of hearing acuity, swallowing and speech disorders, abducens,
phrenic and facial paralysis, sometimes with loss of sensitivity as well); in persons
40 years old or more meningoencephalomyelitis or meningoencephaloradiculitis are
more common: severe forms seen more often in adults than in children; prognosis:
10 % –20 % of the symptoms are only transitory and regress mostly within days or
weeks; permanent neurological losses are possible with incomplete recovery from
encephalitic or/and myeloradiculitic disorders; in cases of radiculitis the monoparesis (especially arms), paraparesis, tetraparesis, monoplegia, paraplegia or quadri-
plegia regresses almost completely; in cases of myelitis the chances of improvement
in the delayed paralysis (especially of the neck, thoracic girdle, upper extremities)
are less; fatalities in cases with CNS involvement 1 %–2 %, (Europe), 20 %–30 %
(Far East).

5   Special medical examination

Detection of infectious agent
Virus isolation (blood, liquor) only during first viraemic phase, detection of nucleic
acid by reverse transcription PCR and sequencing.

Detection of antibodies
To establish vaccination status/susceptibility to infection, anamnesis of illnesses and
vaccinations is not sufficient, inspection of vaccination documents required; ELISA,
neutralization test, complement fixation reaction, haemagglutination inhibition test,
indirect immunofluorescence test, Western blot; antibodies detectable mostly only for

a few weeks, in exceptional cases for up to 18 months; a temporal association with a CEE vaccination (IgM-antibodies) must be excluded anamnestically.

6   Specific medical advice

Before exposure
Exposure prophylaxis: in areas where the organism is endemic avoid low vegetation; repellents (protection for short periods); clothing that covers the body, e.g. long trousers, long-sleeved shirts, socks, closed shoes;
Disposition prophylaxis (vaccination): vaccination possible for children aged 3 years or more; indication to vaccinate is potential contact with ticks in a high risk area and seronegative status; basis vaccination and boosters according to the producer's instructions with a vaccine authorized for use in adults or children; rapid vaccination possible; note seasonal occurrence April–November; the person is to be informed of potential post-vaccination side effects on the central and peripheral nervous systems especially given an autoimmune disease; critical evaluation of indications for pregnant women because of lack of data.

After exposure
Searching the body for ticks: immediate mechanical removal (do not twist! do not squash! use no oil or glue!) with subsequent disinfection; specific antiviral therapy not available, possibly anti-CEE human immunoglobulin (controversial, not generally recommended, only to be considered for persons more than 14 years old), only within 96 hours of tick contact, otherwise less favourable course of the disease possible; observe 4-week interval after CEE vaccination; combination of passive and active immunization (so-called simultaneous vaccination) not recommended at present, lower seroconversion rate, less increase in specific antibodies; after every tick bite tetanus vaccination status should be checked.

7   Additional notes

Any national notification regulations are to be observed.

Chlamydophila pneumoniae, Chlamydophila psittaci (avian strains)

1   Infectious agent
Chlamydia species
a)   *C. trachomatis* with 15 serovars
b)   *C. psittaci*
c)   *C. pneumoniae*
Pleomorphic, non-motile, Gram-negative, obligate intracellular bacteria; classification in group 2 as defined in the Directive 2000/54/EC.
Has been placed in category B (*C. psittaci*) on the list of potential bioterrorism agents by the US Center for Disease Control and Prevention (CDC).

G 42

2   Occurrence
General
Worldwide, reservoir of infection man for *C. trachomatis* and *C. pneumoniae* and animal for *C. psittaci* (wild birds and poultry).

Occupational
Research institutes, laboratories, consulting laboratories, risk of ornithosis/psittacosis in poultry farming and the poultry processing industry, animal-keeping and veterinary medicine;
C. pneumoniae in the health service (paediatrics), in overseas service;
C. trachomatis mainly in ophthalmology (serovars A–C) and gynaecology (serovars D–K).

3   Transmission route, immunity
a)   *C. trachomatis:* transmission via infectious secretion from the eyes (indirect infection), serovars D–K via all kinds of sexual contact and during birth to the baby, Chlamydia transmission in cases of lymphogranuloma venereum (LGV) also sexual, but much less common.
b)   *C. psittaci:* zoonosis, transmission via the faeces of infected birds (dust inhalation), transmission from person to person unusual but has been described.
c)   *C. pneumoniae:* droplet infection person to person.

4   Symptoms
a)   *C. trachomatis* serovars A–C: *incubation period:* gradual begin, about 1–3 weeks; trachoma, bilateral chronic follicular conjunctivitis with pannus formation, keratitis and corneal scarring, causing blindness in 10 % to 20 % of cases; serovars D–K1: infection of the urogenital tract, non-gonorrhoeal urethritis (NGU), cervicitis-salpingitis (pelvic disease), inclusion conjunctivitis, pneumonia;

serovars L1–L3: lymphogranuloma venereum, inguinal bubo formation with high temperature, shaking chills, arthralgia and fistula formation.
b) *C. psittaci:* ornithosis, psittacosis; *incubation period:* 1–3 weeks, an influenza-like form (raised temperature, headaches, myalgia) and atypical pneumonia.
c) *C. pneumoniae: incubation period:* a few days; relatively mild cases of pneumonia in young adults, atypical airway disorders in children (bronchitis, tracheo-bronchitis); suggested to be an etiological agent for arteriosclerosis.

5 Special medical examination

Throat swab, bronchoalveolar lavage typical inclusion bodies (Giemsa stain, direct immunofluorescence test with monoclonal antibodies); *culture:* culture of permanent cell lines (requires a lot of time and work), for *C. psittaci* only in laboratories with safety level III; *molecular biology:* PCR, gene probes, ligase chain reaction, *antigen detection:* direct immunofluorescence test, ELISA (low sensitivity and specificity).

Detection of antibodies
To establish the susceptibility to infection; in exceptional cases if clinically indicated; procedures (ELISA, complement fixation reaction) with recombinant lipopolysaccharide often detect only strain-specific antibodies; microimmunofluorescence test as standard procedure for species-specific antibodies.

6 Specific medical advice

Before exposure
Exposure prophylaxis: Personal protective equipment, perhaps particle filtering half mask (FFP3); general hygienic and disinfection measures;
Disposition prophylaxis (vaccination) not available.

After exposure
In infected persons (trachoma) local medicinal therapy, isolation of patients with *C. pneumoniae* infections; otherwise for all *Chlamydia* infections systemic application of doxycycline for at least 3 weeks, alternatively erythromycin.

7 Additional notes

Any national notification regulations are to be observed.

Clostridium tetani

1   Infectious agent

Clostridium (*C.*) *tetani*, Gram-positive, rod-shaped bacterium which forms a terminal spore, strictly anaerobic, motile; family Bacillaceae; spores are highly resistant to environmental factors (heat, disinfectants); produces exotoxins: tetanospasmin (neurotoxic), tetanolysin (haemolytic, cardiotoxic); classification in group 2 as defined in the Directive 2000/54/EC.

G 42

2   Occurrence

General
Worldwide, large regional differences, most common in warm damp climates in countries with a low vaccination frequency, low socio-economic status; incidence in Asia, Africa 10–50 cases/100000 inhabitants, estimated (WHO) annual deaths worldwide >1 million cases; low incidence in industrial countries (Europe, North America) because of high proportion of people vaccinated; in Germany in recent years <15 cases annually.

Occupational
Work where injuries are common and where wounds may come into contact with soil, road dust, wood, dung, wounds made with contaminated objects; contact with animals (e.g. bites), consulting laboratories.

3   Transmission route, immunity

Reservoir (pathogen, spores) soil, intestines of herbivorous animals (mainly the horse, sometimes also man); via grazes and scratches (minor wounds) or bites (anaerobic, deep necrotic wounds) contaminated with soil or faeces; severe burns, foreign bodies (e.g. splinters of wood, nails, thorns) favour toxin production; no antitoxic immunity after natural infection or after recovering from the disease.

4   Symptoms

Generalized disease
Most common form (adults); *incubation period* 3 (1) days to 3 weeks (several months); not *contagious* from person to person; prodromes, e.g. sweating, slight tension in muscles near the wound, hyperreflexia, beginning stiffness, afebrile or subfebrile course; progressive tonic spasms (skeletal muscles): jaw and masticatory muscles with lockjaw (trismus), facial muscles with whining expression or fixed smile (risus sardonicus/cynic spasm), neck and back muscles with painful, over-stretched (opisthotonic) posture with stomach muscles as hard as a board, intercostal muscles/diaphragm in (life-threatening) inspiration position; fractures (spine) caused by simultaneous spasms of flexors and extensors; extremities generally not involved; at

the same time clonic convulsions: painful paroxysmal contractions of whole groups of muscles (30–40 spasms/h) amplify the opisthotonus, sometimes pharynx and tongue muscles (dysphagia), larynx muscles (laryngospasm) with risk of asphyxiation; often induced by optic, acoustic or tactile stimuli, patient remains conscious, respiratory insufficiency as a result of airway obstruction, congestion; fatal in 10 %–20 % of cases in intensive care, untreated 30 %–90 %; dependent on incubation period (the shorter, the less favourable is the prognosis), level of toxin production.

Neonatal disease
Newborn babies of not immunized mothers e.g. after unhygienic treatment of the umbilical cord; begins with restlessness, poor feeding, then the typical symptoms of the generalized form (rigidity, spasms).

Localized tetanus
Rare, mild, abortive form; in partially immune persons manifestations restricted to muscles around the point of entry; only muscle stiffness, no spasms; good prognosis, mostly on the head (cephalic tetanus) after tooth extraction, otitis media; fatal in 1% of cases.

5 Special medical examination
Diagnosis is made essentially on a clinical anamnestic basis.

Detection of infectious agent
Mouse-protection study: excised wound material (30 min., 80°C), characteristic tonic muscle spasms in the back legs; detection of toxin in culture medium or suspension of wound material with specific anti-tetanus toxin antibodies; *culture:* anaerobic culture in media such as blood agar medium (filmy growth with ring of haemolysed cells); deep soft glucose agar, liver broth, thioglycolate broth; identification by microscopy after staining (rod with terminal spore "drumstick" form), determination of biochemical characteristics.

Detection of antibodies
To establish the vaccination status/susceptibility to infection: anamnesis of illnesses and vaccinations is not sufficient, inspection of vaccination documents required; serological anti-toxin detection is possible to prevent unnecessary revaccination.

6 Specific medical advice
Before exposure
Exposure prophylaxis is not possible.
Disposition prophylaxis (vaccination) with tetanus toxoid as standard vaccine: one dose of vaccine at ages 2, 3, 4 and 11–14 months, booster at age 5–6 and 9–17 years; with polyvalent combination vaccine; vaccination status must be tested at age 15–23 months, no sure protection from infection if the IgG antitoxin level is <0.01 IU/ml, if necessary complete the vaccination series; in adults boosters

generally after 10 years, not sooner than 5 years after the previous dose (in combination with diphtheria vaccine), children under 6 years old T, older persons Td (i.e. tetanus-diphtheria combination vaccine with reduced diphtheria toxoid content), at each appointment for a Td booster the indication for a whooping cough vaccination should be checked and, if necessary, this included in the combination vaccine (Tdap); vaccination of persons who have recovered from an infection is recommended.

After exposure
For wounded persons immediate immunoprophylaxis as shown in the table; vaccinations missed from the basis immunization series should be given; passive immunization with high doses of human anti-tetanus immunoglobulin (HTIG) i.m., up to 10000 IU, no absolute protection.

G 42

Surgical cleansing of the infected area, antibiotic application according to the antibiogram, generally penicillin G, tetracycline (super-infection); metronidazole reduces amount of circulating toxin. Limited possibilities for symptomatic treatment: intensive care for maintenance of vital functions, muscle relaxants (curare-type medication), keeping the airways open (if necessary tracheotomy), long-term artificial ventilation; no particular anti-epidemic measures necessary for persons with the disease or contact persons.

7   Additional notes

Any national notification regulations are to be observed.

Tetanus immunoprophylaxis for injured persons (as of 7/2006)

History of tetanus vaccination (number of vaccinations)	Clean minor wounds		All other wounds[1]	
	Td[2]	TIG[3]	Td[2]	TIG[3]
unknown	yes	no	yes	yes
0 to 1	yes	no	yes	yes
2	yes	no	yes	no[4]
3 or more	no[5]	no	no[6]	no

[1] Deep and/or dirty wounds (contaminated with dust, earth, saliva, stool), wounds with crushed tissue and reduced oxygen supply or containing foreign bodies (e.g. crushed or torn tissue, bites, stings, shot wounds); severe burns and frost-bite, tissue necrosis, septic abortions
[2] Children under 6 years old: T, older persons: Td, (i.e. tetanus-diphtheria vaccine with reduced content of diphtheria toxoid)
[3] TIG = tetanus immunoglobulin, generally 250 IU are administered, the dose can be increased to 500 IU; TIG is used simultaneously with Td/T vaccine.
[4] Yes if the wound is more than 24 hours old.
[5] Yes (1 dose), if it is more than 10 years since the last vaccination.
[6] Yes (1 dose), if it is more than 5 years since the last vaccination.

Corynebacterium diphtheriae

1   Infectious agent

Corynebacterium diphtheriae, Gram-positive, non-sporulating rods, Order Actino-
mycetales; virulence factors: diphtheria toxin (exotoxin) and diphtheria toxin gene
(dtx), haemolysin (cytotoxic effects); classification in group 2, T: toxin production as
defined in the Directive 2000/54/EC.

2   Occurrence

General
Mainly in temperate climatic regions, seasonal morbidity peak in autumn/winter; endemic in the Third World; the frequency of infections in Europe has been decreasing
since the year 1995, during the same period there were large regional epidemics in
the ex-USSR states (about 50000 cases, 1500 deaths); in Germany in the year 1958
there were still 10000 cases, in 1964 <1000 cases ; since 1984 only sporadic single cases infected with toxinogenic strains, often imported after visits to countries
where the organism is endemic; contact infections of unprotected persons limited by
the high proportion of vaccinated infants (about 95 %); immunity among young persons only about 45 %, adults about 30 %, which is indicative of neglected booster
vaccination.

Occupational
The health service, especially ENT and dental services, laboratories, communal facilities (accommodation for emigrants, refugees and persons seeking political asylum
from areas where the organism is endemic), work abroad in areas where the organism is endemic.

3   Transmission route, immunity

Man is the only source of infection (pathogen reservoir), mostly droplet infection
(face-to-face), contact infection, indirect infection (rare); temporary antitoxic immunity, prevents illness but not infection or colonization.

4   Symptoms

Toxin synthesis necessary for clinical manifestation; *incubation period* 2–5 (8) days;
contagious as long as the pathogen is detectable, 2–4 weeks without treatment, 2–4
days with antimicrobial therapy; course of the illness more often benign than malignant (mainly effects of the toxin); uncharacteristic prodromal symptoms (characteristic discomfort during swallowing, temperature not above 38°C).

Localized forms (tonsillo-naso-pharyngeal)
Characteristic lesion: pseudomembranous deposits (extensive greyish whitish fibrin exudate), firmly attached, removable only by force and with bleeding.
Pharyngeal diphtheria: severe pharyngitis with pseudomembrane formation, often spreads to the tonsils (tonsillitis), palate and uvula, indistinct speech, typical sweet-smelling breath, painful swelling of the cervical lymph nodes; bleeding into the pseudomembrane because of toxic vessel damage, sometimes progressive oedema ("bull neck").
Nasal diphtheria: sanguineous-serous unilateral or bilateral nasal discharge, encrustations (mainly in babies and infants).
Unusual localizations: conjunctiva, vulva, umbilical cord; skin/wounds (typical of tropical countries).
Laryngeal diphtheria (progressive form): hoarseness, barking cough, obstruction, inspiratory stridor ("diphtheritic croup"); descent of the pseudomembrane into the trachea and bronchi is possible; respiratory insufficiency with risk of asphyxia.

Post-infection toxin-induced complications
Cardiotoxicity: myocarditis (conduction system disorders and dysrhythmia), early deaths (week 1), late deaths (after about 6 weeks during convalescence);
Neurotoxicity: polyneuritis (n. facialis, n. recurrens, paresis generally with spontaneous recovery);
Nephrotoxicity: glomerulonephritis; also (rare): endocarditis, encephalitis, cerebral infarction, pulmonary embolism; lethal in 5 %–10 % of cases.

5   Special medical examination

Detection of infectious agent
Given clinical indications, laboratory diagnostic tests to be carried out: sub-pseudomembranous swab to detect pathogen *before* administration of antibiotics; demonstration of toxin-secreting strains in culture by means of toxin-PCR, followed by immunoprecipitation reaction (Elek immunoprecipitation test).

Detection of antibodies
To establish the vaccination status/susceptibility to infection: anamnesis of illnesses and vaccinations is not sufficient, inspection of vaccination documents required; demonstration of anti-diphtheria toxin antibodies in neutralization test.

6   Specific medical advice

Before exposure
Exposure prophylaxis: personal protective equipment: inhalation protection with filtering half mask (FFP2).
Disposition prophylaxis (vaccination): adsorbed diphtheria vaccine (i.m.); one dose at age 2, 3, 4 and 11–14 months, booster at age 5–6 and 9–17 years; preferably with combination vaccine (TD/Td), from age 5 or 6 years (according to the manufacturer's

instructions) boosters and basic vaccination with vaccine containing less diphtheria toxoid (d), generally in combination with tetanus toxoid and pertussis vaccine or other indicated antigens; booster for adults without titre control generally after 10 years, not sooner than 5 years after the previous dose; persons who have not been vaccinated should be given two doses at an interval of 4–8 weeks and a third dose 6–12 months after the second; protection is given at the earliest after the second vaccination dose; for persons with face-to-face contact with infected persons: booster as early as 5 years after the last vaccination; at each appointment for a Td booster the indication for a whooping cough vaccination should be checked and, if necessary, this included in the combination vaccine (Tdap); vaccination of unvaccinated adults who care for children is recommended.

After exposure
Isolation of infected persons; given clinical indications immediate administration of diphtheria antitoxin; available at present only from international apothecaries; never wait for the microbiological laboratory results; *medicinal prophylaxis* independent of vaccination status, e.g. with erythromycin for persons in close contact with contagious infected persons, for symptom-free carriers of toxin-producing strains, not before taking a swab, does not alter the effects of the toxin, but stops toxin synthesis (eradication), promotes antitoxin effect in persons with the disease.

7   Additional notes

Any national notification regulations and rules for avoiding infection are to be observed.

Dermatophytes (Mycosporum spp., Trichophyton spp., Epidermophyton floccosum)

1   Infectious agent

Infectious keratophilic Deuteromycetes, class Hyphomycetes, clinically relevant are *Microsporum* (M.) *audouinii, M. canis, M. gypseum, Trichophyton* (T.) *rubrum, T. mentagrophytes, T. tonsurans, T. verrucosum, T. schoenleinii, Epidermophyton* (E.) *floccosum;* classification in group 2 (A: potential allergenic effects), as defined in the Directive 2000/54/EC.

2   Occurrence

General
Ubiquitous in man and animals (mycozoonosis), e.g. pets, animals in animal shelters, laboratory animals, farm animals, animals bred for their fur (chinchilla, mink),

game, zoo animals, hedgehogs, wild birds (see table); *M. gypseum* (occurs naturally in soil) in swimming pools, saunas, sport and fitness centres.

Occupational
Farming, forestry, timber industry, gardening, animal dealers, the health service, reference centres, consulting laboratories, geriatric centres, body and beauty care (cos-
metic salons), hairdressing, centres for medical examinations, treatment and nursing
of children, care of pre-school children and young persons, and other communal facilities.

G 42

3   Transmission route, immunity

Pathogens with affinity for the skin (horny layer) and its appendages (hair, hair follicles, nails); transmission by *direct* contact with animals or *indirectly* via contaminated objects, soil or vectors such as arachnids (mites), insects (nits, fleas, flies); hair
follicles, dermal (micro-)lesions as entry points, favoured by alkaline skin pH/insuffi-
cient evaporation from the skin, increased sweating; no *immunity* but immune response in the form of a skin reaction of delayed type.

4   Symptoms

Incubation period 10–14 days (*M. audouinii*), for the other species probably a few
days; *contagious* until the foci have healed (skin scales, hair roots, nail chippings,
pus, blistered skin); hyphae and spores are infectious for years away from the body;
various kinds of dermatophytes can induce similar efflorescences; clinically they are
generally called "tinea" with the location.

Tinea corporis
Surface trichophytosis
Infection with, e.g., *T. rubrum* (40 %), *T. mentagrophytes* (14%), *T. verrucosum* (8%),
T. tonsurans (6%); disc-shaped sharply delimited, itching, red inflamed skin on body
parts with vellus hair, scaling at the edges.

Deep trichophytosis
Infection especially with *T. rubrum*, *T. mentagrophytes*, *T. verrucosum* most often in the
area of the scalp and beard (tinea barbae); deep follicular pustules; infiltration with
colliquations; tumour-like foci with scabs and purulent secretion from the follicles; local lymph node swelling.

Tinea pedis/manus
Infection especially with *T. rubrum*, *T. mentagrophytes*, *T. verrucosum*, *E. floccosum*
(rare);
Intertriginous form: infection of the clefts between the toes or fingers with weeping,
maceration, rhagades, itching; spreads to skin on the extensor side with blisters
along the edges;

squamous hyperkeratotic form: infection of the arch of the foot, palm of the hand and edges on both sides, tips of the toes and fingers; yellow-brownish scaling together with hyperkeratosis, rhagades formation, itching;
dyshidrotic form: infection of the arch of the foot, palm of the hand, spreading to neighbouring skin areas; very itchy blisters, sometimes coalescing, on reddish skin, with scaly edges.

Tinea inguinalis/cruris
Infection with, e.g., *E. floccosum, T. rubrum, T. mentagrophytes;* begins with brownish red spots which merge to form sharply delimited itching foci with weeping, scaly edges; inner sides of the thighs, other body regions which sweat (excessively) (genitoanal, axillary, submammary).

Tinea unguium (onychomycosis)
Infection with, e.g. *T. rubrum* (70 %–80 %), *T. mentagrophytes* (about 20 %), *T. tonsurans, E. floccosum* (about 2 %); begins distally/laterally at the free edge of the nail (toes, fingers); subungual hyperkeratosis (colonization of the nail matrix): whitish-yellowish keratin masses under splintering, crumbling nail plate.

Tinea capitis
Infection with *M. audouinii* (anthropophilic), *M. canis* (zoophilic) in cases of *microsporia;* particularly on the scalp of children: sharply delimited foci, with highly infectious, flour-like flaking scales ("as if covered in ash"), merging to polycyclic areas with broken hairs ("like a badly mown meadow"); heals spontaneously at the beginning of puberty; skin without hair, nails affected less often, also adults; in infections with *T. mentagrophytes, T. verrucosum,* for example, disc-shaped, inflamed, reddened scaly foci with single broken hairs, also purulent, spongiform infiltration (kerion).

Tinea favosa (favus/St. Aignon's disease)
Infection with *T. schoenleinii;* mostly localized on the scalp of children, occasionally on other sites (skin, nails); sulfur-yellow, crumbly, scutiform crusts (scutula), merging to flat, squamous scaly foci, penetrating mouse-like odour, hair follicle destruction, healing with scars and alopecia.

5   Special medical examination
Detection of infectious agent
In unclear cases material from skin eruptions can be examined in special laboratories; microscopy and identification of cultured fungi and their reproductive organs (spores).

Detection of antibodies
No serological methods for local mycosis in skin compartments, cutaneous test with group-specific antigens (trichophytin test) of no use in practice.

Dermatomycosis in man an animals (Microsporum spp.)

G 42

Localization	Microsporum audouinii	Microsporum canis	Microsporum gypseum	Trichophyton mentagrophytes	Trichophyton rubrum	Trichophyton tonsurans	Trichophyton verrucosum	Trichophyton schoenleinii	Epidermophyton floccosum
Comments	Central Europe, North America, West Africa, epidemic in schools and other communal facilities for children and young persons	30% of all cases of microsporia,	15% of all cases of dermatophytosis found worldwide, in the soil, common in gardeners	Central and Western Europe, North America; occurs naturally (also) in the soil	Central and Western Europe, North America	North and South America	The Balkans, North America, Near and Far East	Central and Eastern Europe, North America, Near East	rare everywhere in the world
other zoo animals		●		●			●		
goat		●		●			●		
game				●		●			
pig		●	●	●					
sheep		●		●			●		
cattle		●		●		●	●	●	
rat	●		●	●					
horse		●	●	●	●	●	●	●	
animals bred for fur		●		●					
poultry				●					
guinea pig	●	●	●	●	●	●	●		
mouse	●		●	●				●	
cat	●	●	●	●	●		●	●	
rabbit	●	●		●	●	●	●	●	
hedgehog		●		●					
dog	●	●	●	●	●		●	●	
golden hamster	●	●		●					
monkey	●	●	●	●					
man	●	●	●	●	●	●	●	●	●

6   Specific medical advice

Before exposure
Exposure prophylaxis: personal protective measures (protective clothing which covers the body) when handling animals (see table), especially if they have skin disorders; hygiene and pest control in buildings used for keeping animals; disinfection with fungicidal preparations, control of milieu factors (hyperhidrosis);
Disposition prophylaxis (vaccination) not available.

After exposure
For infected persons antimycotic therapy, topical (skin cream, nail varnish, lotion, spray, powder) and/or systemic with orally administered antibiotics with antimycotic activity.

7   Additional notes

Any national notification regulations are to be observed.

Ebola virus (viral haemorrhagic fever)

1   Infectious agent

Ebola virus, RNA virus, family Filoviridae; classification in group 4 as defined in the Directive 2000/54/EC.
Has been placed in category A on the list of potential bioterrorism agents by the US Center for Disease Control and Prevention (CDC).

2   Occurrence

General
Sporadic and epidemic appearances in the regions where it occurs; regionally restricted, especially in tropical areas; natural reservoir unknown; epidemics in Central Africa and Sudan; last outbreak December 2002 to May 2003 in Congo with 143 cases, of whom 129 died (53 % men); here gorillas and antelopes suspected as source of infection; infections described in primates and other mammals;

Occupational
Specialist centres (examination, treatment, nursing), pathology, research institutes, consulting laboratories, reference centres, animal keeping (monkeys), work in areas where the virus is endemic (during an outbreak antibodies found in about 30 % of physicians, 11 % of technical assistants, 10 % of nurses).

3   Transmission route, immunity

Transmission from monkey to man, otherwise very readily from person to person given close contact; aerogenic via infectious faecal particles in dust; also via contaminated objects, nosocomial and laboratory infections are possible; in survivors immunity persists probably for life.

4   Symptoms

Incubation period 7 days, very contagious; rapid temperature increase to 40°C, myalgia, endocardial bleeding, haemorrhage caused by direct involvement of the vessel endothelia, clotting disorders, bleeding in many organs including the CNS, relatively late in the gastrointestinal tract, pneumonia, shock caused by cardiocirculatory failure; fatal in about 90 % of cases (Zaire).

G 42

5   Special medical examination

Detection of infectious agent
Biopsy or autopsy specimens, blood (days 3–16 after the appearance of clinical symptoms); virus isolation (cell culture, animal tests) best method of diagnosis; rapid test by electron microscopy and serologically with the direct immunofluorescence test; antigen detection with capture-ELISA (antigen capture method), with molecular biological methods (reverse transcription PCR).

Detection of antibodies
ELISA (method of choice), immunofluorescence test, Western blot; IgM antibodies appear sometime between day 7 and day 30 (or later) of the illness, IgG antibodies between days 6 and 18, persist for years; proof of infection is a 4-fold increase in IgG antibody titre.

6   Specific medical advice

Before exposure
Exposure prophylaxis: waterproof protective clothing, particle-filtering half mask (FFP3); *Disposition prophylaxis* (vaccination) not available.

After exposure
Treatment of persons with the disease in special infection wards; disinfection with a new generation of disinfectants, so-called nanoemulsions (ATB). Specific hygienic measures during nursing and handling the pathogen laid down by specialists; when handling the pathogen intentionally maximum safety precautions (laboratories).

7   Additional notes

Any national notification and quarantine regulations are to be observed.

Epstein-Barr virus

1   Infectious agent

Epstein-Barr virus (EBV), DNA virus, family Herpetoviridae; classification in group 2 as defined in the Directive 2000/54/EC.

2   Occurrence

General

Infectious mononucleosis (glandular fever) worldwide, in Germany endemic infection level in young adults >95 %, in countries with low socio-economic status, the population is almost entirely infected with EBV in early childhood; EBV-associated Burkitt's lymphoma during childhood; endemic in regions where malaria is prevalent in Africa (incidence 0.3/100000), Latin America, New Guinea; spontaneous infections in adults in Europe and North America; EVB-associated nasopharynx carcinoma (Schmincke tumour), in Southeast Asia (incidence 10/100000), rare in Europe, in Germany 4 % of all malignant tumours; EBV-associated B cell lymphoma associated with immunosuppression.

Occupational

The health service, consulting laboratories, care of handicapped persons, facilities for medical treatment and nursing of children, care of pre-school children and young persons, geriatric facilities.

3   Transmission route, immunity

Excretion with saliva, semen, vaginal secretion of infected persons, in some cases life-long (20 %–30 %); transmission direct (kissing disease), aerogenic (droplet infection), via transplants, transfusions (EBV-containing B lymphocytes); risk of nosocomial infection; pathogenesis of tumour development not understood; long-lasting immunity, endogenic reactivation possible.

4   Symptoms

Incubation period (infectious mononucleosis) about 10–60 days in young people, 4–8 weeks in adults; contagious as long as virus is excreted, virus carriers with persistent EBV in the parotid gland (B lymphocytes); primary infection during childhood (younger than 5 years) rare (1:2000), later every second infection apparent; raised temperature, pharyngitis, tonsillitis, lymph node swelling (glandular fever), increased T lymphocyte count (mononuclear cells), more rarely hepatitis; complications include pneumonia, meningitis, meningoencephalitis, myocarditis, pericarditis, glomerulonephritis, polyradiculitis (Guillain-Barré syndrome); severe course (fatal in 70 % of cases) in persons with inherited or acquired immune defects; embryopathy possible, also reactivation as a side effect of other infections: Burkitt's lymphoma with EBV-specific components in tumour cells (cofactors); characteristic chromosome trans-location, B lymphocyte proliferation associated with defective proto-oncogene re-arrangement; Schmincke tumour with environmental cofactors (food components, microbiogenic substances); EBV-associated B cell lymphoma after application of cyclosporin A (organ transplantation), HIV infection, genetic immunosuppression with EBV-DNA in tumour cells (analogous situation in biopsies of Hodgkin lym-phomas), in this case the chromosome translocations typical of B lymphocytes are ab-sent.

5   Special medical examination

G 42

Detection of infectious agent
Direct detection (biopsy material, leukocytes) with Southern blot, molecular biologi-cal methods (PCR), *in situ* hybridization; from saliva via cultured umbilical cord lym-phocytes (rare).

Detection of antibodies
EBV infection detectable routinely only by serological methods, indirect immunofluo-rescence test (method of choice), ELISA; antibodies against various groups of virus antigens: virus capsule antigen (VCA), "early antigen" (EA), "Epstein-Barr nuclear antigen" (EBNA), make it possible to differentiate between new, past and reactivat-ed infections; may also be used to provide evidence of EBV-associated tumours, e.g. nasal pharynx carcinoma; course of the infection may be observed with molecular biological methods, with quantitative EBV-PCR.

6   Specific medical advice

Before exposure
Exposure prophylaxis: general hygienic and disinfection measures;
Disposition prophylaxis (vaccination) not available; subunit vaccine is being tested (animal model).

After exposure
Medicinal therapy (nucleoside analogues) affects productive infection, does not re-duce the number of circulating B lymphocytes.

7   Additional notes

Any national notification regulations are to be observed.

Escherichia coli

1   Infectious agent

Escherichia (E.) coli, Gram-negative rods, motile, sometimes with capsule; non-pathogenic strains or facultative pathogens (opportunists) (physiological intestinal flora); enterohaemorrhagic strains (EHEC) are obligate pathogens; also other strains are intestinal pathogens (*E. coli* enteritis), classification as defined in the Directive 2000/54/EC in group 2: *E. coli* (apart from non-pathogenic strains); group 3: *E. coli* (EHEC).
Has been placed in category B on the list of potential bioterrorism agents by the US Center for Disease Control and Prevention (CDC).

2   Occurrence

General
E. coli strains which are facultative pathogens (opportunists) (outside the intestines):
ubiquitous, animals, man, all age groups especially babies, immunodeficient persons, in persons with obstructions of the efferent urinary passages or bile duct, paraplegics, persons with indwelling bladder catheters (after 3 days urinary tract infections in 90 % of cases), cholelithiasis cases, artificially ventilated patients (pneumonia), after burns, colon surgery (peritonitis) or other operative measures (wound infection).

Enterohaemorrhagic E. coli strains (EHEC infection):
pathovar EHEC: worldwide, endemic in industrial countries, ruminants as reservoir, pathogens enter the human food chain via foodstuffs and drinking water; *outbreaks* in communal facilities, homes; in the year 2000 in Germany 1088 registered EHEC cases, of those 764 persons with the illness and 324 carriers; *nosocomial infection* (multiresistant strains),

Other E. coli strains which are intestinal pathogens (E. coli enteritis):
endemic, epidemic in warm climatic zones, regions with low socio-economic/hygienic standards, frequent infections in babies and infants, sporadic in tourists (travellers' diarrhoea); man is the only carrier.

Occupational
The health service, care of handicapped persons including supply and service areas of these institutions (e.g. room cleaning services), research institutes, laboratories, consulting laboratories, reference centres, paediatrics, care of pre-school children, food industry, canteens, waterworks, water supply and distribution, sewage works, sludge usage, work in areas where the organism is endemic; veterinary medicine, animal breeding units, zoological gardens (EHEC).

3   Transmission route, immunity

E. coli strains which are facultative pathogens (opportunists):
indirect infection, formation of chains of infection also for nosocomial infections, i.e.
via hands/objects as vehicle; no *immunity.*

Enterohaemorrhagic E. coli strains (EHEC infection):
pathovar EHEC *alimentary infection* via contaminated foodstuffs, drinking water; *indirect infection* via hands, objects, faecal-oral via bathing in contaminated water; via
contact with carriers, infected animals (children's zoos), on farms; no *immunity.*

G 42

Other E. coli strains which are intestinal pathogens (E. coli enteritis):
alimentary infection, faecal-oral, *indirect infection.*

4   Symptoms

E. coli strains which are facultative pathogens (opportunists):
Localized processes: most common agent of urinary tract infections, infections pre-
venting wound healing, pneumonia (artificially ventilated persons), cholangitis, cholecystitis, appendicitis, peritonitis; especially in immunodeficient persons.
Generalized processes: septicaemia (in 30 % of the Gram-negative isolates from
blood culture); spread from infected urinary passages, bile ducts, abscesses; septic
endotoxin shock: raised temperature, blood clotting disorders, drop in blood pressure, vessel and tissue damage, irreversible organ failure *(Waterhouse-Friderichsen
syndrome);* often fatal.

Enterohaemorrhagic E. coli strains (EHEC infection):
Incubation period 1–3 (8) days; *contagious* as long as the pathogen is detectable in
the stool, generally 5–10 (20) days; infections range from inapparent to manifest illness (about 30 %): mild watery diarrhoea (duration 7–10 days); in 10 % to 20 % of
cases (babies, infants, immunodeficient persons) severe course with raised temperature, blood in the watery stools (enterohaemorrhagic colitis); extra-intestinal (5 % to
10 % of cases) haemolytic-uraemic syndrome (HUS), fatal in 2 % to 10 % of cases;
thrombotic-thrombocytopenic purpura (TTP).

Other E. coli strains which are intestinal pathogens (E. coli enteritis):
EPEC (enteropathogen); *incubation period* 12 hours to 6 days; *contagious* as long
as the agent is detectable in the stool, acute sometimes life-threatening diarrhoea
with mushy/watery stool, risk of desiccation, fatal in 25 % to 50 % of cases.
ETEC (enterotoxigenic): *incubation period* 6–48 hours, *contagious* as long the agent
is detectable in the stool, all age groups, travellers' diarrhoea, watery diarrhoea
(cholera-like), course limited to a few days, may be self-limiting.
EIEC (enteroinvasive): *incubation period* 2–4 days; *contagious* as long the agent is
detectable in the stool, all age groups, enterocolitis, generally febrile, milder than
Shigella dysentery, often self-limiting (after some days).

EAggEC (enteroaggregative): *contagious* as long as the agent is detectable in the stool, frequently the course is prolonged (> 14 days), watery or slimy diarrhoea rarely containing blood.
DAEC (diffuse adherent): *contagious* as long as the agent is detectable in the stool, watery diarrhoea (> 14 days).

5 Special medical examination

Detection of infectious agent
Depending on the pathovar involved, culture from stool, urine, aspirate, wound swab, sputum; blood culture, nutrient broth and solid medium, biochemical differentiation, antibiotic resistance pattern.

Detection of toxin
Shiga toxin ELISA (EHEC), Shiga toxin PCR, Vero cell cytotoxicity assay (for screening at least two methods; Shiga toxin detection essential).

Detection of antibodies
Indicated in cases of systemic infection (suspected haemolytic-uraemic syndrome, thrombotic thrombocytopenic purpura).

6 Specific medical advice

Before exposure
Exposure prophylaxis: hygienic measures during care of patients, production/consumption of food and drinks; explanation of chains of infection (highly infectious), isolation of patients (infected with EHEC), identification of carriers; hygienic disinfection of hands; antibiotic prophylaxis (controversial), e.g. with fluoroquinolone antibiotics (brief period in an area where the organism is endemic); appropriate technical and organizational protective measures (laboratories and similar establishments);
Disposition prophylaxis (vaccination) not available.

After exposure
E. coli strains which are facultative pathogens (opportunists): *medicinal therapy* according to the antibiogram; aminopenicillins, ureidopenicillins, cephalosporins, carbapenems, quinilones, co-trimoxazole; in cases of sepsis initial treatment with wide spectrum antibiotics (cephalosporins (3rd generation), aminoglycosides, carbapenems), then further treatment according to the results of the antibiogram.
Enterohaemorrhagic E. coli strains (EHEC infection): pathovar EHEC: *medicinal therapy* (antibiotics) not indicated, makes the illness worse, can stimulate toxin formation, increases the frequency of haemolytic-uraemic syndrome, can delay elimination of the bacteria; replace lost fluids and electrolytes; in haemolytic-uraemic syndrome, thrombotic thrombocytopenic purpura symptomatic treatment: forced diuresis, haemodialysis, peritoneal dialysis.

Other E. coli strains which are intestinal pathogens (E. coli enteritis): illness (gastroenteritis) generally self-limiting; replace fluids and electrolytes as recommended by the WHO; if necessary additional *medicinal therapy* if the pathovar is EPEC, in severe cases administration of antibiotics (antibiogram); for infections with the pathovar ETEC antibiotics (e.g. fluoroquinolones) shorten the diarrhoeal phase; for the pathovar EIEC generally no antibiotic therapy; pathovar EAggEC rare, fluid replacement necessary, danger of development of multiple antibiotic resistance; for the pathovar DAEC no antibiotic therapy.

7   Additional notes

Any national notification regulations and restrictions on activities and employment are to be observed.

Hantavirus, Hantaan virus (Korean haemorrhagic fever virus)

1   Infectious agent

Hantavirus, RNA virus, various genetically characterized groups (species) correspond to defined serotypes (Hantaan, Puumala, Seoul, Dobrava); family Bunyaviridae; classification in group 3 (Hantaan, Seoul, Dobrava, Sin Nombre serotypes) and group 2 (Puumala serotype) as defined in the Directive 2000/54/EC.
Has been placed in category C on the list of potential bioterrorism agents by the US Center for Disease Control and Prevention (CDC).

2   Occurrence

General
Worldwide (Seoul serotype); in individual countries sporadic, endemic, epidemic; haemorrhagic fever with renal syndrome (HFRS), about 90 % of Hantavirus infections are in Asia (Russia, China, Korea), about 10 % in Europe; Hantaan serotype mainly in Southeast Asia, Southern Europe, Eastern Russia; Puumala serotype in Central and Northern Europe up to 3 % of Hantavirus infections, Dobrava serotype mainly in South-eastern Europe, the Balkans (coexists with the Puumala serotype); HFRS, HPS (hantavirus pulmonary syndrome) annually in the world a total of 200000–300000 cases; in Germany seroprevalence between 1 % and 2 % (normal population) and about 6 % (farmers), 143 cases (2003); areas where the virus is endemic: Baden-Württemberg, North Rhine-Westphalia, Mecklenburg-West Pomerania, Berlin-Brandenburg, Bavaria; in Southern and Western Germany mainly Puumala, in Northern and Eastern Germany Dobrava. Natural hosts (pathogen reservoir) rodents in the wild (also laboratory animals): inapparent, persistent infections in the striped field mouse *(Apodemus agrarius)*, yellow-necked mouse *(Apodemus flavicollis)* (Hantaan serotype), bank

vole *(Clethrionomys glareolus)* or red-backed vole *(Myodes glareolus)* (Puumala sero-type), brown rat *(Rattus norvegicus)*, black rat *(Rattus rattus)* (Seoul virus), yellow-necked mouse (Dobrava serotype), white footed mouse (Peromyscus leucopus) (Sin Nombre serotype), population dynamics subject to a 3-year to 4-year cycle, with periodic out-breaks of the disease; serotypes specifically associated with certain species of rodent.

Occupational
Farming, forestry, wool spinning mills, animal-keeping (rodents), sewage works, waste disposal and recycling, laboratories, consulting laboratories.

3   Transmission route, immunity

Excretions, secretions (faeces, urine, saliva) from infected rodents infectious for some days; aerogenic infection mostly as dust infection, alimentary via contaminated food-stuffs, rarely via bites; antibody response with maximum within a few weeks, persis-tence for many years, probably for life.

4   Symptoms

Haemorrhagic fever with renal syndrome (HFRS)
Incubation period 4–42 days; *contagiousness* from person to person unclear, only 5 % to10 % of cases clinically apparent; most common in the age group between 20 and 40 years, more often in men; severe disease caused by the serotypes Han-taan, Seoul, Dobrava; acute initial febrile phase (duration 3–4 days, influenza-like symptoms), after 3–6 days colic-like pain, functional renal disorder progresses to re-nal insufficiency requiring dialysis; hypotensive phase results from increased vessel permeability and can lead to shock symptoms; with the Hantaan serotype haemor-rhage, in 80 % of cases visceral, intravascular clotting with diffuse intravascular co-agulation; fatal in 4 %–6 % of cases; convalescence characterized by polyuric phase (daily max. 6 litres, duration up to 3 months); extrarenal manifestations possible: concomitant hepatitis, myocarditis, thyreoiditis, involvement of the lungs and CNS.

Nephropathia epidemica
Incubation period 2–5 weeks; mostly mild HFRS variants in Central Europe (Puumala serotype), morbidity 20 cases/100000 inhabitants (Finland); haemorrhage-related complications are rare, fatal in <1 % of cases, but severe pulmonary syndrome-like disorders are possible.

Hantavirus pulmonary syndrome (HPS)
Incubation period 10–21 days, severe manifestation form of the hantavirus infection without involvement of the kidneys; no asymptomatic or mild cases; prodromal phase 2–3 days, sudden increase in temperature, feeling severely ill, myalgia, gastroin-testinal symptoms, rapidly developing bilateral interstitial pneumonia, hypoxaemia, non-cardiac pulmonary oedema; blood count triad: leukocytosis with shift to the left, atypical blast cell-like lymphocytes, thrombocytopenia; fatal in 60 %–70 % of cases.

5   Special medical examination

When infection is suspected, confirmation requires a positive result with at least one of the following methods:

Detection of infectious agent
Virus isolation, detection of virus genome-specific sequences, e.g. by reverse transcription PCR (during the acute phase of the illness).

Detection of antibodies
Serological detection of IgG antibodies, e.g. with the indirect haemagglutination test, ELISA; if necessary subsequent serotype-specific serodiagnosis (neutralization test); marked cross-reactions between Hantaan and Dobrava serotypes, rarely with Puumala serotype.

G 42

6   Specific medical advice

Before exposure
Exposure prophylaxis: in regions where the disease is endemic, rigorous control especially of rodents, avoid contact (gloves, particle filter mask FFP2); when handling the pathogen in laboratories observance of appropriate safety measures;
Disposition prophylaxis (vaccination): inactivated whole virus vaccine (Southeast Asia) and recombinant vaccine (Europe, USA) are being developed or tested.

After exposure
Therapy only possible when persons become ill: for HFRS mainly symptomatic treatment: maintain stability of circulatory system, short-term haemodialysis, in cases of HPS also oxygen supply; in severe cases of HFRS early antiviral medicinal therapy (ribavirin).

7   Additional notes

Any national notification regulations and restrictions on activities and employment are to be observed.

Helicobacter pylori

1   Infectious agent

Helicobacter pylori, Gram-negative, motile, non-sporulating bacillus, binds to blood group 0 antigen (parietal cells in the stomach);
Classification in group 2 as defined in the Directive 2000/54/EC.

2   Occurrence

General
Worldwide, man is the only pathogen reservoir, habitats are stomach compartments (mucous membranes, mucous); infection during childhood, persists (without treatment) life-long; in developing countries high endemic infection (80 % in 20-year-olds); in Germany prevalence increases continually with age, reaches a peak of 50 %–60 % among 60 to 70-year-olds; high population density and crowding favour infection.

Occupational
Research institutes (where stomach biopsy specimens, stomach aspirates and faeces are handled), reference centres, laboratories, endoscopy units in gastroenterology departments; dental medicine.

3   Transmission route, immunity

Presumably faecal-oral (indirect infection) and/or oral-oral; stomach secretions, stomach biopsy specimens, dental plaque, faeces are considered to be infectious materials; local and systemic immunity develops without effective elimination of the pathogen.

4   Symptoms

Incubation period and duration of *contagiousness* unknown; mostly no symptoms or uncharacteristic epigastric symptoms, for which reason acute infections are rarely diagnosed.

Chronic active (atrophic) gastritis
Persistent infection of the mucosa associated with atrophic (antral) gastritis, in 80 % of cases caused by *H. pylori*; granulocytic, later monocytic epithelial infiltration, favoured by: genetic predisposition (blood group 0), environment (diet, stress).

Gastroduodenal peptic ulcer
75 %–80 % of all stomach ulcers and 95 % of all duodenal ulcers are caused by *H. pylori* infection.

Malignant gastric tumour
55 %–60 % of gastric adenocarcinomas result from chronic *H. pylori* infection; in combination with ulcus ventriculi the risk factor is 1.8, with ulcus duodeni 0.6; development of a B cell lymphoma (MALT lymphoma) is possible.

5   Special medical examination

Detection of infectious agent
If necessary, PCR to detect *H. pylori* DNA; biopsy material: rapid urease test, culture of pathogen (makes it possible to determine antibiotic resistance); further tests for screening and follow-up: ^{13}C-urea breath test, stool antigen test (to check the success of eradication therapy).

Detection of antibodies
To establish susceptibility to infection, detection of anti-Helicobacter IgG antibodies in serum with an immunoblot technique (Western blot) or ELISA as the most reliable screening and rapid diagnosis method, diagnostic significance of IgM and IgA detection is low.

G 42

6   Specific medical advice

Before exposure
Exposure prophylaxis: personal protective equipment: waterproof protective clothing, particle-filtering half mask (FFP2); general hygienic and disinfection measures; *Disposition prophylaxis* (vaccination) not available.

After exposure
Eradication therapy as 7-day combined (triple) therapy: antisecretory (proton pump inhibitor), antimicrobial (macrolide antibiotic and aminopenicillin or metronidazole preparation); follow-up of eradication success: ^{13}C-urea breath test, stool antigen test, serological test methods not suitable.

7   Additional notes

Any national notification regulations are to be observed.

Hepatitis A virus (HAV)

1   Infectious agent

Hepatitis A virus (HAV), RNA virus, family Picornaviridae;
classification in group 2 as defined in the Directive 2000/54/EC.

2   Occurrence

General
Worldwide, sporadic and epidemic outbreaks; high endemic infection level in Mediterranean countries and in the Third World (100 % at age 10 years); in Western, Central and Northern Europe infection levels have been sinking for years; currently <4 % in Germany in persons under 30 years of age.

Occupational
Homes for the handicapped, children's wards, stool laboratories, consulting laboratories, sewage works, sewers, research institutes, the health service (especially paediatrics, treatment of infections, other specialist staff and nurses, kitchen staff, cleaners), prisons, work in areas where the organism is endemic.

3   Transmission route, immunity

Faecal-oral; contagious from 7–14 days before the beginning of the illness until the symptoms begin to abate, life-long immunity.

4   Symptoms

Incubation period 20–40 days; *contagious* from 7–14 days before the beginning of the illness until it reaches its peak; uncharacteristic prodromes, primarily cholestatic course possible in adults, increased transaminase levels for about 2 months, does not become chronic, fulminant forms <1 %, rarely fatal; risk of abortion, early births, and stillbirths.

5   Special medical examination

Detection of infectious agent
HAV antigen in stool (ELISA), molecular biological methods (PCR) possible but not significant in routine diagnosis.

Detection of antibodies
To determine vaccination status/susceptibility to infection, anamnesis of illnesses and vaccinations not sufficient, inspection of vaccination documents required; virological diagnosis generally by means of anti-HAV determination in persons over 40 years of age or from areas with increased incidence; HAV-antigen (ELISA) in stool or HAV-RNA (PCR) in stool and blood demonstrate new infection, antibody assays after vaccination not necessary.

6   Specific medical advice

Before exposure
Exposure prophylaxis: personal protective equipment: if necessary, waterproof protective clothing, general hygienic and disinfection measures;

Disposition prophylaxis (vaccination) with killed vaccine recommended if indicated by risk situation, vaccination of previously unvaccinated adults caring for children or older persons recommended; basis vaccination and booster (HA) according to the manufacturer's recommendations; a previous test for anti-HAV antibodies makes sense in persons born before 1950, in persons for whom anamnesis suggests HA or who have lived for longer periods in areas where the organism is endemic.

After exposure
Disposition prophylaxis (vaccination) also makes sense immediately after exposure; administration of standard immunoglobulin is possible (passive immunization) as prophylaxis during outbreaks of hepatitis A or when (contact) persons are exposed; if necessary, immunoglobulin preparations can be given at the same time as the first vaccination dose (active-passive immunization); mass vaccinations appropriate especially in homes and schools.

G 42

7   Additional notes

Any national notification regulations and restrictions on activities and employment are to be observed.

Hepatitis B virus (HBV)

1   Infectious agent

Hepatitis B virus (HBV), DNA virus, family Hepadnaviridae;
classification in group 3(**) as defined in the Directive 2000/54/EC.

2   Occurrence

General
Worldwide, endemic infection level (anti-HBc positive) in Central Europe 5 %–10 %, in Germany 7 %, medical personnel in high risk areas up to 30 %, in Third World countries, in Southern and South-eastern Europe >50 %; chronic infections 0.6 % (HBsAg positive) in Central Europe up to 2 %, in Third World countries up to 20 %, in Southern and South-eastern Europe up to 5 %; groups with higher levels of infection include:
- i.v. drug addicts up to 80 %
- mentally retarded persons in institutions
- homosexuals
- prisoners up to 60 %
- prostitutes up to 30 %.

Occupational
The health service, care of handicapped persons including supply and service areas of these institutions, emergency and rescue services, pathology, research institutes, consulting laboratories, prisons; homes and day care centres for the elderly, outpatient nursing services, especially when handling body fluids and working with tools which can cause injuries or handling aggressive patients; work in sewage works if there is a danger of injury from injection needles (drug addicts' equipment); manufacture of medical products.

3   Transmission route, immunity
Parenterally via body fluids (mainly blood and blood products from virus carriers), occupationally mainly via pricks and cuts, in about 10 % virus resistance, otherwise life-long immunity.

4   Symptoms
Incubation period 2–6 months; duration of *contagiousness* variable, correlates with detectable HBs antigen (persistent in 10 % usually for years), in many cases few or no symptoms;
acute cholestatic, but also fulminant courses with liver failure, fatal in 1 %–2 % of cases;
progresses to chronic hepatitis in 10 % of cases (also when the disease is not clinically manifest);
Forms of chronic hepatitis B:
• asymptomatic carrier of HBsAg
• chronic persistent hepatitis B
• chronic active hepatitis B
• HBV-associated liver cirrhosis
• primary liver cell carcinoma.
HDV super-infection of the HBsAg carrier is possible.

5   Special medical examination
Detection of infectious agent
Direct electron microscopy (Dane particles); culture of virus difficult; detection of virus components: HBsAg, HBeAg (biopsy material/serum) by means of ELISA; DNA hybridization; by *molecular biological methods:* amplification techniques (PCR, ligase chain reaction).

Detection of antibodies
To establish the susceptibility to infection, anamnesis of illnesses and vaccinations not sufficient, inspection of vaccination documents required; determination of anti-HBc; if anti-HBc negative, no further diagnostics; if anti-HBc positive, determination of HBsAg and anti-HBs (quantitatively); if HBsAg positive, determination of HBeAg and

anti-HBe; to check the success of vaccination quantitative determination of anti-HBs (via vaccination documents or antibody assay).

6   Specific medical advice

Before exposure
Exposure prophylaxis: safe sharps; goggles when there is a risk of blood spattering, hygienic and disinfection measures, impenetrable safety boxes for disposal of contaminated injection needles, scalpels, etc;
Disposition prophylaxis (vaccination): hepatitis B vaccination according to the recommendations of the manufacturer, generally after serological tests; if the person is anti-HBc negative, basis vaccination at intervals of 0, 1 and 6 months recommended; 4 weeks after completed basis vaccination the success of the immunization should be checked (anti-HBs quantitative), also in immunodeficient persons; booster according to the antibody titre achieved at this time, for anti-HBs levels ≥100 IU/l a booster (1 dose) generally 10 years after completion of the basis vaccination is sufficient; for anti-HBs levels <100 IU/l repeat vaccination (1 dose) immediately, check antibody titre after 4 weeks (60 %–75 % of non-responders and low responders react with a sufficient increase in antibody titre after up to 3 additional vaccinations or combination vaccinations with other vaccines).
Record anti-HBs titre in the vaccination document; vaccination against hepatitis B protects simultaneously against hepatitis D infection; refusal to be vaccinated should be recorded in writing but is not a cause for occupational medical concern.

After exposure
For pricks and cuts with injection needles: promote bleeding, clean the wound immediately under running water and with soap, then disinfect the area with a skin disinfectant effective against viruses or alternatively clean the contaminated area of skin or mucous membrane thoroughly with water or a 20 % to 30 % alcoholic solution (oral mucosa).

Active-passive immunization

Postexposure Hepatitis B immunoprophylaxis

| current anti-HBs value | neccesary is the administration of | |
	HB vaccine	anti-HB-immunglobulin
≥ 100 IU/l	no	no
≥ 10 to < 100 IU/l	yes	no
< 10 IU/l	yes	yes
not to be determined within 48 hours	yes	yes

G 42

Estimation of the infection risk associated with HBsAg carriers: the presence of HBeAg is indicative of high infectivity, presence of anti-HBe is indicative of low infectivity, it is also possible to determine HBV-DNA; infective employees should be advised as to their behaviour at the workplace and the risk of infection of associates; infectivity plays no role in the occupational medical assessment.

7   Additional notes

Any national notification regulations are to be observed.

Hepatitis C virus (HCV)

1   Infectious agent

Hepatitis C virus (HCV), RNA virus, family Flaviviridae;
classification in group 3(**) as defined in the Directive 2000/54/EC.

2   Occurrence

General
Anti-HCV prevalence up to 1.5 % in Western Europe and North America, about 0.4 % in Germany, 1 %–3 % in the Middle East and parts of Asia, 10 %–20 % in Central Africa and Egypt; groups with higher endemic infection levels: haemophiliacs up to 90 %, haemodialysis patients 10 %–40 %, i.v. drug addicts up to 80 %; also prisoners 12 %, sexual partners, medical personnel 0.8 %; preliminary data reveal higher prevalence of seropositive results among dialysis personnel.

Occupational
The health service, care of handicapped persons including supply and service areas of these institutions, emergency and rescue services, pathology, research institutes, laboratories, reference centres, prisons; homes and day-care centres for the elderly, outpatient nursing services, especially when handling body fluids and working with tools which can cause injuries or handling aggressive patients; work in sewage works if there is a danger of injury from injection needles (drug addicts' equipment); manufacture of medical products.

3   Transmission route, immunity

Parenteral via body fluids (mainly blood and blood products from virus carriers, sexual contact), via pricks and cuts at the workplace, contamination of eyes and mucous membranes (the virus can actively penetrate mucosa). In 30 %–40 % of cases the transmission route is unknown.

4   Symptoms

Incubation period about 50 days (21–84 days); almost all anti-HCV positive persons are *contagious*;
Forms of the disease:
- clinically inapparent hepatitis C
- acute infection with influenza-like symptoms
- icterus rather unusual
- chronic hepatitis C (up to 80 %), mostly insidious with mild symptoms;

Cases of chronic hepatitis C have a high risk of developing liver cirrhosis (about 20 %, latency period 20 to 30 years) with progression to primary liver cell carcinoma even for inapparent infections.

G 42

5   Special medical examination

Detection of infectious agent
To date no known way of culturing the virus; detection of virus components: PCR to detect (sections of) the RNA in serum/EDTA-blood, blood lymphocytes, biopsy material (liver); branched DNA (bDNA, reverse transcription PCR (quantitative methods); genome typing by restriction fragment length polymorphism (RFLP); anti-HCV antibody confirmation test (antibody populations against various HCV proteins).

Detection of antibodies
To establish the susceptibility to infection: ELISA, Western blot.
Note: in the acute phase infection not detectable serologically (diagnostic window period).

6   Specific medical advice

Before exposure
Exposure prophylaxis: safe sharps; goggles when there is a risk of blood spattering, hygienic and disinfection measures, impenetrable safety boxes for disposal of contaminated injection needles, scalpels, etc;
Disposition prophylaxis (vaccination) or passive immunization not available.

After exposure
For pricks and cuts with injection needles or sharps: promote bleeding, clean the wound immediately under running water and with soap, then disinfect the area with a skin disinfectant effective against viruses or alternatively clean the contaminated area of skin or mucous membrane thoroughly with water or a 20 % to 30 % alcoholic solution (oral mucosa).
In persons who are anti-HCV positive, HCV-RNA determination by PCR is possible; PCR and determination of the HCV genotype for diagnosis and for checking success of therapy with alpha-interferon.

Antiviral therapy combined with peginterferon in the early phase of the illness results in permanent virus elimination in up to 80 % of cases. Not suitable for post-exposure prophylaxis.

7 Additional notes

Any national notification regulations are to be observed.

Hepatitis D virus (HDV)

1 Infectious agent

Hepatitis D virus or delta virus (HDV), defective RNA virus, family Hepadnaviridae; for replication requires HBsAg of the hepatitis B virus (HBV); classification in group 3(**) as defined in the Directive 2000/54/EC.

2 Occurrence

General
Worldwide, occurs only together with HBV; high prevalence in Eastern and Southern Europe (especially Italy), the countries along the Nile and northern South America (especially the Amazon region) and Asia; in Germany prevalence under 1 %; in drug addicts about 40 %, dialysis patients 0.4 %, in persons with chronic HBV infection 1.7 %, to date detected rarely in persons with acute hepatitis B infection.

Occupational
The health service, care of handicapped persons including supply and service areas of these institutions, emergency and rescue services, pathology, research institutes, consulting laboratories, prisons; homes and day care centres for the elderly, outpatient nursing services, especially when handling body fluids and working with tools which can cause injuries or handling aggressive patients; work in sewage works if there is a danger of injury from injection needles (drug addicts' equipment); manufacture of medical products.

3 Transmission route, immunity

Analogous to hepatitis B, transmission route parenteral, sexual and perinatal; direct body contact has been suggested, immunity to HBV also protects from HDV.

4   Symptoms
A defective virus which is dependent on the presence of HBV for replication;
Co-infection: initially HBsAg detectable, three weeks later as a sign of the simultaneous infection HD-Ag; suppression of HBV replication in some cases of simultaneous infection can give the impression of an HbsAg-negative hepatitis; often biphasic course, fulminant in up to 5 % of cases, becomes chronic in 5 % to 10 %; course of the coinfection generally more complex and protracted.
Super-infection: HD-Ag detectable about three weeks after infection;
Total *incubation period* for co-infection 12 to 15 weeks, 3 weeks for super-infection of a person suffering from chronic hepatitis B; *contagious* for HBsAG-positive persons with super-infection or co-infection; fulminant in 30 % to 60 %, becomes chronic in 70 % to 90 %; when screening blood donations residual risk of HDV infection 1:3000 (HBsAg-negative hepatitis B).

G 42

5   Special medical examination
Detection of infectious agent
Detection of virus components: in persons coinfected with HBV detection of HDV-RNA by hybridization (Northern blot), reverse transcription PCR; during acute phase more reliable than anti-HDV (serum); detection of HDV-RNA to monitor chronic HDV infections and antiviral therapy not usual as routine methods: detection of HDV-antigen in liver biopsy material (direct immunofluorescence test), serum (ELISA) after destruction of the HBsAg-envelope with detergents.

Detection of antibodies
To establish the susceptibility to infection: as for hepatitis B. If HbsAg positive, HD-Ag and anti-HDV should be determined by means of radioimmunoassay or ELISA; RNA hybridization to detect the HDV genome, Western blot to determine the HDV antigenicity; repeat regularly in HBs-positive persons to exclude the possibility of a superinfection.

6   Specific medical advice
Before exposure
Exposure prophylaxis: personal protective equipment; hygienic and disinfection measures;
Disposition prophylaxis (vaccination) for persons negative for anti-HBc, hepatitis B vaccination;

After exposure
As for hepatitis B including HDV diagnosis; specific therapy not available.

7　　　　Additional notes

Any national notification regulations and restrictions on activities and employment are to be observed.

Human cytomegalovirus (HCMV)

1　　　　Infectious agent

Human cytomegalovirus (HCMV) synonym human herpesvirus type 5 (HHV-5), DNA virus, family Herpetoviridae, mainly cell-bound virus; classification in group 2 as defined in the Directive 2000/54/EC.

2　　　　Occurrence

General
Worldwide, prevalence in industrial countries (40 %–70 %), in the Third World up to 100 %, levels of infection increase with age, infection levels in industrial countries increase in two phases: during the first 2–3 years of life as a result of perinatal and early postnatal infection, in youths and adults as a result of sexual contacts.

Occupational
The health service, consulting laboratories, care of handicapped persons, facilities for medical examination, treatment and nursing of children, care of pre-school children, geriatric facilities.

3　　　　Transmission route, immunity

Indirect infection, contact infection (mucosa), sexual transmission; transplacental, most frequent intrauterine infection (1 % of all newborn babies), mostly latent infection (virus persists in the body mostly for life in 40 %–50 % of all women); iatrogenic/parenteral (transmitted during 0.4 %–4 % of transfusions and 28 %–57 % of transplantations); transmission via blood, blood products, secretions, semen, saliva, urine, mother's milk; life-long virus persistence, reactivation possible at any time.

4　　　　Symptoms

Incubation period variable, after blood transfusion 2–6 weeks, after primary infection 4–12 weeks; mostly clinically inapparent course after acquired, not intrauterine infection; when clinically apparent, mononucleosis-like symptoms: clinical manifestation dependent on age and immune status of the person; progression to latent phase, illness as primary infection or reactivation; connatal CMV syndrome, especially in cases of primary infection of the mother during pregnancy; foetal infection in 40 %

of first infections during pregnancy, foetal damage in 10 % of these; in young persons mononucleosis-like course, lymphadenopathy for 1–4 weeks; after transfusions, posttransfusion mononucleosis syndrome (haemolytic anaemia, monocytosis, increase in transaminase levels); in the age group between 25 and 35 years often only local infections in immunocompetent persons.

Generalized cytomegaly, especially in immunosuppressed patients (AIDS-defining conditions 1993), then high temperature, pharyngitis, cervical adenopathy, hepatosplenomegaly, hepatitis, lymphocytosis, myocarditis, encephalomeningitis, interstitial pneumonia, leukocytopenia, thrombocytopenia, oesophagitis, colitis, retinitis; reactivation factors not well known, mainly associated with immunosuppression, during pregnancy in 10 %–30 % of infected seropositive women. Reactivation results in virus excretion (saliva, urine), in immunocompetent persons no symptoms; children infected after reactivation of the infection in the mother (10 % of all seropositive mothers) in 1 % of children (only 1 % of infected children have symptoms, mostly only mild).

G 42

5   Special medical examination

Detection of infectious agent
Urine, blood, throat lavage fluid; *culture:* cell culture, perhaps rapid culture (within 24–72 hours), *molecular biological methods:* DNA detection; in infected pregnant women or immunosuppressed patients primary infections can be distinguished from reactivated infections by determination of anti-HCMV IgG avidity.

Detection of antibodies
To establish the susceptibility to infection of blood and organ donors, immunosuppressed patients, women of child-bearing age, pregnant women (ELISA, neutralization test, immunofluorescence test); IgM antibodies in primary infections/reactivated infections and IgG antibodies after infection (note: passively transmitted antibodies) offer no protection from endogenous reactivation or exogenous new infection.

6   Specific medical advice

Before exposure
Exposure prophylaxis: avoid close contact with small children, repeated titre checks during pregnancy of seronegative mothers;
Disposition prophylaxis (vaccination): vaccine currently being tested; in pregnant women working in the health service determination of antibody status in the 1st trimester recommended, check-up during trimester 2–3 (by the woman's gynaecologist); anti-CMV-negative pregnant women and immunosuppressed persons should be informed about the potential risk when handling dialysis and immunosuppressed patients.

After exposure
Hyperimmunoglobulin, perhaps antiviral substances (aciclovir).

7   Additional notes

Any national notification regulations are to be observed.

Human immunodeficiency virus

1   Infectious agent

Human immunodeficiency virus (HIV-1 and HIV-2), RNA virus, family Retroviridae; classification in group 3(**) as defined in the Directive 2000/54/EC.

2   Occurrence

General

HIV-1 worldwide, HIV-2 endemic all over the world, 40 million infected persons, 72 % of those in Africa south of the Sahara, in Germany about 49000, of whom about 750 die annually (data from January 2006).

Risk groups:

- homosexuals (about 61 % of new infections)
- i.v. drug adducts (about 15 % of new infections)
- heterosexual contacts (about 4 % of new infections)

Occupational

The health service, reference centres, care of handicapped persons including service sector (e.g. cleaning), emergency and rescue services, pathology, prisons.

3   Transmission route, immunity

During sexual contact (about 71 % of new infections), via blood and blood products, transplacental and during birth; among drug addicts via communally used injection needles.

4   Symptoms

Incubation period: generally viraemia develops after a few weeks (max. 12 weeks), but it is several years until the clinical picture is fully developed; *contagiousness* of persons who are anti-HIV positive depends on the HIV subtype; seroconversion period 1–6 months, contagiousness already present during this time and generally persists for life, being highest when the AIDS symptoms are fully developed; occasional mononucleosis-like symptoms at the end of the seroconversion period are followed by a latency period which lasts for months to years and finally progresses to the actual AIDS syndrome.

Without treatment, 10 years after infection about 50 % of the infected persons have severe immunodeficiency. The clinical pictures resulting from the immunodeficiency are classified according to CDC 1993:
a) asymptomatic acute HIV infection or persistent generalized lymphadenopathy (PGL)
b) HIV-associated clinical symptoms and disorders, which do not fall into the category of AIDS-defining clinical conditions
AIDS-defining conditions (especially pneumocystis carinii pneumonia, candidiasis, toxoplasmosis, and also cytomegaly, *herpes simplex* virus infection, cryptococcosis, aspergillosis, tuberculosis, atypical mycobacterium tuberculosis, cryptosporidiosis and microsporosis; Kaposi's sarcoma)

G 42

5   Special medical examination

Detection of infectious agent
Detection of antigen or part of the antigen in plasma/serum (ELISA), no statement as to infectiousness possible; *culture:* culture on mitogen-stimulated lymphocytes from healthy donors; *molecular biological methods:* PCR with detection of integrated pro-virus (DNA-PCR) or viral mRNA (reverse transcription PCR).

Detection of antibodies
Only for the exclusion of an HIV infection: blood sample immediately after occupational exposure (especially injuries with blood contact); screening tests: rapid HIV test, ELISA for anti-HIV antibodies, if the results are positive, confirmation with Western blot, indirect immunofluorescence test; more control tests after 6 weeks, 3 and 6 months; PCR-detection of proviral HIV DNA.

6   Specific medical advice

Before exposure
Exposure prophylaxis: personal protective equipment, perhaps waterproof clothing; hygienic and disinfection measures;
Disposition prophylaxis (vaccination) not available.

After exposure
After pricks or cuts with injection needles or sharps: promote bleeding, cleanse the wound immediately under running water and with soap followed by disinfection with a virus-inactivating disinfectant; after declaration of consent, blood sample from the person affected and the patient with serological tests (care because of potential HBV or HCV infection).
Because of the risk of side effects of post-exposure medical prophylaxis, this is only to be recommended if the HIV-exposure was associated with a clear risk of transfer of the HIV virus, e.g. after parenteral contact with blood and/or body fluids from an HIV-positive person.

Stages of HIV infection (CDC classification)

Stage	Duration	Clinical symptoms	Diagnostics/ laboratory findings
acute infection	3 days to 4 weeks	occasional transient mono-nucleosis-like symptoms	detection of antibodies after 4–16 weeks
asymptomatic HIV infection	months to years	occasional indolent, persistent, generalized lymph node swellings	anti-HIV antibody detection
symptomatic HIV infection	months to years	*mild forms with slight effects on the general state of health* weight loss (<10 % of normal weight) mucocutaneous changes: • seborrheal eczema, • local recurring herpes simplex, • segmental herpes zoster, • mild recurring respiratory infections (e.g. bacterial sinusitis)	
		more severe forms with marked effects on general state of health weight loss (>10 % of normal weight) chronic diarrhoea, intermit-tently or constantly increased temperature (>1 month), oral candidiasis, oral hair leukoplakia, severe bacterial infections (e.g. bacterial pneumonia)	increase in IgG and IgA, increased erythrocyte sedimentation rate, during the course of the illness gradual reduction in leukocyte, lymphocyte and T helper cell (CD4$^+$) counts, occasional thrombo-cytopenia
severe immuno-deficiency (AIDS)	months to years depending on the manage-ableness of the complications	recurring infections with opportunistic pathogens and parasites (e.g. *pneumocystis carinii* pneumonia, thrush oesophagitis, cerebral toxo-plasmosis) and/or Kaposi's sarcoma (aggressive, dis-seminated form) and/or neoplasms mostly of the lymphoreticular system (non-Hodgkin's lymphoma), HIV encephalopathy, HIV cachexia	frequent anti-HIV anti-body detection detection of p24 anti-gen, leukopenia, lymphopenia, T helper cell count markedly reduced (generally <200/mm^3) or zero, occasional anaemia and thrombocytope-nia, anergy (intracuta-neous test repeatedly negative)

Stages of HIV infection (WHO, 1993) according to the CD4 lymphocyte count

CD4 lymphocytes per mm³	Asymptomatic HIV infection	Symptomatic HIV infection	Severe immuno-deficiency (AIDS)
≥ 500	A1	B1	C1
200–499	A2	B2	C2
≤ 200	A3	B3	C3

G 42

HIV-positive employees must be advised as to their increased risk of developing in-fections, depending on the stage of the infection/illness, and also as to their behav-iour at the workplace and the risk of HIV-infection for associates.

7   Additional notes

Any national notification regulations are to be observed.

Influenzavirus A and B

1   Infectious agent

Influenzavirus types A, B, C; family Orthomyxoviridae, RNA viruses with a lipid-con-taining envelope, types A and B of epidemiological significance in Europe, subtypes classified according to haemagglutinin and neuraminidase markers; influenza A viruses frequently produce variants by antigen shift (exchange of gene segments by reassortment during mixed infections), influenza A and B viruses by antigen drift (point mutations in the base sequence); classification in group 2 as defined in the Di-rective 2000/54/EC.

2   Occurrence

General
Influenza pandemics in 1918/1919 (more than 20 million people died), 1958/9 and 1968/9; less extensive epidemics; in Germany, excess deaths up to several ten-thousands of persons led to the establishment of an influenza surveillance system sup-ported by medical practitioners; annual incidence of infections (excluding pan-demics) 10 % to 20 %; type A also in mammals (pigs, horses) and birds.

Occupational
Research institutes, reference centres, consulting laboratories, handling/contact with swab material and body fluids from the nose and throat area by persons in the health

service (paediatrics, ENT, ophthalmology, dentistry, rescue services; clinicochemical, virological, dental laboratories), work involving extensive contact with the public, work with the influenzavirus in production of medical products and medicines, e.g. diagnostics, vaccines, travellers in areas where the virus is endemic, persons at high risk because of direct contact with infected poultry and wild birds.

3 Transmission route, immunity

Droplet infection

4 Symptoms

Incubation period 1 to 5 days; *contagious* for up to a week after the appearance of clinical symptoms; manifest illness in about every second infected person with exhaustion, headaches, pains in the limbs, sudden high temperature, pharyngitis, laryngitis, tracheitis, bronchitis, bradycardia, low blood pressure and haemorhagic diathesis.

Complications: pneumonia, myocarditis; bacterial superinfections caused by streptococci, staphylococci, *Haemophilus influenzae*, etc; much less frequent are encephalitis, meningoencephalitis, myelitis; in children and young people Reye syndrome with liver failure and brain oedema can develop and is fatal in every third case; at particular risk are pregnant women, persons older than 60 years, diabetics, persons with chronic kidney, heart and lung disorders, babies and infants.

5 Special medical examination

Detection of infectious agent
When clinically indicated, virus culture from nose and throat swabs or lavage fluid; identification of the pathogen with the haemadsorption virus test, indirect immunofluorescence test, ELISA (also as a rapid test) or more recently with the aid of reverse transcription PCR, differentiation of virus types with the haemagglutination inhibition test.

Detection of antibodies
complement fixation test, ELISA

6 Specific medical advice

Before exposure
Exposure prophylaxis: avoid being sneezed at, coughed at, shaking hands; when handling infected animals respiratory protection with a particle filtering half mask (FFP1, FFP2); hygienic and disinfection measures; medicinal prophylaxis with oral amantadine.
Disposition prophylaxis (vaccination) preferably between September and November; plan for an influenza pandemic recommended.

After exposure
For unvaccinated and non-immune persons, vaccination and/or treatment with neuraminidase inhibitors especially for unvaccinated persons in close contact with those infected.

7   Additional notes
Any national notification regulations are to be observed.

G 42

Japanese B encephalitis virus (JEV)

1   Infectious agent
Japanese B encephalitis virus, single stranded RNA virus with a bilayer envelope, 4 genotypes, family Flaviviridae; classification in group 3 as defined in the Directive 2000/54/EC.

2   Occurrence
General
Endemic in considerable areas of Asia, Pacific Siberia, West Pacific USA, Australia; in tropical and subtropical countries during the rainy season, seasonal in moderate climatic regions depending on the activity of vectors (June to September), rice-growing regions, pig farming areas; *epidemics* associated with biocyclic occurrence of appropriate conditions, annual incidence up to 20/100000 inhabitants, increasing (low socio-economic status); 30000 to 50000 cases annually, fatal in about 20 % to 30 % of cases (Asia); imported infections have been described.

Occupational
Research institutes, laboratories, farming, forestry (areas where the pathogen is endemic), the health service (consulting laboratories), work in areas where the pathogen is endemic.

3   Transmission route, immunity
Mosquito bites (*Culex* spp., *Aedes* spp.), *virus reservoir:* domesticated and wild host animals, mainly pigs, horses, birds; man as primary host; *immunity* life-long (after illness or inapparent infection); cross-protection may result from other flavivirus infections.

4 Symptoms

Incubation period 6–16 days; not *contagious* from person to person; severe course of the disease more common in children, young people and adults more than 50 years old; various forms of the disease: mostly *asymptomatic*, otherwise (0.3 % to 2 %) uncharacteristic mild *febrile illness* from which the persons recover without sequelae, *aseptic meningitis* or typical acute *meningomyeloencephalitis* (0.2 % to 5 % of cases); after a 2-day to 4-day prodromal phase sudden rise in temperature, vomiting, stiff neck, photophobia, rigor (mask-like face), nystagmus, coarse tremor, generalized or localized (brain nerve) paresis, convulsions (in 10 % of adults); marked refractory hyperthermia, cardiopulmonary decompensation; disorientation, stupor, coma; fatal in 25 % of cases; recovery with variously severe neurological-psychiatric defects (80 % of adults, 45 % of children): motor, mental and extrapyramidal defects; infections during early pregnancy can lead to abortion, connatal damage; virus persistence in about 5 % of cases.

5 Special medical examination

Detection of infectious agent
Culture by virus isolation in primary/permanent cell lines, *molecular biology:* reverse transcriptase PCR with serum, liquor; unambiguous identification in spite of high level homology (flaviviruses); *immunohistochemical* identification of JEV antigens in brain tissue;

Detection of antibodies
Serological diagnosis carried out routinely only in reference centres or consulting laboratories: shortly after the beginning of the illness specific IgM and IgG antibodies may be identified with the indirect immunofluorescence test, haemagglutination inhibition test, ELISA, perhaps with recombinant JEV antigens; blotting test (Western blot), neutralization test; high level of cross reactions with other flaviviruses.

6 Specific medical advice

Risk of infection of unprotected persons depends on the place, season and duration of stay: 1:5000 per month of exposure, for shorter visits (< 4 weeks) 1:1000000.

Before exposure
Exposure prophylaxis: in areas where the pathogen is endemic vector control, vaccination of host animals; personal protection from ectoparasites (clothing which covers the body and is suitable for the tropics, repellents, mosquito screens, mosquito nets); personal protective equipment (laboratories, firms): gloves, protective clothing, particle filtering half mask (FFP3), eye protection (goggles); hygienic and disinfection measures; appropriate technical and organizational measures for persons handling the virus in laboratories and industry;
Disposition prophylaxis (vaccination): possible in principle, vaccines not approved for use in Germany, indication (CDC) for persons planning to stay for at least one

month in an area where the pathogen is endemic; Japanese inactivated vaccine (BIKEN®, JE-VAX®), basis immunization from age 2 years (3 doses of vaccine i.m.): days 0, 7, 14 or 30, booster after 2 (3) years; 80 % protection after the second dose, practically 100 % after the third; available from international chemists; in China live vaccine, in Japan a genetically engineered vaccine is being tested.

After exposure
With febrile illnesses, think of Japanese B encephalitis in time (travel anamnesis!); when JEV is suspected transfer the patient to a hospital for tropical medicine; specific antiviral therapy not available; supportive treatment according to the symptoms; recombinant alpha-interferon effective in some cases.

G 42

7   Additional notes
Any national notification regulations are to be observed.

Lassa virus (viral haemorrhagic fever)

1   Infectious agent
Lassa virus, Machupo virus, Junin virus, Guanarito virus, Sabia virus, RNA viruses, inactivated in 1 hour at 60°C; family Arenaviridae; classification in group 4 as defined in the Directive 2000/54/EC.
Has been placed in category A on the list of potential bioterrorism agents by the US Center for Disease Control and Prevention (CDC).

2   Occurrence
General
Sporadic and epidemic occurrence in each of the regions where the viruses occur: Lassa virus in Africa, especially West Africa, regional differences in levels of endemic infection (1 % to 27 %), annually about 200000 cases of which 5000 are fatal, in Germany 4 imported cases, 2 fatal; rodents in the wild (do not become ill) as pathogen reservoir, especially the rat *(Mastomys natalensis)*; Junin virus in Argentina, Guanarito virus in Venezuela.

Occupational
Specialized medical centres (examination, treatment, nursing), pathology, research institutes, laboratories, reference laboratories, work in areas where the pathogen is endemic.

3   Transmission route, immunity

Contact with rodents, perhaps primates (life-long pathogen excretion by asymptomatic infected animals) generally faecal-oral, otherwise indirect or aerogenic infection; person to person via body fluids, especially blood, laboratory infections possible; after recovery immunity probably lasts for life.

4   Symptoms

Incubation period 3 to 21 days; *contagious* as long as the body fluids contain virus (urine infectious for up to 9 weeks); 80 % of cases subclinical or mild, slow appearance of symptoms, high temperature, unspecific symptoms, life-threatening haemorrhagic fever only in some cases; typical signs from day 7 of illness: oedema (eyelids, face), conjunctivitis, severe myalgia, proteinuria, retrosternal pain, ulcerative pharyngitis, sometimes with glottis oedema; poor prognosis in cases with high SGOT values, sometimes multi-organ failure; particularly severe course of the disease in pregnant women; fatal in 10 %–20 % of hospitalized cases, otherwise 90 %–95 %.

5   Special medical examination

Detection of infectious agent
For persons suspected of having the disease: diagnostics in specialized laboratories, blood sample (serum, whole blood with citrate) to be taken at once by the doctor in attendance, nucleic acid detection (reverse transcriptase PCR) and if necessary sequencing for rapid virus isolation from blood, urine, liquor; differentiation with monoclonal antibodies; electron microscopic virus detection (liver biopsies, post mortem).

Detection of antibodies
From week 2 of the illness antibody detection (IgM, IgG) via the indirect immunofluorescence test and ELISA (4-fold increase in titre).

6   Specific medical advice

Before exposure
Exposure prophylaxis: in regions where the disease is endemic rigorous rat control; appropriate safety measures during relevant activities in laboratories; hygienic and disinfection measures;
Disposition prophylaxis (vaccination) not available.

After exposure
Persons with the disease to be isolated strictly until they can be transferred to a specialized medical centre; intensive search for all contact persons, if necessary isolation, medicinal prophylaxis (ribavirin), if asymptomatic, molecular biological and serological tests not indicated.

7   Additional notes

Any national notification regulations and restrictions on activities and employment are to be observed.

In cases of infectious (person to person) haemorrhagic fever, persons suspected of having the disease and persons suspected of being infected, immediate isolation in an appropriate hospital (quarantine).

G 42

Legionella pneumophila

1   Infectious agent

Legionella (L.) pneumophila, the species causing most Legionella infections in man (90 %), obligate aerobes, motile, non-sporulating, Gram-negative bacteria,18 serogroups, family Legionellaceae; in all 41 species with 62 serogroups, e.g. L. micdadei, L. feeleii;

classification in group 2 as defined in the Directive 2000/54/EC.

2   Occurrence

General

Worldwide, in natural streams, lakes and ponds, also intracellular in free-living amoebae and other protozoans, and in damp soil nearby (primary reservoir); survive in inadequately maintained or only intermittently used (stagnant) low-temperature water supplies or household water systems, room ventilation and air-conditioning systems and other systems in which aerosols are formed, optimum replication temperatures 35–45°C; occurrence sporadic or as outbreaks, more frequent in late summer/autumn, in the year 2001 (in Germany) 328 cases, incidence 4 cases per 1 million inhabitants; in USA about 10000 cases annually, endemic infection level 5 %–10 % (30 %).

Occupational

Work handling aerosol-producing devices in old or poorly maintained heating, cooling and air-conditioning systems (heat exchangers, ventilation, air filtration, humidification, e.g. wet scrubbers, evaporators, atomizers), plumbing, e.g. hot water systems, mechanical or natural draught cooling towers in industry, the health service, e.g. physiotherapy, hydrotherapy (hot whirlpool), dental practices (water cooled turbine drills), consulting laboratories.

3   Transmission route, immunity

Droplet infection, rarely dust infection, survival time 3 minutes (at 30 % relative humidity) or 15 min (80 %); in immunocompetent individuals high bacterial count necessary, persons in the age group over 50 years are mostly affected, men 2–3 times as often as women; infection favoured by: chronic cardiac, pulmonary, or metabolic disorders (diabetes mellitus), neoplasms (hairy cell leukaemia), immunosuppression (treatment with corticosteroids, cytostatics, AIDS), alcohol and nicotine abuse (reduced ciliary function); probably T cell mediated cellular immunity.

4 Symptoms

Pulmonary legionellosis (classical legionellosis/legionnaire's disease)
Incubation period 2–10 days; *contagiousness* from person to person has not been demonstrated; influenza-like prodromal symptoms, temperature 39–40.5°C, chills, initially unproductive, later productive cough; gastrointestinal symptoms; rarely CNS involvement (lethargy, dazed feeling, confusion); severe atypical pneumonia with infection of the interstitium/alveoli (unilateral, bilateral infiltrates, mostly lower fields), pleuritis, about one third nosocomial, 1 % to 5 % (10 %) of all cases of pneumonia treated in hospital, slow convalescence; reduced lung function, pulmonary fibrosis possible; fatal in 15 % of cases, untreated up to 80 %.

Pontiac fever
Incubation period 1–2 days; mild cold-like syndrome without pulmonary infiltration, dizziness, photophobia, occasionally confusion; regresses spontaneously within 5 days.

Extrapulmonary infections
From the primary lesion (lung) septic metastasis: pleural empyema, pericarditis, myocarditis, endocarditis, pancreatitis, pyelonephritis, peritonitis, wound infections/cellulitis, gastrointestinal and liver abscesses, contamination of intravascular prostheses; also non-infectious skin exanthemata, arthritis, acute kidney failure, myoglobulinaemia.

5 Special medical examination

When infection is suspected, early diagnosis by detection of *Legionella* antigen in urine (ELISA, radioimmunoassay); detection after as little as 24 hours;

Detection of infectious agent
Isolation of the pathogen from sputum, bronchoalveolar lavage fluid, lung biopsy samples, demonstration of *Legionella* DNA (PCR) in airway samples, urine, serum, pleural fluid with subsequent differentiation (direct immunofluorescence test), radioactive cDNA-probe; detection of antigen (ELISA).

Detection of antibodies
Indirect immunofluorescence test, ELISA, Western blot; titre increase from about day 10 after the start of the illness, occasionally not until after 4–9 weeks.

6   Specific medical advice

Before exposure
Exposure prophylaxis: use of steam humidifiers in air-conditioning systems; water temperatures in hot water boilers and pipes for drinking water must be = 55°C; if necessary thermal (70°C), chemical (chlorination) or physical (UV irradiation) decontamination or appropriate cleaning of air-conditioning systems; water temperature should be adjusted by mixing hot and cold water immediately before exiting the system at the tap to minimize the level of any *Legionella* in the aerosol; if aerosol formation cannot be avoided, particle filtering half mask (FFP2).
Disposition prophylaxis (vaccination) not available.

G 42

After exposure
Isolation of infected and contact persons not necessary; antibiotic therapy (duration at least 10–12 days) with erythromycin (macrolide antibiotic) as the drug of choice, perhaps (in severe cases) also rifampicin, in cases with immunosuppression further macrolide antibiotics (azithromycin, clarithromycin), gyrase inhibitors, ciprofloxacin.

7   Additional notes

Any national notification regulations are to be observed.

Leishmania major

1   Infectious agent

Leischmania (L.) major (L. tropica complex), flagellate protozoa, 2 forms: obligate intracellular (in the host) oval amastigote (withdrawn flagellum) form and spindle-shaped promastigote form (in the vector); 12 species pathogenic for humans (*L. donovani, L. tropica, L. mexicana, L. braziliensis* complexes); family Trypanosomatidae; classification of *L. donovani* and *L. braziliensis* complexes in group 3(**) as defined in the Directive 2000/54/EC, *L. tropica* and *L. mexicana* complexes in group 2.

2   Occurrence

General
Worldwide, endemic: Africa, Middle East, Asia, Latin America, Central America; infections in the area from the European Mediterranean north to the southern edge of the Alps; 12 million persons infected in 80 countries, 2 million new cases annually (WHO); increasing number of cases imported into Germany, 17 reported in 2005, estimated 100–200 annually.

Life cycle: amastigote form in the monocyte/macrophage system of infected persons is transferred after an insect bite into the insect stomach and intestines, develops into the infectious flagellated promastigote (5–8 days); inoculated into man when the insect sucks blood again (via vomited stomach contents), on infection of the monocyte-macrophage system, the protozoa are converted to the amastigote form.

Occupational
Work in areas where the pathogen is endemic, research institutes, reference centres.

3   Transmission route, immunity

Pathogen reservoirs in animals on almost all continents (not Australia); small wild rodents, dogs, human host; rarely congenital, transmitted via blood transfusions, wounds from injection needles, sexual contact, but mainly via vectors: dusk and night active (female) sand flies, *Phlebotomus* spp. vector for species from the *Leishmania donovani* complex (*L. d. donovani*, *L. d. infantum*, *L. d. chagasi*) and *Leishmania tropica* complex (*L. t. tropica*, *L. t. major*, *L. t. aethiopica*); *Lutzmyia* spp. (mainly Latin America, Central America) vector for species from the *Leishmania mexicana* complex (*L. m. mexicana*, *L. m. pifanoi*, *L. m. amazonensis*, *L. m. venezuelensis*) and *Leishmania braziliensis* complex (*L. b. braziliensis*, *L. b. peruviana*, *L. b. guyanensis*, *L. b. panamensis*).
Immunity (cell mediated) after inapparent infection, inapparent illness.

4   Symptoms

Visceral leishmaniasis (kala azar)
Caused (Mediterranean region) mostly by organisms of the *Leishmania donovani* complex, otherwise by *L. t. tropica*, *L. m. amazonensis; incubation period* 2 to 20 weeks; also *contagious* from person to person (e.g. via blood transfusions); mainly subclinical course; in the initial phase 2 temperature peaks daily, later dermal hyperpigmentation (black fever, kala azar), marked hepatosplenomegaly, pancytopenia: haematopoiesis reduced by the increased proportion of macrophages in hyperplastic bone marrow; hypergammaglobulinaemia, hypoalbuminaemia, ascites, oedema; severe cachexia, untreated generally fatal within 3 years: sepsis: pulmonary and gastrointestinal superinfection; complications: post-kala azar dermal leishmanoid (*L. d. donovani*) with diffuse nodular skin lesions; in rare cases (acute infection) mucosal, mostly oropharyngeal lesions (nasal septum not affected); opportunistic infection (AIDS-defining condition).

Cutaneous leishmaniasis (oriental sore)
Caused (Southern Europe, Asia, Africa) by *L. d. infantum*, *L. t. tropica*, mild form (dry urban form, reservoir man); *L. t. major*, severe form (moist rural, reservoir small rodents); *L. t. aethiopica*, *L. m. mexicana*, *L. m. amazonensis*, disseminated form; caused (Central and South America) especially by *L. m. mexicana*, *L. m. pifanoi*, *L. m. amazonensis*, *L. m. venezuelensis*, *L. b. braziliensis; incubation period*

5–10 weeks, also contagious from person to person; at the site of entry (face, forearm, lower leg) inflammation (solitary, multiple papules), progression to delimited flat-centred necrotic lesions with livid parasite-containing raised edges; heal generally spontaneously within a year leaving atrophic scarring, sometimes (*L. t. tropica*) recurrent; uta (*L. b. peruviana*) local slow-healing lesion resembling oriental sore (pathogen reservoir: dog).

Mucocutaneous leishmaniasis
Caused (Central and South America) by all the species of the *Leishmania mexicana* and *L. braziliensis* complexes; *incubation period* 5–10 weeks, also *contagious* from person to person; primary lesions can disseminate even after years with disfiguring, sometimes life-threatening tissue destruction (oral mucosa, cartilage); heals spontaneously or disseminates with progressive infiltrating ulcer formation or polypiferous mucosal growths (nose, nasal septum, "tapir nose") sometimes with involvement of the eyes and even loss of sight, prognosis unfavourable, sometimes with fatal bacterial superinfections; *complications:* ulceration of the external ear with cartilage destruction caused by *L. m. mexicana* (chicleró's ulcer) or otonasopharynx caused by *L. b. braziliensis* (espundia).

G 42

5   Special medical examination

Detection of infectious agent
Microscopy: in blood, spleen, bone marrow, lymph nodes, liver (visceral form); in swabs (also wound secretions), thick smears from the edge of lesions; *culture:* reliable only for the visceral form, culture in special media, promastigotes in the supernatant; species differentiation by electrophoretic isoenzyme analysis; false negative results for immunosuppressed patients; *histology* haematoxylin-eosin stain: oval amastigote nucleus, rod-shaped, DNA-containing mitochondrial structured kinetoplast, *molecular biology:* PCR for species identification.

Detection of antibodies
Indirect immunofluorescence test, ELISA, indirect haemagglutination test; high antibody titre in cases of visceral leishmaniasis; in persons with cutaneous infections antibody titre generally lower than in those with mucocutaneous lesions; absence of antibodies does not exclude the possibility of infection; cross reactions in cases of trypanosomiasis; cell-mediated allergy may be demonstrated in a skin test for delayed type hypersensitivity, positive results are obtained after 2 to 3 days in about 90 % of cases.

6   Specific medical advice

Before exposure
Exposure prophylaxis: insecticides, protective measures against mosquitoes (impregnated clothing which covers the skin, repellents);
Disposition prophylaxis (vaccination) not available; vaccines are being tested.

After exposure
Medicinal therapy according to the pathogen species; for (uncomplicated) cutaneous lesions rarely necessary; systemic (i.m./i.v.) therapy with pentavalent antimony preparations (drug of choice) in cases of extensive cutaneous or mucocutaneous processes, several cycles of treatment; Pentostam, Glucantime perhaps in combination with interferon-γ; alternatively (resistance) pentamidine, amphotericin B, allopurinol, paromomycin, ketoconazole, recently also miltefosine (visceral form); local paromomycin-urea ointment, paromomycin methylbenzethonium chloride ointment, perilesional subcutaneous injections of antimony preparations; cryotherapy, excision, curettage, plastic surgery.

7   Additional notes
Any national notification regulations are to be observed.

Leptospira spp.

1   Infectious agent
Leptospira (L.) interrogans, Gram-negative spirochaete, 19 serogroups with > 200 serovars, *L. icterohaemorrhagiae, L. grippotyphosa,* etc.; family Leptospiraceae; classification in group 2 as defined in the Directive 2000/54/EC.

2   Occurrence
General
Worldwide (rural and urban regions), epidemic, endemic, sporadic in animals and man (incidental host); especially in tropical/subtropical countries, also in damp temperate (European) climatic zones; seasonal summer to autumn (Germany 48 reported cases in the year 2001, considerable number of unreported cases); natural pathogen reservoir comprises 160 species of rodents (up to 50 % of animals infected), other wild, domesticated and farm animals; generally persistent asymptomatic infection with leptospiruria (rats life-long, dogs up to 6 months); also symptomatic infections (shorter period as carrier).

Occupational
Research institutes, laboratories, sewage and effluent technology (sewer and sewage plant workers), waste disposal and utilization, veterinary medicine, farming, gardening, livestock keeping, breeding and production, working the soil, hunting, abattoirs, zoological gardens.

3   Transmission route, immunity

Direct contact with animals, contact with infectious excrement (urine), secretions (saliva, milk, amniotic fluid, semen), infected tissue; indirect via damp alkaline material contaminated with *Leptospira* (where the pathogen remains infective for up to 3 months), natural bodies of water, meadows, woods, fields; entry thought to be through intact mucosa in the facial area, skin wounds (microlesions); homologous serovar-specific immunity.

4   Symptoms

G 42

Incubation period: 7–13 (26) days; *contagiousness:* man as the source of infection extremely rare, in 90 % of cases self-limiting, otherwise biphasic febrile course (38–41°C).

1st phase (transitory leptospiraemia): sudden begin with chills, headaches, pains in the limbs, conjunctivitis/episcleritis, pharyngolaryngitis, lymphadenitis (throat, neck, groin lymph nodes), arthralgia, neuralgia, transient measles-like, scarlet-fever-like exanthema with bran-like scaly (maculopapulous) efflorescences (days 3–7).

2nd phase (organ manifestations): meningism/non-suppurative (concomitant) meningitis (especially in anicteric forms); pericarditis, endocarditis, myocarditis (rare); encephalomyelitis/radiculitis with transient paresis (rare); apathy, possibly disorders of consciousness; as secondary illness (50 % of cases); sometimes recurring iridocyclitis, sometimes with opacity of the vitreous humour.

Icteric leptospirosis
Prototype Weil's disease (*L. icterohaemorrhagiae*); dramatic course because, in addition to the symptoms described above, a hepatorenal syndrome develops (begin between days 2 and 7): hepatitis (cholestatic icterus), hepatosplenomegaly, interstitial nephritis (acute renal insufficiency); typical muscle pains (especially calf, abdomen, thorax, neck), bronchitis, cardiovascular disorders (relative bradycardia), haemorrhagic diathesis (petechia, purpura, epistaxis, haematemesis, intestinal haemorrhage, haematuria); complications (rare): pancreatitis, bronchopneumonia, phlebitis, subacute protracted chronic meningitis/encephalomyelitis (weeks to months); fatal in up to 20 % of cases.

Anicteric leptospirosis
Prototype "mud fever" (*L. grippotyphosa*); influenza-like illness with, in addition to the symptoms described above, gastrointestinal syndrome (constipation/watery diarrhoea); often self-limiting illness (without complications, 2–4 weeks), hepatomegaly (rare), splenomegaly (10 %–15 % of cases), hair loss; sometimes symptoms of acute febrile illness without organ involvement; as secondary illness choroiditis possible; fatal in less than 1 % of cases.

5   Special medical examination

Detection of infectious agent
From blood, liquor, liver, kidney, spleen (week 1 of the illness) by *culture* or directly by dark field *light microscopy;*

Detection of antibodies
To establish susceptibility to infection: detection of IgG antibodies; if infection is suspected also detection of IgM-antibodies, e.g. ELISA, microagglutination reaction, complement fixation reaction with serum (from week 2 of illness).

6   Specific medical advice

Before exposure
Exposure prophylaxis: personal protective equipment: appropriate (waterproof) protective clothing, goggles, e.g. when wiping up urine, during care and treatment of sick animals, of those thought to be infected, and game, during work in stagnant, muddy water or water contaminated with animal urine, flooded areas, swamps; during direct/indirect contact with animals on farms or in animal shelters, etc., avoid being licked or bitten; medicinal prophylaxis with doxycycline (tetracycline) possible in regions where the pathogen is endemic and common (rainy season), immunization of pets and farm animals with inactivated whole pathogen vaccine (locally endemic serovars);
Disposition prophylaxis (vaccination): French vaccine, use in Germany currently not permitted

After exposure
Antibiotic therapy (duration 5–7 days): in severe cases penicillin G is the drug of choice, alternatively ampicillin, in less severe cases doxycyclin, amoxycillin, therapy begin before day 4 affects the outcome of the illness, after day 4 only avoids complications (eye).

7   Additional notes

Any national notification regulations are to be observed.

Marburg virus (viral haemorrhagic fever)

1   Infectious agent
Marburg virus, RNA virus, family Filoviridae; classification in group 4 as defined in the Directive 2000/54/EC.
Has been placed in category A on the list of potential bioterrorism agents by the US Center for Disease Control and Prevention (CDC).

2   Occurrence
General
Sporadic and epidemic occurrence in Africa, pathogen reservoir not known with certainty (monkeys, bats).

Occupational
Specialized medical centres (examination, treatment, nursing), pathology, research institutes, laboratories, consulting laboratories, reference centres, animal houses (monkeys), work in areas where the pathogen is endemic.

3   Transmission route, immunity
Transmission by close contact (splashes of blood, wounds, skin contact) from person to person, from monkey to man; aerogenic via infectious faeces particles in dust; nosocomial and laboratory infections possible; after recovery immunity presumably for life.

4   Symptoms
Incubation period 7 days, *contagious* as long as the virus is excreted (pharynx secretions, urine); rapid temperature increase to 40°C, myalgia, bleeding, apathy, haemorrhage with bleeding in the organs (CNS, gastrointestinal tract relatively late), pneumonia, cardiocirculatory failure; fatal in up to 50 % of cases.

5   Special medical examination
Detection of infectious agent
In high security laboratories virus detection in cell culture, directly by electron microscopy.

Detection of antigens
Direct immunodiffusion test, nucleic acid detection by means of nested reverse transcription PCR with sequencing of the amplification product.

Detection of antibodies
ELISA, Western blot.

6   Specific medical advice

Before exposure
Exposure prophylaxis: waterproof protective clothing, particle-filtering half mask
(FFP2, FFP3);
appropriate hygienic and disinfection measures
Disposition prophylaxis (vaccination) not available.

After exposure
Treatment of persons with the disease in specialized infection wards; specific hygienic measures during nursing and when handling the pathogen to be defined by specialists; maximum safety precautions when handling the pathogen in laboratories; therapy of persons with the disease should be attempted with convalescent's serum.

7   Additional notes

Any national notification regulations and restrictions on activities and employment are to be observed.
In cases of infectious (person to person) haemorrhagic fever, persons suspected of having the disease and persons suspected of being infected, immediate isolation in an appropriate hospital (quarantine).

Measles virus

1   Infectious agent

Measles virus, RNA virus pathogenic only for man, family Paromyxoviridae, 21 genotypes, dominant genotypes C2, D6 (Central Europe), D7 (Germany) – antigenically stable (1 serotype); classification in group 2 as defined in the Directive 2000/54/EC.

2   Occurrence

General
Worldwide, incidence 31 million (WHO 1997), most frequent in countries with low socio-economic status (there among the ten most frequent infectious diseases), high proportion of fatal outcomes, fatal in 2 %–6 % of cases; in Germany frequency of wild virus infections (illness/complications) reduced in the last 30 years (measles vaccination!), peak frequency has been shifted into the adult age group, outbreaks in areas with suboptimum vaccination frequency, currently 85 % of the 16 to 20-year-olds and 90–95% of the 21 to 30-year-olds are immune, 5780 cases were reported in the year 2001, at the current immunity status estimated illnesses per year could rise

to about 80000; fatal in 0.01 %–0.02 % of cases; currently a national intervention program aims to eliminate measles.

Occupational
Facilities for medical examination, treatment and nursing of children and for care of pre-school children, research institutes, reference centres, laboratories, oncology clinics, care of immunodeficient patients, children's homes.

3   Transmission route, immunity

G 42

Infected or acutely ill persons form a natural reservoir, droplet infection via infectious secretions during the catarrhal prodromal stage, contact infection; exposed non-immune persons are almost always infected, >95 % unprotected infected persons develop the disease (manifestation index); no risk of contagion in cases of mitigated measles (the transient high temperature and rash which can follow measles vaccination); nosocomial measles infections feared; life-long immunity after natural infection.

4   Symptoms

Measles
Incubation period 8–10 days until beginning of catarrhal stage, 14 days until the rash appears; *contagious* from 5 days before appearance of the rash until up to 4 days afterwards; systemic infection with biphasic course.
Catarrhal prodromal stage: duration 2–5 days, temperature >39°C with conjunctivitis (photophobia), rhinitis, bronchitis, dark red enanthema (palate), pathognomonic: so-called Koplik spots (before rash).
Exanthema stage: duration up to 10 days, maculopapulous efflorescences 3–7 days after the first symptoms, visible for 4–7 days, appear with the second increase in temperature (brownish-pink, confluent/disseminated, macropapular), first behind the ears, then spread over the whole body, skin peels on abatement; temperature decreases on days 5–7 of the illness.
Complications: Transient immunodeficiency (duration 6 weeks) favours bacterial superinfections, e.g. otitis media (7 %–9 %); pseudocroup (laryngotracheitis, ulceration, glottis oedema), (peri-)bronchitis, bronchopneumonia (1 %–6 %), epithelial necrosis in the intestinal mucosa (diarrhoea/appendicitis/ileocolitis) and cornea (ulcerations/malacia); myocarditis (20 % of cases); hepatitis; para-infectious/post-infectious acute measles encephalomyelitis presumably as autoimmune reaction (against brain antigens) in immunocompetent persons 4–7 days after appearance of the rash, fatal in 10 %–40 % of cases; residual CNS damage (20 %–30 %), rare transverse myelitis; subacute sclerosing panencephalitis (rare) after a latency period of 6–15 years (classical slow virus infection), high anti-measles antibody titre (serum, liquor): neurological disorders or deficits, e.g. myoclonia, ataxia, spasticity or even loss of cerebral cognitive functions: abnormal psychic behaviour, mutism, intellectual personality changes, unfavourable prognosis.

Mitigated measles
Milder course of the infection, reduced viraemia, measles rash not fully developed; virus replication reduced as a result of incomplete vaccination immunity, maternal antibodies (newborn babies), transfused antibodies (antibody substitution therapy).

Measles in immunosuppressed patients
In persons with immunosuppression or cellular immunodeficiency (e.g. leukaemia) the clinical measles symptoms persist for weeks; progressive giant cell pneumonia, measles inclusion body encephalitis, fatal in 30 % of cases. Note: measles rash atypical or absent.

Atypical measles syndrome
In spite of immunization with a killed measles virus vaccine (now obsolete) a later infection with the wild virus produces a marked immune response including high temperature, myalgia, lobar or segmental pleuropneumonia, atypical measles rash (distal extremities).

5 Special medical examination

To establish the vaccination status/susceptibility to infection: anamnesis of illnesses and vaccinations is not sufficient, inspection of vaccination documents required;

Detection of infectious agent
To distinguish between vaccine and wild virus in exceptional cases (complex process) virus isolation with differentiation (direct immunofluorescence) from cells (swabs, lavage fluid, biopsy material) from the nose and throat, conjunctiva, bronchial secretion, blood lymphocytes, urine, liquor, perhaps reverse transcription PCR.

Detection of antibodies
IgG antibody detection (neutralization test, haemagglutination test, ELISA), negative results are an indication for vaccination, vaccination success to be tested after 4 weeks at the earliest; perhaps detection of IgM antibodies (absent in 30 % during the first three days of the rash), persist for at least 6 weeks. Note: vaccinated persons who have been re-infected often have no marked IgM response, therefore two tests at an interval of 7–10 days by means of IgG ELISA, complement fixation reaction.

6 Specific medical advice

Before exposure
Exposure prophylaxis: hygienic and disinfection measures;
Disposition prophylaxis (vaccination) with live vaccine, e.g. monovalent vaccine, preferably as a combination vaccine (measles-mumps-rubella, MMR vaccine); *first vaccination* when the child is 11–14 months old, immune response detectable after 4–6 weeks; in week 2 after the vaccination mitigated, transient measles (5 % of

cases); *second vaccination* when child is 15–23 months old ensures maximum immunity; booster recommended for young people; vaccination of previously unvaccinated adults who care for children is recommended.

After exposure
When a person has developed measles, an outbreak of the infection among non-vaccinated immunocompetent contact persons may be prevented by vaccination; single vaccination preferably with MMR vaccine for persons in contact with measles cases in institutions; if possible within 3 days after exposure (mass vaccination); in immunocompromised persons with a high risk of complications and seronegative pregnant women immediate administration of standard human immunoglobulin (up to 3 days after exposure); symptomatic therapy depending on organ manifestations; antiviral therapy not available.

G 42

7   Additional notes
Any national notification regulations and restrictions on activities and employment are to be observed.

Mumps virus

1   Infectious agent
Mumps virus, enveloped RNA virus, family Paramyxoviridae; classification in group 2 as defined in the Directive 2000/54/EC.

2   Occurrence
General
Endemic worldwide, man the only pathogen reservoir, most frequent in children and young people (unvaccinated populations), and in winter and spring; in Germany 90 % of the population protected by vaccination of pre-school children, for persons who are not immune the peak of infections has been moved into the adult age group, sporadic cases without seasonal peak, epidemics in areas with low levels of endemic infection, annual incidence currently 2/100000.

Occupational
Facilities for medical examination, treatment and nursing of children and for care of preschool children, research institutes, laboratories, reference centres.

3   Transmission route, immunity

Droplet infection, rarely indirect infection (saliva, urine), after clinically apparent illness and inapparent infection persons are generally immune for life (98 %), no manifest second illness, but inapparent re-infection possible.

4   Symptoms

Incubation period 16–18 (max. 25) days; *contagious* from 7 days before until 9 days after the beginning of the illness (swelling of the parotid glands), also in clinically inapparent or subclinical disorders (30 %–50 %); occasionally acute respiratory disorder on its own, systemic self-limiting infection; severe forms more frequent in older persons.

Parotitis: raised temperature (to 40°C), unilateral or in succession bilateral (two thirds of cases) inflammation of the salivary glands which become tender to pressure (raised lobe of the ear), sometimes only glandula (g.) submandibularis, g. sublingualis (duration 3–8 days).

Complications: Complications also possible without recognizable manifest parotitis; in 3 %–10 % of cases meningitis (recovery usually without sequelae), of which 50 % are without parotitis, sometimes with acoustic nerve neuritis or labyrinthitis (inner ear deafness 4 %); meningoencephalitis with residual defects; postpubertal pancreatitis, in some cases with type I diabetes, unilateral or bilateral orchitis, testicular atrophy (infertility), epididymitis, prostatitis; oophoritis, mastitis; arthritis, hepatitis, keratitis, myelitis, myocarditis, nephritis, retinitis, thrombocytopenic purpura, thyreoiditis; spontaneous abortion (rare), congenital malformations (embryopathy) not known, if the mother is seronegative: postnatal, perinatal pneumonia, meningitis.

5   Special medical examination

Detection of infectious agent
Virus isolation in cell culture or detection of virus RNA (reverse transcription PCR) from throat swab, liquor, saliva, urine.

Detection of antibodies
To establish vaccination status and susceptibility to infection, an anamnesis of illnesses and vaccinations is not sufficient, inspection of vaccination documents required, if necessary IgG antibody detection; vaccination success can be checked at the earliest after 4 weeks, given seronegativity the vaccination is to be repeated (max. 2x); in atypical cases perhaps specific IgM antibody detection; demonstration of IgG antibodies is also indicative of a fresh infection (only given $\geq$4-fold increase in titre between two samples), e.g. ELISA (method of choice), neutralization test, indirect immunofluorescence test, haemagglutination test, complement fixation reaction.

6   Specific medical advice

Before exposure
Exposure prophylaxis: hygienic and disinfection measures
Disposition prophylaxis (vaccination) with live vaccine, preferably with a trivalent combination vaccine (measles, mumps, rubella: MMR-vaccine), seroconversion 90 % to 95 %; single dose for unvaccinated adults; vaccination of previously unvaccinated adults who care for children recommended.

After exposure
For unvaccinated or other endangered persons in contact with measles cases in institutions a single vaccination preferably with MMR vaccine, if possible within 3 days after exposure (mass vaccination); administration of standard human immunoglobulin appropriate for unvaccinated pregnant women to prevent or mitigate complications associated with mumps; if necessary therapy according to the symptoms.

G 42

7   Additional notes

Any national notification regulations and restrictions on activities and employment are to be observed.

Mycobacterium tuberculosis complex: M. tuberculosis/M. bovis

1   Infectious agent

Mycobacterium tuberculosis/M. bovis, acid resistant rods; increased incidence of multidrug-resistant tuberculosis (MDR-TB) and of extensively resistant strains (XDR-TB); classification in group 3 as defined in the Directive 2000/54/EC.

2   Occurrence

General
Worldwide, 8–9 million new infections annually in the world, incidence in Germany 7.3/100000 inhabitants, among foreign residents in Germany 27.4/100000 inhabitants; age distribution in the German population: mainly in older persons (median 56 years); in immigrants mainly among younger persons (median 35 years); mortality 0.2/100000 inhabitants (data from 2005).

Occupational
Tuberculosis clinics and other institutions for pulmonary medicine, research institutes, laboratories, reference centres, institutions for retarded persons, prisons, animal-keeping; work in areas with high tuberculosis incidence.

3   Transmission route, immunity

Droplet infection, rarely infection via contaminated dust particles.

4   Symptoms

Incubation period 4–8 weeks, *contagious* as long as the pathogen is excreted.

Primary tuberculosis: initial infection of the respiratory tract with specific pneumonic infiltration (primary infiltrate), infiltration and swelling of regional lymph nodes (primary complex).

Postprimary tuberculosis: progression after primary tuberculosis via the following routes:

a) *per continuitatem* from initial pulmonary site (rare),
b) by haematogenic and lymphogenic distribution of the tuberculosis bacteria in the whole organism with subsequent organ tuberculosis (most common form),
c) by canalicular spread (bronchogenic tuberculosis)

Meningeal tuberculosis: earliest manifestation of generalization.

Miliary tuberculosis: lymphogenic haematogenic dissemination.

Inoculation tuberculosis: inoculation of tuberculous material into the skin (laboratory personnel, pathologists, animal keepers).

5   Special medical examination

Before carrying out the tuberculin test, the vaccination status should be determined, anamnesis of vaccinations is not sufficient, inspection of vaccination documents required.

Detection of infectious agent

Microscopy: sputum, bronchial secretion, gastric juice, urine, pleural exudate, liquor, biopsy samples (Ziehl-Neelsen stain, auramine staining); *culture:* liquid media (incubation for 6 weeks), solid media (incubation for 6 weeks); *molecular biology:* when infection is suspected and microscopy yields negative results, not suitable for checking effects of therapy, also detects DNA/RNA of non-viable pathogens; species determination especially with gene probes, antibiogram from each initial isolate (repeat after 2–3 months).

Blood test

Interferon-γ detection (ELISA) given clinical signs of a *M. tuberculosis* infection (florid, latent), also for screening contact persons; sensitivity 90 % for florid infection, 80 % for latent infection, specificity 98 %, negative after BCG vaccination or with atypical mycobacteria (no cross-reaction).

Intracutaneous test

In unvaccinated persons, Mantoux test with increasing concentrations of tuberculin.
In vaccinated persons or persons known to produce a positive tuberculin reaction: after a BCG vaccination a positive tuberculin reaction must generally be expected for

a period of 5–10 years; in the German Democratic Republic BCG vaccination was compulsory for newborn babies and for tuberculin-negative 16-year-olds; in West Germany general voluntary vaccination of newborn babies was replaced in 1975 by vaccination only when indicated; posterior-anterior chest x-ray examination only when medically indicated.

Detection of antibodies
Anti-mycobacterium antibody test (antigen A60) only for florid infections, not suitable for screening, cross-reactions with ubiquitous mycobacteria (MOTT), *M. leprae* and *Nocardia* spp.; *TB IgG/IgM rapid test* for screening, IgM positive in florid infections (sensitivity 93 %, specificity 97 %), IgG positive in latent infections (sensitivity 94 %, specificity 97 %) and after BCG vaccination, cross reactions with *M. bovis*, *M. africanum*.

G 42

6   Specific medical advice

Before exposure
Exposure prophylaxis: during close contact particle filtering half mask (FFP2/FFP3); hygienic and disinfection measures
Disposition prophylaxis (vaccination): BCG vaccination can not prevent infection/illness; vaccination with the currently available BCG vaccine is not recommended.

After exposure
The currently preferred therapy: treatment with a combination of four tuberculostatic agents (rifampicin, isoniazid, pyrazinamide, ethambutol); and then during the further course of the disease with two (e.g. rifampicin, isoniazid); scheme of treatment dependent on whether cavitary processes or haematogenic dissemination is involved.

7   Additional notes

Any national notification regulations are to be observed.

Mycoplasma pneumoniae

1   Infectious agent

Mycoplasma (M.) *pneumoniae*, *M. hominis*, *Ureaplasma* (U.) *urealyticum;* family Mycoplasmataceae, pleomorphic bacteria·without a cell wall, sensitive to environmental factors (drying out); classification in group 2 (*M. pneumoniae*, *M. hominis*) as defined in the Directive 2000/54/EC.

2   Occurrence

General
Respiratory tract (M. pneumoniae): worldwide, man is the natural pathogen reservoir, sporadic infections during the whole year, endemic in densely populated areas and/or outbreaks, epidemic cycles (late summer until spring) every 2–5 years; seroprevalence >50 % (among adults).
Urogenital tract (M. hominis, U. urealyticum): worldwide, man is the natural pathogen reservoir, colonization with *U. urealyticum* in 40 %–80 % of women, with *M. hominis* in 30 %–70 %, colonization with *U. urealyticum* in 5 %–20 % of men, with *M. hominis* in 1 %–5 % depending on age, number of partner changes, socio-economic status.

Occupational
The health service, care of handicapped persons, children, pre-school children, hostels (for asylum seekers, emigrants, refugees), consulting laboratories, prisons.

3   Transmission route, immunity

Respiratory tract (M. pneumoniae): droplet infection, indirect infection (rare), contact infection (oral); limited immunity from age 5 years mainly because of local IgA antibodies; re-colonization/re-infection possible.
Urogenital tract (U. urealyticum, M. hominis): contact infection (sexual), intrapartal by indirect infection (≥50 %); injection needle pricks, transmucosal via the conjunctiva, uncertain immunity after urogenital infections.

4   Symptoms

Respiratory tract (M. pneumoniae)
Incubation period 12–20 days; *contagiousness* low, 1 week before appearance of the clinical symptoms until and including convalescence; mostly inapparent, subclinical course (in 3 to 5-year-olds); most frequent in 5 to 20-year-olds; about 35 %–50 % of all treated cases of pneumonia; initially upper airway infection, later tracheobronchitis, bronchiolitis; in 5 %–25 % interstitial (atypical) pneumonia, mostly prolonged illness with raised temperature, headaches, persistent, non-productive cough, sometimes sputum tinged with blood; recovery within 2–6 weeks; discrepancy between inconspicuous pathological auscultation results and abnormal x-ray results: extensive, frequently peribronchial infiltrates; fatal outcome rare; severe course in immunodeficient patients; second infection is often clinically more severe than the first.

Extrapulmonary locations (M. pneumoniae)
Rare complications/sequelae, sometimes without previous pulmonary manifestation: pleuritis, otitis media; arthritis, diarrhoea, erythema exsudativum multiforme majus, erythema nodosum, haemolytic anaemia (cold agglutinins), thrombocytopenic purpura, hepatitis, pancreatitis, myocarditis, pericarditis, myelitis, polyradiculoneuropathy, focal encephalitis.

Urogenital tract (M. hominis, U. urealyticum)
Infection of the lower urinary tract and the genital tract, favoured by obstruction, by instrumental intervention.

Extra-urogenital locations (M. hominis)
Bacteraemia possible after extensive operative intervention or intensive β-lactam therapy.

5   Special medical examination

Detection of infectious agent
Respiratory tract (M. pneumoniae): swab, throat lavage fluid, retronasal aspirate, sputum, bronchoalveolar lavage fluid; culture: on agar medium and identification by epifluorescence; *molecular biology:* PCR, hybridization analysis (gene probe).
Urogenital tract (U. urealyticum, M. hominis): blood, liquor, smear material, secretions, bladder puncture; culture semiquantitative, differentiation on special nutrient media, antigen detection (ELISA); *molecular biology:* PCR, gene probe.

Detection of antibodies
to determine the susceptibility to infection after exposure; antibody detection (seroconversion) only of significance for *M. pneumoniae:* ELISA (note: cross-reactions), complement fixation reaction, for confirmation detection of unspecific cold agglutinins (autoantibodies).

6   Specific medical advice

Before exposure
Exposure prophylaxis: particle filtering half mask (FFP2, FFP3) for acute untreated mycoplasma infections; hygienic and disinfection measures
Disposition prophylaxis (vaccination) not available (vaccines are being tested).

After exposure
No therapy if person colonized without symptoms (*M. hominis, U. urealyticum);* given clinical manifestations antibiotic therapy with doxycycline (drug of choice for *M. pneumoniae*), macrolide antibiotics for *M. hominis, U. urealyticum.* Note: resistant strains, with *M. pneumoniae* occasional persistence of the pathogen in spite of improved clinical condition.

7   Additional notes

Any national notification regulations are to be observed.

Neisseria meningitidis

1   Infectious agent

Neisseria meningitidis, Gram-negative diplococcus, family Neisseriaceae; highly sensitive to environmental factors; serogroups A, B, C, X, Y, Z, 29 E, W 135, H, I, K, L; 8 serotypes, 14 serosubtypes; classification in group 2 as defined in the Directive 2000/54/EC.

2   Occurrence

General
Man is the only pathogen reservoir; 90 % of all the infections in the world involve the serogroups A, B, C, Y; other serogroups in carriers (excreters); epidemics at intervals of 5–10 years involving mostly serogroup A almost exclusively in the "meningitis belt" of Africa (Sahel), South America, Asia; especially serogroup B and increasingly C in North America, Europe: most frequent in winter and spring; in industrial countries generally as single infections or local outbreaks; annual incidence 1–4 cases per 100000 inhabitants; in Germany (2001) 829 registered cases; half of cases in children and young people; pathogen carriers (nasopharyngeal colonization) 5 %–10 %, during epidemics up to 30 %, in institutions up to 90 %.

Occupational
The health service, institutions for medical treatment and nursing of children, centres for care of pre-school children, children's homes, reference centres, laboratories (work where there is a risk of exposure to a meningococcus aerosol); work in areas where the pathogen is endemic.

3   Transmission route, immunity

Droplet infection, generally on close contact with carriers of the pathogen or persons with the disease; indirect infection of secondary importance; immunity for a limited period.

4   Symptoms

Clinically apparent meningococcus infections (purulent meningitis) about 40 % of infections, fulminant sepsis about 25 %, Waterhouse-Friderichsen syndrome about 10 %–15 %, mixed forms about 25 %.

Purulent meningococcal meningitis (epidemic meningitis)
Incubation period 2–5 (max. 10) days; *contagious* 4 weeks to 14 months, no longer contagious 24 hours after starting therapy; in >50 % of cases prodromal symptoms (upper airway infections) one week before the beginning of the systemic illness; otherwise illness develops from a completely healthy state: sudden high temperature,

chills, meningeal symptoms (75 % of cases), photophobia, hyperaesthesia, failures in the nervus oculomotorius/n. facialis area, changes of consciousness; macu-lopapular rash; in 50 %–70 % of cases endothelial cell damage with extravasation of blood: petechiae, purpura fulminans, large haemorrhagic infiltrates in skin and mucosa (ecchymoses). Note: virulent pathogen! Fatalities: treated 10 % and untreat-ed 85 %; residual organic brain damage in up to 30 %: epileptic fits, dementia, psy-chic defects.

Waterhouse-Friderichsen syndrome
Fulminant course (septic endotoxic shock), massive parenchymal bleeding, dissemi-nated intravascular clotting with haemorrhagic necroses in the skin, mucosa, inner organs (bilateral adrenocortical insufficiency, acute interstitial myocarditis, peri-carditis with pericardial tamponade), consumption coagulopathy, circulatory col-lapse within a few hours; age-dependent fatalities, on average 10 % (to 40 %), can heal leaving residual defects.

G 42

Mixed forms
Local or systemic infections of the sinuses, conjunctiva, middle ear, upper and lower airways, urogenital tract (urethra, cervix); in 7 % of cases post-infectious allergic complications as a result of circulating antigen-antibody complexes: arthritis, epi-scleritis, cutaneous vasculitis, pericarditis.

5   Special medical examination

Detection of infectious agent
When clinical symptoms suggest an infection: examination of liquor, blood (smear culture), possibly biopsy samples from skin efflorescences or infiltrates, throat swab, sputum, tracheal secretion, urine; culture: pathogen isolation, if unsuccessful PCR.

Detection of antibodies
To establish susceptibility to infection/vaccination status: anamnesis of illnesses and vaccinations not sufficient, inspection of vaccination documents required; detection of specific anti-meningococcus antibodies possible, but not for serogroup B; it is not necessary to check vaccination success (seroconversion up to 97 %).

6   Specific medical advice

Before exposure
Exposure prophylaxis: during close contact particle filtering half mask (FFP2/FFP3); hygienic and disinfection measures.
Disposition prophylaxis (vaccination) against pathogens of the serogroups A, C, W135, Y with conjugated MenC vaccine in children more than twelve months old, second vaccination with tetravalent polysaccharide (PS) vaccine 6 months later; the meningococcal conjugate vaccine should not be given simultaneously with pneumo-coccal conjugate vaccine or MMR and varicella vaccine or MMRV; seroconversion

in 97 % of cases; immunization protection for 2–5 years; if risk of infection persists booster generally after 3 years with PS vaccine; vaccine against serogroup B is not yet available. Note: vaccination of laboratory personnel indicated; vaccination of previously unvaccinated adults who care for children under 6 years old is recommended; school children and students before they spend long periods in countries where the vaccination is generally recommended.

After exposure
Initial therapy of infected persons with penicillin G (drug of choice), alternatively third generation cephalosporins, e.g. ceftriaxone, for meningococcus sepsis in combination with aminoglycoside or carbapenem; shock therapy, treatment of clotting disorders, brain oedema, epileptic fits; *prophylactic medicinal treatment* of persons in close contact with a person with an invasive meningococcus infection (all serovars) recommended 7 to 10 days after the last meeting in institutions (e.g. establishments for pre-school children, boarding schools, homes), rifampicin (drug of choice), except for pregnant women (in this case ceftriaxone).

7 Additional notes
Any national notification regulations and restrictions on activities and employment are to be observed.

Orthopoxvirus, Parapoxvirus

1 Infectious agent
Orthopoxvirus (O.): primarily human pathogens *O. variola* (variola major virus), *O. alastrim* (variola minor virus), *O. vaccinia* (vaccinia virus), animal pathogens which can be transmitted to man *O. bovis* (cowpox virus), *O. simiae* (monkeypox virus); *Parapoxvirus (P.):* primarily animal pathogens *P. bovis 1* (BPSV, bovine pustular stomatitis virus), *P. bovis 2* (milker's nodule virus), *P. ovis* (orf virus); DNA viruses, family Poxviridae;
classification in group 4 (variola major, variola minor viruses), group 3 (monkeypox virus) and group 2 (vaccina virus, other animal pox viruses) as defined in the Directive 2000/54/EC.
Has been placed in category A on the list of potential bioterrorism agents by the US Center for Disease Control and Prevention (CDC).

2   Occurrence

General
Last registered (Germany) imported case of smallpox 1972, worldwide last known case of *variola major* infection 1977 (Somalia), until the 1950s >5 reported (WHO) cases annually per 10^5 population, WHO eradication program 1967, since the 1980s outbreaks in Central Africa increasingly caused by monkeypox virus: 1996/1997 >500 cases in USA, 93 cases since 1993, 33 cases in May–June 2003, since then it has been suggested that a renewed zoonotic dissemination of members of the family Poxviridae is taking place within the population.

G 42

Occupational
Specialized medical centres (examination, treatment, nursing), pathology, research institutes, reference centres, consulting laboratories;
Variola major virus, variola minor virus (alastrim virus): specialized medical centres (examination, treatment, nursing), pathology, research institutes, laboratories, (emergency and rescue services, nursing staff, high security laboratories).
Vaccinia virus: specialized laboratories (genetically modified *Vaccinia* viruses).
Animal pox viruses: veterinary medicine (veterinary surgeons, obduction assistants), zoological gardens (zoo-keepers), circuses, farming (breeders, shepherds, milkers, shearers), specialized laboratories, reference centres, consulting laboratories.

3   Transmission route, immunity

Variola major, variola minor virus: persons infected with the poxvirus are the only reservoir, healthy carriers unknown; in contrast with the once widespread assumption, chains of infection form slowly(!); in initial phase via expired droplets (*droplet infection*); less often via contact (contact infection), later via dry pustule and scab material (dust infection), contaminated material (*indirect infection*); no reliable life-long natural immunity, later partial immunity, life-long postvaccination immunity probably not attainable, complete protection probably lasts only for 1–2 years.
Vaccinia virus: transmission from man to animals possible (droplet and contact infection).
Animal pox viruses: (mostly) animal to man; man to man or man to animal (contact infection) cannot be excluded (e.g. cow pox, milker's nodules); indirect infection possible; immunity uncertain.

4   Symptoms

Variola (smallpox, variola vera, pestis variolosa)
Spreads systemically in two phases: from the respiratory tract via regional lymph nodes, on day 4 after infection appears in the blood stream (primary viraemia), spreads into the spleen, lymph system, bone marrow, liver, lungs (secondary viraemia) with metastases in the skin and mucosa, associated with enanthema (oropharynx), highly contagious; severe course in 90 % of cases, fatal haemorrhagic course in 5 %, mild smallpox in 5 %.

Incubation period (min. 7 days) 12–14 (max.19) days; *contagious* from the beginning of the febrile phase until the skin and mucosal efflorescences have scabbed and
healed (3 weeks), highly contagious during outbreak of the rash (week 1); the feeling of being very ill develops from a state of feeling completely well: abrupt biphasic temperature increase to 40°C, catarrhal symptoms, muscle pain, backache,
swelling of the lymph nodes; skin efflorescences appear simultaneously (all in one
stadium), mainly on the face (first eruptions on the forehead and nose), spread over
the whole body. Stages: macula (initial erythema), papules with reddish edges,
unilocular(!) vesicles, filled with pus becoming cloudy as pustules, after 4–6 weeks
forming scabs; scarring especially on the face; fatalities 20 %–30 %; sometimes re-
infection or variola mitigata/varioloid (5 % of cases): milder form but still with the
characteristic centrifugal distribution of the rash (differentiation from varicella); sometimes a fulminant haemorrhagic, confluent form (black smallpox); in partially immunized persons sparse efflorescences, but still highly febrile and infectious (variola mi-
nor/alastrim); fatal in about 1 % of cases.

Vaccinia

Weaker vaccination/vaccinia virus with properties of variola and cowpox virus;
postvaccinal (p.v.) in sequence from day 4: papules, vesicles, drying scabbing pustules which leave a scar on healing (3 weeks p.v.), axillary lymphadenitis, slightly
raised temperature (day 9).
Complications: progressive vaccinia/vaccinia necrosum, eczema vaccinatum, ocular vaccinia infection; generalized vaccinia (immunodeficient persons), postvaccinal
encephalitis; fatal in 25 %–50 % of cases; vaccination in Germany no longer compulsory (since 1974); recommended only for persons handling recombinant vaccinia
virus (reference centres, consulting laboratories).

Animal pox infections

Cowpox: primary host small rodents (not cattle); recent infections of persons via cats;
lesions localized on the thumb, forefinger, forearm and face; isolated hazelnut-sized
livid reddish, sometimes haemorrhagic nodules, occasionally associated with feeling
very ill, encephalitis rare, no generalized rash.
Milker's nodules: primary host cattle; incubation period in man 5–7 days, on the
hands reversible, benign skin tumours (persist for 4–8 weeks): pea-sized, half spheri-
cal, bluish red nodules, with pale red edges.
Orf : primary hosts sheep and goats; incubation period in man 5–7 days; raised temperature, joint pains; mostly on the hands and arms papulopustular, reddish, weeping, hard, painful nodules of 3–4 cm diameter (ecthyma contagiosum), occasional efflorescences in the head area, rarely permanent blindness.
Catpox: primary host cats, either clinically inapparent infection or local skin ulceration or generalized (systemic) illness (immunosuppressed persons): formation of pustules and subsequent ulcers in the head area.
Monkeypox: primary host monkeys; incubation period in man 8–17 days; course of
the disease almost indistinguishable from that of variola major infection with scarring; severe nuchal lymphadenopathy; fatal in 1 % of cases.

5   Special medical examination

Direct diagnosis (usual); otherwise in special laboratories:

Detection of infectious agent
For example, electron microscopic particle detection (rapid diagnosis, virus culture obligatory).

Detection of antibodies
Detection of virus-specific antibodies in serum: anti-variola antibody detection by ELISA, immunodiffusion, indirect immunofluorescence test, complement fixation reaction, haemagglutination test, neutralization test, Western blot, for fine differentiation PCR, DNA hybridization, restriction enzyme analysis.

6   Specific medical advice

Before exposure
Exposure prophylaxis: particle-filtering half mask (FFP3), gloves, overall with head covering, galoshes, goggles, hygienic and disinfection measures;
Disposition prophylaxis (vaccination) formally discontinued (1991); (inter)national reserves of vaccine exist; intradermal first vaccination produces high reactivity; in general, therefore, pre-exposure vaccination currently not recommended.

After exposure
Variola major
Therapy: symptomatic, specific therapy unknown; infected persons to be isolated in competent centres; segregation/quarantine (infected and exposed persons, nursing personnel) for 19 days;
Active immunization (for employees in high security laboratories and in cases of smallpox alarm/ bioterrorism): live vaccine to be given as early as possible and certainly within 4 days of exposure; illness cannot always be prevented (less severe course, reduced virus excretion); passive immunization: consider injection of anti-vaccinia immunoglobulin (i.m.) in several doses (0.6 ml/kg body weight) distributed over a 24 to 36-hour period (especially in cases of eczema vaccinatum), repeat after 2–3 days possible; medicinal therapy: no data available for the effectiveness of virustatic agents in man.

Animal pox infections
In man active immunization (i.m.) with attenuated deletion mutants; MVA vaccine for protection of dogs/cats (in households with immunosuppressives); passive (man): specific, polyclonal anti-vaccinia immune serum, for monkeypox hyperimmune gamma-globulin, medicinal therapy with cidofovir (i.v. infusion).

7   Additional notes

Any national notification regulations are to be observed.

Parvovirus B 19

1 Infectious agent

Human parvovirus B19 (HPV-B19), environmentally stable DNA virus, family Parvoviridae; classification in group 2 as defined in the Directive 2000/54/EC.

2 Occurrence

General
Worldwide, man is the pathogen reservoir, endemic especially in children, young people; regional epidemic outbreaks at intervals of 3–7 years, seasonal peaks in temperate climates (late winter to early summer); seroprevalence (industrial countries) 2 %–10 % (<5-year-olds), 40 %–60 % (>20-year-olds), over 85 % (>70-year-olds), nosocomial infections possible.

Occupational
The health service (paediatrics), consulting laboratories, facilities for medical examination, treatment and nursing of children and for care of preschool children, obstetrics, treatment of infectious diseases.

3 Transmission route, immunity

Droplet infection; parenteral via blood/blood products; infections during pregnancy result in transplacental transmission in one third of cases; after an infection life-long immunity.

4 Symptoms

Erythema infectiosum (fifth disease)
Incubation period 4–20 days, highest *contagiousness* during asymptomatic, viraemic phase before the rash appears (5 days); inapparent infections (20 %–30 %), self-limiting illness; prodromal influenza-like symptoms, butterfly-shaped rash on the face; descending maculopapular, ring-shaped, reticular rash on the trunk and extremities (extensor surfaces), can change its form and colour, perhaps lymphadenopathy, arthralgia (small joints); generally recovery without sequelae.

Transient aplastic crisis (TAC)
Life-threatening acute anaemia, associated with thrombocytopenia, neutrocytopenia, reticulocytopenia (possibly pancytopenia/necrosis in the bone marrow); disorders which predispose to TAC include chronic haemolytic disorders such as sickle cell anaemia, thalassaemia, hereditary sphaerocytosis, autoimmune haemolytic anaemia, persistent or remittent anaemia with immunosuppression, inherited or acquired immune defects or immunodeficiency (AIDS); virus persists sometimes for years in the bone marrow.

Congenital infections/hydrops fetalis
Risk of prenatal toxicity in one third of infections of non-immune pregnant women: hydrops fetalis intrauterine (possibly postpartal) early death, spontaneous abortion, after congenital infections sometimes virus persistence.

Other manifestations
Peripheral, persistent (weeks to months) polyarthropathy (also after inapparent infection); juvenile vascular purpura, Henoch-Schoenlein purpura (can be life-threatening); erythroblastopenia (pure red cell aplasia) in persons with acquired/inherited immunodeficiency; rarely diarrhoea, encephalopathy, glomerulonephritis, fulminant hepatitis, meningitis, myocarditis, pneumonia, pseudoappendicitis, uveitis.

G 42

5   Special medical examination

Detection of infectious agent
Blood, blood products, serum, bone marrow, amnion cells, saliva, amniotic fluid, cord blood, (foetal) tissue/synovia (fine-needle biopsy), autopsy material; *immunoelectron microscopy:* detection of virus particles; *culture:* virus isolation (cell culture); detection of antigens with monoclonal antibodies; *molecular biology:* genome detection with dot blot hybridization, perhaps nucleic acid amplification techniques, e.g. PCR; restriction enzyme analysis.

Detection of antibodies
To establish the susceptibility to infection or for diagnosis of unclear rash, e.g. during pregnancy, chronic-haemolytic disorders, AIDS: detection of specific antibodies with radioimmunoassay, ELISA, indirect immunofluorescence test, Western blot, in special cases PCR.

6   Specific medical advice

Before exposure
Exposure prophylaxis: hygienic and disinfection measures;
Disposition prophylaxis (vaccination) not available (vaccines are being tested).

After exposure
For erythema infectiosum symptomatic therapy, blood transfusions for aplastic crises, chronic haemolytic disorders, immunoglobulin preparations with high anti-HPV-B19 titre, intrauterine transfusion of erythrocyte concentrate for foetal infection.

7   Additional notes
Any national notification regulations are to be observed.

Poliomyelitis virus

1   Infectious agent

Poliovirus, entero-neurotropic, environmentally stable, RNA virus without an envelope, serotype 1 (Brunhilde, 85 %), serotype 2 (Lansing, 3 %), sporadic cases with serotype 3 (Leon); genus Enterovirus, family Picornaviridae; classification in group 2 as defined in the Directive 2000/54/EC.

2   Occurrence

General
Wild viruses are found today only in African (sub-Saharan region, Horn of Africa) and Southeast Asian countries; before the introduction (1954) of the "first" parenteral inactivated poliomyelitis vaccine (IVP, Salk vaccine) worldwide there were about 500000 registered cases of poliomyelitis annually, afterwards about 5000 (WHO, 1998); there were 12 vaccine-associated paralytic poliomyelitis cases (VAPP) in Germany in the years 1985–1996, until the introduction of the "second" parenteral IVP (1998) 1–2 VAPP cases annually; currently a Global Polio Eradication Initiative (WHO, 1988) is attempting to eradicate the disease.

Occupational
Research institutes, reference centres, laboratories (regular work and contact with infected animals/samples, samples and animals suspected of being infected, other contaminated objects or materials containing the infectious agent given a practicable route of transmission), facilities for medical examination, treatment and nursing of children and for care of pre-school children, hostels (e.g. for asylum seekers, refugees, emigrants), work in areas where the pathogen is endemic.

3   Transmission route, immunity

Man the only source of infection (virus reservoir); mainly faecal-oral (indirect infection) via contaminated objects, drinking water, sewage, foodstuffs, occasionally via flies; rare droplet infection via saliva possible during the early phase of the infection (primary virus multiplication in the pharynx); permanent humoral type-specific immunity (IgG antibodies): only certain with antibodies against all 3 serotypes.

4   Symptoms

More than 95 % of infections are inapparent, clinically manifest illness can end during any phase; *incubation period 5–14 (35) days*; *contagious* as long as virus is excreted, 36 hours to 1 week (throat), 72 hours to several weeks (stool), serotype-dependent low contagion index; local virus multiplication in the mucosa of throat and intestines (Peyer's patches), secondary viraemia with organ manifestations (skin, myocardium, meningeal space), infection or damage of vessel endothelia and ganglion cells, mainly of α-motoneurons of the anterior horn cells of the spinal cord and centres in the hind brain; usually complete virus elimination.

Abortive poliomyelitis (initial stadium)
Uncharacteristic general symptoms for 1–2 days ("minor illness") such as raised temperature, sore throat, headaches, pains in the limbs.

Non-paralytic poliomyelitis
3–7 days after minor illness, aseptic meningitis with severe meningeal syndrome (high temperature, stiff neck), back pains, transient muscle weakness; complete recovery after a few days.

G 42

Paralytic poliomyelitis ("major illness")
After aseptic meningitis in about 1 % of infected persons; about 80 % *spinal form:* lytic defervescence, sudden flaccid, asymmetrical paralysis of the leg (most frequent), arm and intercostal muscles, diaphragm; *bulbopontine form:* affects the brain nerves X (n. vagus), XI (n. accessorius), XII (n. hypoglossus), the pons and medulla oblongata (respiratory centre); *encephalitic form:* encephalitis (rare) with clouding of consciousness, hyperkinesia, convulsions, vegetative disorders (hyperhidrosis), personality changes; generally after 2 years irreversible state of paralysis; recovery possible with all forms leaving residual defects, deformation of the extremities and spinal column.

Post-poliomyelitis syndrome (PPS)
In 20 %–80 % of cases of the spinal form, after a symptom-free interval of decades, new progressive symptoms: sleepiness, fatigue, pain, insomnia, temperature regulation disorders, general muscle weakness; frequently wrongly diagnosed because the symptoms are unspecific.

5   Special medical examination

Detection of infectious agent
Perhaps virus isolation, e.g. from faeces, throat lavage fluid or swabs.

Detection of antibodies
To establish the susceptibility to infection: anamnesis of illnesses and vaccinations is not sufficient, inspection of vaccination documents required; specific antibody detection (serum) with complement fixation reaction, ELISA, neutralization test (method of choice): in acute infections IgM antibodies (7–10 days after infection) and/or two serum samples showing significant ($\geq$4-fold) increase in IgG titre.

6 Specific medical advice

Before exposure
Exposure prophylaxis: hygienic and disinfection measures;
Disposition prophylaxis (vaccination) generally recommended with IPV (inactivated polio vaccine) as standard vaccination for children, booster at the age of 9–17 years, in adults booster with IVP if basis immunization is incomplete or when vaccination indicated.

After exposure
Specific antiviral therapy not available; symptomatic treatment, perhaps artificial respiration in cases with bulbar paralysis, subsequent physiotherapeutic, orthopaedic treatment; without delay vaccination of contact persons with IVP, independent of vaccination status; "secondary cases" (infected contact persons) indicative of a requirement for mass vaccinations, tests for virus excretion.

7 Additional notes

Any national notification regulations and restrictions on activities and employment are to be observed.

Prions

1 Infectious agent

Prion (proteinaceous infectious agent), pathological folded prion protein (PrP^{Sc}), a form of the endogenous prion protein which is expressed on cell surfaces (PrP^{C}); highly resistant to heat, ionizing radiation, UV radiation, listed disinfectants and proteases; classification in group 3(**) as defined in the Directive 2000/54/EC.

2 Occurrence

General
Endogenous genetic manifestation
Somatic mutant PrP gene: Creutzfeld-Jakob disease (CJD), about 10 % familial inherited (autosomal dominant); Gerstmann-Sträussler-Scheinker syndrome (GSS), fatal familial insomnia (FFI).

Endogenous sporadic ("classical") manifestation
Spontaneous mutation of the three-dimensional structure of the cellular cerebral prion protein (PrP^{C}): Creutzfeld-Jakob disease (CJD), about 90 % of cases.

Exogenous infectious acquired manifestation
Transmissible spongiform encephalopathy (TSE); *man:* iatrogenic Creutzfeld-Jakob disease (CJD), new variant of the Creutzfeld-Jakob disease (vCJD), kuru; *animals:* scrapie, bovine spongiform encephalopathy (BSE), chronic wasting disease (CWD), transmissible mink encephalopathy (TME), feline spongiform encephalopathy (FSE), exotic ungulate encephalopathy (EUE).

Sporadic ("classical") and iatrogenic Creutzfeld-Jakob disease (CJD)
Cause largely unknown (CJD); worldwide constant annual incidence $1/10^6$ inhabitants (sporadic CJD), in Germany (from 1994–2002) annually 28 to 84 cases (Robert Koch Institute, RKI); in all 565 "probable" or "confirmed" cases (RKI); iatrogenic after administration of human growth hormone (about 200 cases) and dura mater transplants (about 100 cases).

New variant of Creutzfeld-Jakob disease (vCJD)
The cause is a pathological prion protein from infected/diseased cattle, human form of BSE with comparable biochemical/pathogenetic properties; first appeared in the year 1996 in GB, there by October 2003 143 cases, Germany free of vCJD, occasional cases in France, Ireland, Italy, Hong Kong, USA, Canada (data from 10/2003), symptom-free carriers are not recognized during their lifetimes.

Occupational
Increased workplace-related risk has not been demonstrated in medical studies; potential exposure to the pathological prion protein (CJD/vCJD) in the health service, e.g. for persons employed in neurosurgery/pathology, veterinary medicine and in the animal processing industry, e.g. for persons working at abattoirs, reference centres.

3   Transmission route, immunity

Iatrogenic Creutzfeld-Jakob disease (CJD)
From person to person via injected growth hormone obtained from cadaveric hypophyses, implanted lyophilized dura mater/cornea, occasionally via neurosurgical instruments/deep stereotactic, intracerebral EEG electrodes.

New variant of Creutzfeld-Jakob disease (vCJD)
Pathogen identity of the prion protein of BSE and vCJK; potential alimentary transmission via infected tissue: risk material/critical tissues: brain, spinal cord, posterior part of the eye, terminal ileum, paravertebral ganglia, lymphatic tissue, e.g. appendix, possibly also tonsils, lymph nodes, spleen and also (questionably) beef (products); there is currently no evidence for transmission of vCJK via blood (products); prion-free are certainly milk (products); no detectable immune response in organisms infected with TSE.

4   Symptoms

Iatrogenic Creutzfeld-Jakob disease (CJD)
Incubation period 4 years; *contagiousness* accidental; duration of illness about 7 months; prodromal personality changes (irritability, apathy, depressive moods, paranoid traits), sometimes only dizziness, poor memory, anxiety; later memory disorders and lapses, failure of critical faculty, orientation disorders, cerebellar disorders (ataxia, intention tremor, dysdiadochokinesia), speech and sight disorders (visual field defects, homonymous hemianopia, sometimes cortical blindness); terminal deep-seated dementia, decerebration, inability to move, restriction to vegetative functions; sleeplike state with the eyes open (vigil coma); typical florid plaques mostly absent.

New variant of Creutzfeld-Jakob disease (vCJD)
Incubation period 10–20 (30) years; not *contagious* during normal day-to-day contact, only on direct contact with infected tissue; person-to-person infection conceivable, infected tissues include brain, spinal cord, posterior part of the eye, terminal ileum, paravertebral ganglia, lymphatic tissue, e.g. appendix, perhaps also tonsils, lymph nodes, spleen; clinical course differs from that of CJD, specific, novel pattern of brain changes; prodromal psychiatric symptoms: depressive moods, anxiety, emotional lability, apathy, optic or acoustic hallucinations, behavioural disorders; neurological symptoms: painful paraesthesia and dysaesthesia, later ataxia, myoclonus, chorea, dystonia; prolonged clinical course (1–2 years) with marked ataxia; in the terminal phase (as in sporadic CJD) progressive cognitive defects develop, ends with dementia, akinetic mutism; death about 4 months after beginning of the illness, age at death (median) 30 years.

5   Special medical examination

Man: no preclinical diagnosis; *sporadic CJD:* prion protein in nervous tissue; vCJD: histological/histopathological gliosis, florid plaques in brain tissue; diagnosis generally *post mortem;* EEG changes in the form of periodic spike-wave complexes (*sporadic CJD*); typical MRI (magnetic resonance imaging) changes in 70 % of cases (vCJD); liquor analysis: no information provided by normal routine tests; sometimes cellular breakdown products detectable, e.g. neuron-specific enolase; PrP^{Sc} detectable in brain homogenates (Western blot), but not with any certainty in blood.

6   Specific medical advice

Before exposure
Exposure prophylaxis: risk minimization (alimentary/iatrogenic) by keeping potentially BSE-containing material out of the human food chain, e.g. slaughter/destruction of animals with BSE, testing of cattle intended for slaughter, elimination of animal material infected with prions, prohibition of its import or circulation, and of feeding of animal remains to animal species used for food production.
Hygienic and disinfection measures when handling critical tissues or invasive medical products potentially contaminated with prions, especially surgical instruments;

avoidance of pricks and cuts and splashing of sample materials (work in a closed hood).
Use of disposable instruments; contaminated (liquor) surfaces to be treated effectively with 1–2 M NaOH or 2.5 %–5 % Na hypochloride (NaOCl) for 1 h; dispose of contaminated disposables (injection needles, scalpels) in medical waste, dispose of medical products which have been in contact with critical tissues as C waste which is then incinerated.
Dry heat is inactivating at temperatures of 300°C or more; autoclaving e.g. at 132–136 °C for at least 30 min (3 bar), perhaps combined with alkali-treatment; the problem of decontamination of reusable medical equipment (endoscopes) remains.
No risk of infection during social or intimate contact, daily care, isolation not necessary, normal washing up procedures for dishes and utensils.
Disposition prophylaxis (vaccination): new immunological approaches will perhaps make it possible to immunize against prion diseases.

G 42

After exposure
Treat pricks, cuts, scratches and bites with 1 M NaOH for 10 min, disinfect whole (contaminated) skin for 5 min, then rinse under running water.

7   Additional notes
Any national notification regulations are to be observed.

Rabies virus

1   Infectious agent
Rabies virus, enveloped RNA virus; serotype 1 (classical rabies virus), a. wild type, b. laboratory passaged virus; in bats further antigenetically different serotypes (types 1–4), European (European bat lyssa virus EBLV 1/2) and Australian bat virus, all not resistant to environmental factors (drying out, UV irradiation, acids, alkalis); family Rhabdoviridae; classification in group 3(**) as defined in the Directive 2000/54/EC.

2   Occurrence
General
Endemic, not globally distributed zoonosis, persistent chains of infection in animal stocks; annually about 60000 rabies cases in man (WHO), especially in South and Southeast Asia (>99 % India, China); about 60 countries are free of rabies; incidence in Europe decreasing, annually just a few individual cases in Belgium, Germany, France, Luxembourg, mainly imported infections.

Occupational
Research institutes, laboratories, consulting laboratories, regions with rabies-infected wild animals, the health service (treatment and care of persons with rabies); farming, forestry, the timber industry, gardening, hunting, veterinary medicine, keeping animals (care, buying and selling of animals, animal laboratories); persons distributing vaccination bait (live vaccine!); working in rabies risk areas.

3   Transmission route, immunity

Reservoir in Europe: mainly (carnivorous) wild animals, e.g. fox (80 %); squirrel, roe deer (10 %), badger, red deer, polecat, marten, weasel, wild pig, but also farm animals, e.g. cattle, small ruminants, horse, (straying) pets; *reservoirs in America:* skunk, raccoon; recently in Europe also bats; in Germany chains of infection formed mostly via fox, wild animals and pets, especially cats and dogs; animals first infectious just before clinical symptoms appear and during the whole of the illness; animal cadavers for weeks.

Transmission mainly via infectious saliva (bite), direct mucosal contact (sprayed saliva), or contaminated materials (via skin wounds), via inhaled bat droppings (rare); alimentary via contaminated raw meat; immunity only after vaccination (protection for 3–5 years), against serotype 1 complete, serotype 4, EBLV-1/2 (partial), against serotypes 2, 3 not to be expected.

4   Symptoms

Fatal infection (generally), in the world only 3 cases documented which were not fatal in man;

Incubation period 3–8 weeks, rarely 9 days to several years (individual cases), short incubation given high virus concentration and an inoculation site close to the CNS; after rabies virus contact only about 20 % of not immunized persons develop the illness; *contagiousness:* virus has been detected in saliva and tears, transmission from persons with the illness to contact persons is, however, unknown; infection via corneal transplantation possible.

Prodromal stage
Duration 2–5 days: slightly raised temperature, nausea, vomiting, headaches, salivation; local burning sensation around the bite, itching, hyperaesthesia (not always); anxiety, vegetative disorders.

Excitatory stage (furious rabies)
Duration 2–5 days: painful spasms of pharynx and larynx induced by visual or acoustic awareness of water (hydrophobia), bright light (photophobia), marked salivation, fear of drinking, generalized agitation, tonic-clonic spasms (the whole musculature); mood swings, uncontrolled fits of anger with screaming, aggressiveness (biting, thrashing); sometimes death during spasms (day 3–4).

Paralysis
Duration 3–4 days: spasms diminish, restlessness; 20 % of cases without excitatory stage; ascending flaccid paralysis (mostly brain nerves); death from asphyxiation of conscious patient (usual case) or in coma (max. 7 days after appearance of the first symptoms).

5   Special medical examination

To establish susceptibility to infection, inspection of vaccination documents or determination of antibody titre required; diagnosis clinical, otherwise in specialized laboratories.

G 42

Detection of antigens
Antigen detection first possible towards the end of the incubation period (e.g. direct immunofluorescence test with anti-rabies serum in clinical samples); *intravital:* epithelial cells from corneal impressions (corneal test), nuchal hair follicle gland cells (skin biopsy); virus isolation from saliva (neuroblastoma cells), intracerebral inoculation (mice); *post mortem:* intraplasmatic inclusions (Negri bodies) in the brainstem of man and animals, especially in the thalamus, hypothalamus, limbic system, especially hippocampus with Ammon's horn, cerebellar cortex.

Detection of antibodies (serum, liquor)
After natural infection antibody detection (serum, liquor) not reliable (antibody production begins late), also preterminal of secondary importance, e.g. by means of indirect immunofluorescence test, neutralisation test, ELISA; postvaccination rapid test (within 48 h) by means of rapid fluorescent focus inhibition test; in doubtful cases detection of nucleic acid (e.g. in salivary glands) by reverse transcription PCR together with nucleic acid sequencing.

6   Specific medical advice

Before exposure
Exposure prophylaxis: caution with pets behaving unusually, wild animals without natural fear, when handling animals found dead; when caring for sick people; immunization of pets, wild animals (foxes), farm animals;
Disposition prophylaxis (vaccination) only with inactivated rabies virus (serotype 1), basis immunization on days 0, 3, 7, 14, 30, 90, protection level practically 100 %; indication: handling of animals (including bats) in areas where rabies is endemic, persons in contact with cases; vaccination status of potentially exposed laboratory personnel to be checked twice yearly, booster when level <0.5 IU/ml.

After exposure
Observation of the animal suspected to have rabies (for up to 10 days); if indicated immediate immunoprophylaxis as shown in the table, do not wait until the infection is confirmed; clean contaminated areas/wounds, rinse thoroughly under running

Post-exposure rabies immunoprophylaxis (from 7/2006)

Exposure grade	Kind of exposure		Immuno-prophylaxis[1] (observe Patient Information Leaflet)
	to a wild or pet animal suspected or shown to have rabies[2]	to a rabies vaccination bait	
I	handling/feeding animals being licked on the intact skin	touching vaccination bait with the intact skin	no vaccination
II	being nibbled on un-covered skin, surface scratches which are not bleeding, being licked by an animal on skin which is not intact	contact with the liquid vaccine of a damaged vaccination bait with skin which is not intact	vaccination
III	any bite or scratch, contamination of mucosa with saliva (e.g. by being licked or splashed)	contamination of mucosa or open wounds with the liquid vaccine from a damaged vaccination bait	vaccination and once *simultaneously* with the first vaccination: passive immunization with anti-rabies immunoglobulin (20 IU/kg body weight)

[1] The individual vaccinations and the administration of anti-rabies immunoglobulin should be documented carefully.

[2] A bat is suspected of having rabies if it allows itself to be touched or behaves otherwise in an unusual or aggressive manner or is found dead.

water and then disinfect, likewise after contamination with liquid vaccine (vaccination bait), wounds should not be stitched; after a grade III exposure, spray around the wounds with anti-rabies hyperimmunoglobulin, administer the rest of the dose i.m. (within 3 days); passive immunization as post-exposure prophylaxis as shown in the table; symptomatic therapy in intensive care.

7   Additional notes

Any national notification regulations are to be observed.

Rotavirus

1   Infectious agent

Rotavirus, double-stranded RNA virus without an envelope, *serogroups* A–G, human and animal pathogens, especially group A, family Reoviridae; highly stable to environmental factors (tenacity, acid and heat resistance); classification in group 2 as defined in the Directive 2000/54/EC.

2   Occurrence

General
Worldwide in man (source of infection) and animals (pathogen reservoir); most important cause of acute infantile gastroenteritis (AGE); seroprevalence >90 %, maintained until the adult age range by (subclinical) re-infections; occurs all the year around (developing countries) or in seasonal peaks in winter (temperate climatic zones); nosocomial infections (about 20 %), sporadic cases (travellers), outbreaks; global (especially Africa, Asia, Latin America) about 500 million children develop the illness annually of whom up to one million die (fatal in 1 %–4 % of cases); of the rotavirus infections in Europe 9 %–29 % (Germany 23 %) are AGE, 2.6 % of cases in Germany require hospitalization; 50199 registered cases of the illness (rarely fatal) in the year 2001 (Germany), of those 82 % children.

Occupational
The health service (especially neonatology), consulting laboratories, facilities for medical examination, treatment and nursing of children and for care of preschool children, geriatric establishments.

3   Transmission route, immunity

Mostly classical faecal-oral (indirect infection), alimentary (water, foodstuffs), aerogenic, perhaps via virus particles in the air (dust infection); excreters (also subclinical); transmission from animal to man unclear; short-term mucosal immunity, illness results in serotype-specific humoral immunity.

4   Symptoms

Incubation period 1–3 days, highly *contagious*, often even before diarrhoea begins and as long as the virus is excreted (generally 8 days); in babies up to 3 months old asymptomatic, subclinical course (maternal immunity); in children between 6 months and 2 years of age severe course, sometimes life-threatening desiccation, in adults rare; main symptoms: sudden watery to slimy diarrhoea, vomiting, high temperature, duration generally 2–6 days; complications a result of massive water and electrolyte loss, encephalitis, haemorrhagic shock.

G 42

5   Special medical examination

Detection of infectious agent
Stool, group-specific antigens by means of antigen ELISA (method of choice), perhaps sandwich ELISA, *microscopy:* histochemical focus assay/fluorescent focus assay; *culture:* virus isolation in permanent cell lines; *molecular biology:* detection of RNA by polyacrylamide gel electrophoresis; reverse transcription PCR, in situ hybridization analysis (RNA probe).

Detection of antibodies
To establish susceptibility to infection: detection of IgG, IgM, IgA antibodies with indirect (antibody) ELISA (method of choice) with anti-group-specific antigen antibodies, neutralizing antibodies with a focus reduction assay.

6   Specific medical advice

Before exposure
Exposure prophylaxis: hygienic and disinfection measures;
Disposition prophylaxis (vaccination): two live vaccines available, in both cases 2–3 oral doses between the ages of 6 and 26 weeks.

After exposure
Rehydration therapy, virustatic treatment currently not possible, antibiotics not indicated; for premature babies daily generally oral (rarely i.v.) doses of human IgG.

7   Additional notes

Any national notification regulations and restrictions on activities and employment are to be observed.

Rubella virus (German measles virus)

1   Infectious agent

Rubella virus, RNA virus not resistant to environmental factors, family Togaviridae; classification in group 2 as defined in the Directive 2000/54/EC.

2   Occurrence

General
Endemic worldwide; in temperate climates seasonal pattern of infections with peak in spring (children), in Germany in spite of the introduction of a rubella vaccination (1974) a large proportion of the population is not immune (endemic persistent

circulation of the virus); 0.8 %–3 % of women in the age group 18 to 30 years have no anti-rubella antibodies.

Occupational
Facilities for medical examination, treatment and nursing of children and for care of preschool children, research institutes, laboratories, reference centres, the health service (obstetrics, care of pregnant women).

3   Transmission route, immunity

Man is the only natural host; low susceptibility; droplet, contact and indirect infection, transplacental; persistent, often life-long humoral immunity (88 %–95 % of pregnant women) probably after natural infection; cellular immunity certain, but does not protect from local re-infection (nasal cavity, throat).

4   Symptoms

Postnatal rubella
Incubation period 12–21 days; *contagiousness* in postnatally infected children from 7 days before appearance of the rash until the rash disappears at latest, in prenatally infected children *contagious* until the second year of life; upper respiratory tract as site of entry; 5–7 days *post infectionem* (p.i.) lymphohaematogenic generalization; in about 50 % of cases asymptomatic course (children); prodromal stage (2 days) with catarrhal symptoms; exanthema stage (1–3 days) with high temperature, maculopapular rash of small not confluent spots (absent in 20 % of cases); beginning behind the ears, spreading over the face, neck, trunk, extremities, first local lymphadenitis, later generalized with splenomegaly; *complications* rare (more common with increasing age of patient): rheumatoid arthralgia, bronchitis, otitis media, encephalitis, myocarditis, pericarditis, thrombocytopenic purpura and haemorrhage, haemolytic anaemia.

Congenital rubella
Primary infections during the first 4 months of pregnancy can cause spontaneous abortion, early births or congenital rubella syndrome (CRS, together fatal in 15 %–20 % of cases); damage during the organogenesis stage: generally classical rubella embryopathy with defects in the heart (ventricular septal defect, persistent ductus arteriosus, pulmonary stenosis), eyes (cataracta congenita sometimes with glaucoma, microphthalmia, pseudoretinitis pigmentosa), ears (especially inner ear deafness); sometimes more extensive rubella syndrome with more visceral and/or cerebral sequelae (some reversible) than are normally found in classical rubella embryopathy; late-onset rubella syndrome: from the 4th to the 6th month of life.

Late manifestations
Insulin-dependent diabetes mellitus, (average latency 10–15 years); rarely progressive panencephalitis, presumably a slow virus disease.

5   Special medical examination
Detection of infectious agent
Virus isolation (tissue culture) or detection with methods of *molecular biology* (reverse transcription PCR) not usual in the acute stage, only for connatal infection, e.g. from throat swab, lens aspirate, urine, liquor.

Detection of antibodies
To establish the vaccination status/susceptibility to infection: anamnesis of illnesses and vaccinations is not sufficient, inspection of vaccination documents (perhaps pregnancy records) required; detection of virus-specific IgM and IgG antibodies quantitatively with the haemagglutination test (HHT) as standard; if the HHT titre ≤16, (ELISA) or haemolysis-in-gel test; perhaps Western blot; IgG antibody titre ≥32 (HHT) before the beginning of pregnancy is considered to be sufficient protection from CRS; prenatal diagnostics indicated in cases with questionable or demonstrated rubella infection (cell culture, PCR).

6   Specific medical advice
Before exposure
Exposure prophylaxis: hygienic and disinfection measures;
Disposition prophylaxis (vaccination) with attenuated live vaccine, preferably with combination vaccine against measles, mumps and rubella (MMR vaccine); standard or *mass vaccination: first MMR vaccination* in children 11 to 14 months old, *second MMR vaccination* at 15–23 months, perhaps single vaccination (monovalent, preferably MMR vaccine) for seronegative women without age limits and/or in spite of anamnestically recorded rubella infection, check of vaccination success is necessary; *occupational indication for vaccination* of unprotected persons working in the institutions listed above, check success of vaccination after 4–6 weeks for women; after vaccination at least 3 months contraception; *vaccination is indicated* for seronegative women with a wish to bear children; check success of vaccination after 4–6 weeks; during pregnancy vaccination contraindicated.

After exposure
Note: risk of infection via body fluids – including synovial fluids; unvaccinated children or those only vaccinated once after contact with persons with rubella; if possible within 3 days of exposure (mass vaccination), preferably MMR vaccine; there is no specific therapy.

7   Additional notes
Any national notification regulations are to be observed.

Salmonella enterica (serovar Typhi)

1   Infectious agent
Salmonella (*S.*) *enteritica*, serovar Typhi, Gram-negative bacterium, human patho-
gen, motile, facultative anaerobe; family Enterobacteriaceae; classification in group
3(**) as defined in the Directive 2000/54/EC.
Has been placed in category B on the list of potential bioterrorism agents by the
US Center for Disease Control and Prevention (CDC).

2   Occurrence
General
Worldwide, annual incidence 17 million cases, 600000 deaths, endemic in countries with inadequate hygiene (prevalence in Africa $200/10^5$ inhabitants), after the
Second World War annual incidence (industrial countries) sank from $40/10^5$ inhabitants to 0.1/105 inhabitants, in Germany 57 registered cases in the year 2002;
mainly (80 %–90 %) imported from developing countries.

Occupational
Stool laboratories, the health service (treatment of infectious diseases, pathology),
laboratories for enterobacterial diagnosis, reference centres, institutions (crèches,
kindergartens, day nurseries, schools, other educational establishments, homes, holiday camps and similar), work in areas where the pathogen is endemic.

3   Transmission route, immunity
Pathogen reservoir only man (during incubation, illness, chronic carriers); mostly faecal-oral via contaminated foodstuffs or drinks (alimentary infection), contaminated
objects (indirect infection), via long-term excreters; minimum natural immunity is for
only 1 year, high infection dose ($>10^5$ CFU) can still cause the disease.

4   Symptoms
Incubation period 3–60 (average 10) days; *contagious* 7–21 days, life-long symptom-free excretion of the pathogen (stool) is possible.
Prodromal stage: duration 1 week; uncharacteristic, often wrongly diagnosed influenza-like symptoms (anorexia, nausea, vomiting, headaches, pains in the limbs,
unproductive cough); within 2–3 days step-wise temperature increase to 40°C, abdominal pain, disturbed sensorium.
Febrile stage: duration 1–3 weeks; persistent high temperature; initial constipation
(older persons), later (week 3) pea soup-like diarrhoea (younger persons); conspicuous relative bradycardia, clouding of consciousness, hepatosplenomegaly, pale red
pinhead-sized not itching roseola (mostly on the abdominal skin); organ manifestations (from week 2): typhoid nodules, e.g. in the bone marrow and striated muscles.

End of the febrile stage: while the organ manifestations are regressing (from week 4 of the illness) undulating (remitting) decreasing temperatures, life-threatening lymphoma colliquation; fatal in 15 % of untreated cases, <1 % after antibiotic therapy. *Complications (without antibiotic therapy):* intestinal bleeding and perforation with peritonitis, necrotizing cholecystitis, hepatitis, interstitial pneumonia or bronchopneumonia, rupture of the spleen, metastatic meningitis, abscesses in the spleen, liver, kidneys, bones, rarely osteomyelitis or spondylitis (often not until months or years later); toxic circulatory collapse.

Without antibacterial treatment long period of convalescence; subfebrile temperatures indicate danger of relapse; multiple relapses possible; of persons who survive the illness 2 %–5 % become chronic carriers (mainly older persons and women).

5 Special medical examination

Detection of infectious agent
For differential diagnosis isolation of the pathogen from blood (weeks 1–2) and/or stool (from week 2), also urine (weeks 2–3), bone marrow (weeks 5–6), duodenal secretions;

Detection of antibodies
Widal test at 7–12 day intervals: 4-fold titre increase is diagnostic; anti-Vi antibody test during convalescence and for chronic carriers (ELISA, direct agglutination test).

6 Specific medical advice

Before exposure
Exposure prophylaxis: in areas where the pathogen is endemic care should be taken when eating and drinking ("cook it, peel it or forget it"); in other regions early identification of persons with the illness, contact persons, chronic carriers; hygienic and disinfection measures;
Disposition prophylaxis (vaccination): indicated before travelling to areas where the pathogen is endemic, during outbreaks, catastrophes; vaccines well tolerated: oral live vaccine or parenteral killed vaccine (booster after 3 years); medicinal prophylaxis not indicated.

After exposure
When illness apparent: antibiotic therapy for 2 weeks with ciprofloxacin (drug of choice), alternatively wide-spectrum cephalosporins (ceftriaxone, cefotaxime), trimethoprim-sulfamethoxazole, β-lactam antibiotics (ampicillin, amoxycillin); temperature drops within 4–5 days; combination therapy for chronic carriers with ceftriaxone, gentamycin, marked pathogen resistance (developing countries) with resistance to treatment.

7   Additional notes

Any national notification regulations and restrictions on activities and employment are to be observed.

Schistosoma mansoni

1   Infectious agent

Schistosoma (S.) haematobium, S. intercalatum, S. mansoni, S. japonicum, S. mekongi, blood flukes/trematodes, family Schistosomatidae; classification in group 2 as defined in the Directive 2000/54/EC.

2   Occurrence

General
Endemic in (sub)tropical countries, 200–300 million people infected; *primary host:* man (accidental host); (African) baboon, rat, mouse, water buffalo, horse, cattle, pig, sheep, goat, dog, cat; *interim hosts:* molluscs (fresh water snails); distribution favoured by extensive irrigation programmes, construction of dams.

Occupational
Research institutes, reference centres, laboratories, infection of persons even on single brief contact with infested waters in areas where the pathogen is endemic (e.g. agricultural technologists, fishermen, rice farmers), Voluntary Service Overseas, other work in areas where the pathogen is endemic.

3   Transmission route, immunity

Not transmitted from person to person; transmission only at certain points of the life cycle which involves several generations and obligate host alternation; alternate *sexual* (primary host) and *asexual* (interim host) reproductive forms (adults, larvae): in contaminated surface waters containing eggs (snail biotope) the larvae with bifurcated tails (cercaria) which are released by the interim host invade the primary host percutaneously; the young developing schistosomes mate permanently and migrate in pairs into the lumen of the submucosal venous plexus of the lesser pelvis, or into intestinal or mesenterial veins, portal vein or hepatic vessel branches; after maturation of the females egg-laying is associated with perivascular cytotoxic-allergic inflammatory infiltration; 5–12 days after infection, eggs with well-developed embryos appear in the urine or faeces (prepatent period) and contaminate the biotope of the interim host; others become encapsulated locally in the organs or die; in the infested waters a miracidium hatches from the egg and reproduces asexually in the interim host where differentiation via mother-sporocyst and daughter-sporocyst generations (hepatopancreas) to the cercaria takes place; the cercaria – released into the body of water – infect the primary host *(carriers with egg excretion);* persistence of adult flukes 2–5 (10) years – protection against re-infection without elimination of the pathogen (concomitant immunity) is limited because developing schistosomes produce masking surface coat antigens (immune evasion).

4   Symptoms

Parasitic disease with alternating generations and hosts.

Penetration phase: cercaria of schistosomes pathogenic for man and animals cause within 1 hour (to 24 hours) local urticarial efflorescences (angio-oedema); repeatedly exposed persons develop generalized maculopapular exanthema (cercarial dermatitis).

Acute phase (early stage): *incubation period 3–7* (12) weeks after exposure to cercaria; not *contagious* from person to person without interim host; frequently without clinical symptoms; *Katayama syndrome* as a reaction to antigenic schistosome metabolites which persists for several weeks: raised temperature, shaking chills, fits of perspiration, headaches, pains in the limbs, coughing with haemorrhagic sputum (bronchitis, pneumonia), lymphadenopathy, eosinophilia; can be fatal; in addition, in cases of urogenital schistosomiasis (54 African countries, Eastern Mediterranean region) cystitis (leukocyturia, urge to urinate), haematuria (*S. haematobium,* rarely *S. intercalatum*); in cases of *intestinal* schistosomiasis caused by *S. mansoni* (53 African countries, Eastern Mediterranean region, the Caribbean, South America) acute epigastric symptoms, mucosanguineous diarrhoea, in cases caused by *S. japonicum, S. mekongi* as oriental or Asiatic form (7 countries in South-East Asia and the West Pacific region) hepatolienal involvement; this does not occur in other intestinal forms caused by *S. intercalatum* (10 Central African countries).

Chronic phase (late stage): after local or ectopic egg deposition; cellular-infiltrating tubercles, perhaps formation of calcifying nodules (1–2 mm), so-called pseudotubercles (granulomas) or papillomatous mucosal growths (polyps); fibrosing cirrhotic (cartilaginous) organ changes.

Urogenital bilharziasis: mainly caused by *S. haematobium,* rarely *S. intercalatum;* granulomas in kidneys, testes, mucosa of urinary bladder and vagina (polyps), in the urethra, fallopian tubes, vas deferens; strictures with urinary retention, blockage of the fallopian tubes and seminal vesicles; fibrotic calcifying bladder wall with narrowed orifices; promotion of bladder carcinoma has been suggested; in the USA incidence is higher than that of bladder cancer not associated with bilharziasis.

Intestinal bilharziasis: caused mainly by *S. mansoni, S. japonicum, S. mekongi,* rarely by *S. intercalatum;* frequently in combination with hepatolienal bilharziasis; colorectal mucosa initially granulopapillomatous, later with ulcerous haematogenic alterations with a disposition to colon carcinoma formation; fibrous thickening of the intestinal wall and mesenterium.

Hepatolienal bilharziasis: granuloma formation in liver parenchyma; cartilaginous-scarlike reconstruction, also around the branches of the portal vein, reduced portal vein and intrahepatic circulation, Banti syndrome (splenomegaly, hepatomegaly, haematopoietic disorders, subicterus, urobilinuria, liver cirrhosis, ascites, cachexia); portal hypertension; congestion and drainage via anastomosis areas with dilation of para-umbilical veins (so-called spider belly), oesophagus varices, haemorrhage in the gastrointestinal canal; cardiac insufficiency with arteriitis in branches of the pulmonary arteries and congestion of the pulmonary circulation (cor pulmonale) or caused by coronary artery infarct (blockage with deposited eggs); focal cerebrospinal symptoms e.g. aphasia, epileptiform fits, meningitis, encephalitis, amaurosis (rare), monoparesis, hemiparesis, incomplete paraplegia, dermal fistula formation caused by unusual ovipositions.

G 42

5   Special medical examination
Serodiagnostic intradermal test with cercaria antigen (dilutions 1:100 to 1:10000) to exclude the penetration phase.

Detection of infectious agent
In persons who have returned home from an area in which the pathogen is endemic to detect a supposed infection with cercaria *before* the beginning of egg deposition.

Detection of antibodies
Serum antibody detection (against fluke eggs, cercarian antigens) by means of ELISA, indirect immunofluorescence test, complement fixation reaction, indirect haemagglutinin test to exclude the acute and chronic phases.

6   Specific medical advice
Before exposure
Exposure prophylaxis: avoid contact with natural or artificial bodies of water containing cercaria or alternatively wear protective clothing; control fresh water snails (molluscidal agents); boil, chlorinate and filter drinking water; improve sewage treatment; prevent access to the biotope of the interim host, or drain it (hygienic organizational measures);
Disposition prophylaxis (vaccination) not available.

After exposure
At the earliest 5–12 days after infection, microscopic detection of fluke eggs in fresh stool sample (thick smear), perhaps after concentration (enrichment) of the sample, of native or stained eggs in mid-stream urine (centrifuge sediment) or pooled spontaneous urine samples (filtrate), direct in mucosal biopsy material from the urinary bladder, rectum, liver (crushed preparation); miracidia test with sedimented fluke eggs exposed to light; "cercarianhüllenreaktion" with specific anti-cercaria immune sera; medicinal therapy or medicinal prophylaxis (if necessary mass prophylaxis) of supposedly infected persons; if eggs or specific serum antibodies are detected medicinal treatment with praziquantel as drug of choice, effective against all schistosoma

species, trichlorfon (metrifonate) only against *S. haematobium*, oxamniquine only against *S. mansoni*.

7   Additional notes
Any national notification regulations are to be observed.

Staphylococcus spp. (S. aureus, MRSA strains, CNS-types including S. epidermidis)

1   Infectious agent
Staphylococcus (S.) aureus, Gram-positive, catalase-positive and coagulase-positive cocci which often form clusters, family Micrococcaceae; pathogenicity factors in the cell walls and extracellular factors; single and multiple drug resistance:
Methicillin-resistant Staphylococcus aureus (MRSA) strains
haMRSA (hospital acquired), caMRSA (community acquired)
Penicillinase-negative Staphylococcus aureus
Coagulase-negative staphylococci of clinical relevance (*S. epidermidis* group and *S. saprophyticus* group)
Penicillinase-positive coagulase-negative variants
Penicillinase-negative coagulase-negative variants
Classification in group 2 (*S. aureus*) as defined in the Directive 2000/54/EC; coagulase-negative variants not yet listed.
Has been placed in category B (staphylococcus enterotoxin B) on the list of potential bioterrorism agents by the US Center for Disease Control and Prevention (CDC).

2   Occurrence
General
S. aureus: worldwide in man and animals (pets), strains infecting animals generally not found in man and the other way around; man as main pathogen reservoir, ubiquitous on the skin and mucosa; preferred sites: throat, nasal vestibule, arm pits, perineal region, forehead hairline, less often colon, rectum, vagina; incidence of carriers (adults) 15 % to 40 %, depending on exposure or on the (habitual or chronic) lack of integrity of the skin epithelium, one of the commonest bacterial pathogens causing nosocomial and not nosocomial infections, especially wound infections.
MRSA strains: worldwide (haMRSA, epidemic MRSA): colonization of hospital patients (nosocomial infections), prevalence (Germany 15 %) a function of improper use of wide-spectrum antibiotics, rapid asymptomatic colonization of contact persons, caMRSA rare, spontaneous outbreaks.

Coagulase-negative variants: main part of the normal flora, recent outbreaks of noso-comial infections, contamination of examination materials.

Occupational
Medical and kitchen staff as possible carriers; MRSA strains: medical staff affected particularly frequently (up to 90 %), reference centres, consulting laboratories.

3   Transmission route, immunity

Endogenous infection (normal body flora); exogenous infection (external pathogen which colonizes the body temporarily or permanently); indirect infection especially via contaminated hands, wound and airway secretions, intertriginous skin areas, blood (bacteraemia) or medical equipment; aerogenic dissemination possible but of lesser importance; predisposing factors include impaired cellular defence mecha-nisms (e.g. diabetes mellitus, maintenance dialysis), plastic implants (e.g. venous catheter, joint replacement), immunosuppression, virus-induced cell damage (predis-position to infections, e.g. as with influenza A), mechanically altered barriers (e.g. skin and mucosal wounds), no effective immunity.

G 42

4   Symptoms

S. aureus/MRSA strains
Local surface or/and invasive suppurative inflammation; *incubation period:* 4–10 days, months in cases of colonization and persistence in wounds or operated tissue (sometimes even years later); *contagious* during persistence of clinically manifest symptoms or when transmitted by clinically healthy colonized persons; *manifesta-tions:* furuncles, carbuncles, pyodermia, abscesses (also in other organs), infections of wounds or around foreign bodies, empyema, sepsis (fatal in 15 % of cases).

caMRSA
Deep, complicated, chronic skin and soft tissue infections, necrotic pneumonia, high-ly lethal, also for young and previously healthy people.

Toxin-mediated disorders
Heat-stable toxins formed outside the body cause food poisoning (intoxications most-ly with enterotoxin A), 30 % of all S. aureus strains produce toxins in meat and milk; toxin formation between 7 and 46°C; incubation period: 2–6 hours, nausea, vomit-ing, diarrhoea, circulatory disorders.
Toxins formed in the infected organism cause the syndromes described below.
Staphylococcal scalded skin syndrome (SSSS) (rare with MRSA strains) as bullous im-petigo contagiosa or dermatitis exfoliativa.
Toxic shock syndrome (TSS) – to date not with MRSA strains; disorder which is fre-quently not recognized, follows skin disorders, burns or traumatic operations: raised temperature (>39°C), diffuse macular exanthema, scaling of the skin 1–2 weeks

after the beginning of the illness (palms of the hands, soles of the feet), multiorgan failure; in older adults >90 % of cases with specific antibodies.

Coagulase-negative Staphylococcus strains
S. epidermidis group: severe, sometimes chronic larvate infections, sometimes with metastatic abscess formation in parenchymatous organs; sepsis originating from a venous catheter or cerebrospinal fluid fistula (>30 % of cases).
S. saprophyticus group: urinary tract infections

5 Special medical examination

Detection of infectious agent
If infection is suspected confirmation by culture of the organism; subsequent species identification (commercial test kits); in unclear cases detection of free plasma coagulase (tube test with MRSA screening, fine differentiation by lysotyping, antibiogram, pulsed field gel electrophoresis (macro-restriction fragment analysis); toxin detection with the Ouchterlony test, ELISA, Western blot.

6 Specific medical advice

Before exposure
Exposure prophylaxis: isolation and control measures as soon as the first case is recognized (colonization, infection); systematic hygiene management if MRSA strains are involved; during nosocomial outbreaks check patients and medical staff for MRSA strains; isolation of contact persons not necessary; avoid invasive diagnostic or operative measures.
Disposition prophylaxis (vaccination) not available.

After exposure
Treat infected persons according to the results of the antibiogram: third generation cephalosporins (not ceftazidime), further treatment according to demonstrated sensitivity.

7 Additional notes

Any national notification regulations are to be observed.

Streptococcus spp. (S. pyogenes, S. pneumoniae, S. agalactiae)

1   Infectious agent

Streptococcus (*S.*) *pyogenes*: pathogenic only for man, Gram-positive, β-haemolytic A streptococcus; family Streptococcaceae;

S. pneumoniae (pneumococcus): pathogenic for man and animals, Gram-positive, α-haemolytic streptococcus, sensitive to environmental factors (cold, drying out); family Streptococcaceae;

S. agalactiae: pathogenic for man and animals, β-haemolytic B streptococcus, co-haemolysin (CAMP factor protein), less resistance to environmental factors than A streptococci; family Streptococcaceae; classification in group 2 as defined in the Directive 2000/54/EC.

G 42

2   Occurrence

General
S. pyogenes
worldwide, man the only natural host; throat infections (15 %–30 %): most frequent bacterial infection in children, outbreaks in all age groups (peak at age 4 to 7 years), in Germany annually 1–1.5 million cases of acute streptococcus pharyngitis; scarlet fever 62 cases per 100000 inhabitants (1998).
S. pneumoniae
worldwide, animals and man, asymptomatic carriers (nasopharyngeal space), 50 % of general population, 35 % of school-age children, 60 % of pre-school children.
S. agalactiae
worldwide in man and animals, 7 % of all streptococcus infections in man involve group B streptococcus; urogenital and intestinal tracts affected most; up to 40 % asymptomatic (young) women.

Occupational
The health service (midwives, neonatology), reference centres, institutions for medical examination, treatment and nursing of children, care of preschool children, outpatient nursing services, hostels, mining (*S. pneumoniae*), veterinary medicine (*S. agalactiae*).

3   Transmission route, immunity

S. pyogenes
Asymptomatic colonization (throat), occasionally also intestinal and urogenital tracts; virus infection predisposes to streptococcus infection, usually droplet infection, suppurative skin infections after contact or indirect infection, rarely alimentary infection, wounds or microlesions (erysipelas); immunity via serotype-specific antibodies, multiple infections possible; in the case of scarlet fever immunity involves specific antitoxins.

S. pneumoniae
Exogenous (expired droplets) and endogenous infections (nasopharynx carriers), favoured by previous virus infection, inherited/acquired immunodeficiency, asplenia; humoral serotype-specific immunity.

S. agalactiae
Transmission from person to person but also from animals to man (e.g. udder, milk) possible (rare); increased risk groups: immunodeficient adults, newborn babies of asymptomatic colonized mothers up to 100 % infected; indirect nosocomial infections, sexual transmission possible.

4   Symptoms

S. pyogenes
Incubation period 2–4 days; *contagious* for up to 3 weeks, after effective antibiotic therapy 24 h.
Suppurative local infections (throat, skin): Localized throat infection, acute pharyngotonsillitis (30 %–50 % of all bacterial pharyngitis cases), sometimes with concomitant sinusitis, otitis media, mastoiditis, pneumonia; complications peritonsillar and retropharyngeal abscesses.
Infections of the skin and soft tissues, on the surface as impetigo contagiosa; pustular eruptions on the face and legs; phlegmon, necrotizing fasciitis, myositis; erysipelas (face, abdomen, buttocks).
Generalized and toxin-induced illnesses: Streptococcus toxic shock syndrome caused mainly by superantigen toxins, fatal in about 30 % of cases (multi-organ failure, shock); disseminated foci with sepsis (rare), osteomyelitis, cavernous sinus thrombosis with meningitis.
Scarlet fever as a result of toxin-induced pharyngitis (mostly tonsillitis), then hypertrophied papilla and initially the coated strawberry tongue, later the peeling raspberry tongue; peri-oral pallor, finely spotted exanthema which is not always present (lasts 6–9 days), neck, over the trunk, extremities (flexor sides), not including palms of the hands/soles of the feet, regional lymphadenitis, after 1 week first bran-like, later coarse lamellar skin exfoliation; feared complications are endocarditis, myocarditis, pericarditis.
Sequelae: Acute rheumatic fever (autoimmune disorder) as rheumatism of the soft tissues and joints, only after throat infection (latency period 18 days); acute glomerulonephritis (immune complex vasculitis), after throat (latency period 10 days) and skin infections (latency period 3 weeks).

S. pneumoniae
Incubation period unknown; contagious for up to 3 weeks; lobar pneumonia, focal bronchopneumonia, often with a septic course; most frequent form of non-nosocomial pneumonia.
Complications: Pleural empyema, brain abscess, pericarditis, endocarditis, purulent meningitis, progressive otitis media, mastoiditis, sinusitis, ulcus serpens corneae

(sometimes with endophthalmitis), adnexitis, appendicitis, primary peritonitis, gonarthritis, fulminant sepsis, Waterhouse-Friderichsen syndrome.

S. agalactiae
Primary suppurative inflammation of the cow's udder (mastitis); human infections increasing in neonatology since 1960; during pregnancy intrauterine infection can lead to premature birth, premature rupture of the membranes, ascending infection, septic abortion; connatal infections (*early onset type*) within 1 week *post partum* (fatal in about 50 % of cases): sepsis, meningitis, pneumonia (rare); postnatal late type (indirect infection) during first 3 months of life: mostly meningitis in some cases with residual defects, when fully developed inflammatory brain oedema, fatal in about 25 % of cases; in adults (immunodeficient persons) mainly nosocomial infections of wounds, urinary tract, pyelonephritis, more rarely endocarditis, peritonitis, osteomyelitis, pneumonia, meningitis, arthritis, endometritis.

G 42

5   Special medical examination

S. pyogenes
Detection of infectious agent: culture and identification with determination of the serogroup (C antigen): swab, aspirate, blood culture; typing by sequencing in specialized laboratories; antigen detection (rapid test) currently not sufficiently sensitive.
Detection of antibodies: In 80 % of cases formation of anti-streptolysin O; anti-desoxyribonuclease B indicated only when a non-suppurative secondary infection is suspected, perhaps a tool to diagnose a past Streptococcus A infection.

S. pneumoniae
Detection of infectious agent: to establish the vaccination status/susceptibility to infection: anamnesis of illnesses and vaccinations is not sufficient, inspection of vaccination documents required; microscopic detection of the pathogen in culture;
Antigen detection (rapid test), currently insufficiently sensitive; serodiagnostics of only epidemiological significance.

S. agalactiae
Detection of infectious agent: blood, liquor, swab material, perhaps urine, necessary for appropriate therapy; *microscopy* (Gram-positive cocci, long chains): vaginal, cervical, rectal swabs from pregnant women, ear, throat swabs, stomach fluid for prophylactic screening of newborn babies; *culture:* concentration in liquid media, solid (perhaps selective) nutrient media for screening;
Antigen detection: B group.

6   Specific medical advice

Before exposure
S. pyogenes
Exposure prophylaxis limited by ubiquitous distribution;
Disposition prophylaxis (vaccination) not available.

S. pneumoniae
Exposure prophylaxis: protective clothing; hygienic and disinfection measures;
Disposition prophylaxis (vaccination): standard vaccination with polysaccharide vaccine (1 dose) for persons over 60 years old; booster at 6-year intervals; vaccination of risk groups when indicated: e.g. children from 2 years of age (preferably conjugated vaccine until 5 years old), young people and adults polysaccharide vaccine (1 dose); boosters at 6-year intervals.

S. agalactiae
Exposure prophylaxis: protective clothing; hygienic and disinfection measures;
Medicinal prophylaxis: prepartum treatment with penicillin G/ampicillin (i.v.) at fixed intervals of several hours;
Disposition prophylaxis (vaccination) not available; administration of immunoglobulins to newborn babies controversial.

After exposure
S. pyogenes
Medicinal therapy (antibiogram not necessary):10-day antibiotic therapy with penicillin, erythromycin; carriers without symptoms need not be treated; in cases of severe systemic infections clindamycin as well; for rheumatic fever recurrence prophylaxis with penicillin: for at least 5 years, after a recurrence life-long.

S. pneumoniae
Medicinal therapy: for colonization not necessary; high dose penicillin G; alternatively (pneumonia, meningitis) high dose ceftriaxon, cefotaxim, imipenem; otherwise according to the antibiogram.

S. agalactiae
Medicinal therapy: penicillins are the drug of choice, for invasive B streptococcus infections ampicillins, aminoglycosides (at least 10 days).

7   Additional notes

Any national notification regulations and restrictions on activities and employment are to be observed.

Toxoplasma gondii

1   Infectious agent

Toxoplasma gondii, intracellular (obligate) protozoan, trophozoite (reproductive stage), cysts (resting stage), oocysts (only in the cat); family Sarcocystidae; classification in group 2 as defined in the Directive 2000/54/EC.

2   Occurrence

General

Worldwide in mammals (cat, pig) including man, considered to be the most widely distributed protozoan in the world (>500 million latent infections), natural infection level up to 20 %, increases with age, prevalence higher in the South than in the North.

G 42

Occupational

Butchers, animal keepers (especially for (wild) cats), work involving contact with earth or sand contaminated with cat faeces, consulting laboratories.

3   Transmission route, immunity

Life cycle: oocysts (excreted by the cat) → develop into trophozoites (reproductive stage) → cysts (resting stage) → taken up by the cat → oocysts. Oral intake of infectious oocytes; ingestion of cyst-containing raw meat from pigs, sheep or goats or unpasteurized milk from infected animals; vectors: insects and earthworms, vehicle: precipitation; transplacental infection especially in man; life-long infection (cysts) in man as interim host; immunity in immunocompetent persons does not prevent re-infection with other *Toxoplasma* strains; exacerbation of silent toxoplasmosis during immune deficiency; generally no transmission from person to person except (rarely) by blood transfusions, organ transplantation, mother's milk.

4   Symptoms

Incubation period: a few hours to 21 days;

Postnatal toxoplasmosis: subclinical influenza-like symptoms in immunocompetent persons, lymphadenitis, raised temperature, sometimes exanthema, after the acute phase latent toxoplasmosis infections because of retention of the cysts in the tissues, especially in the muscles and the brain (cerebral toxoplasmosis as AIDS-defining condition; case definition 1993), rupture of cysts can cause local inflammation (eye, brain) (eye toxoplasmosis with infection of the retina and chorioidea, chronic recurring course is possible); in severe cases liver, lungs, heart, colon can be infected.

Postnatal toxoplasmosis in immunodeficient persons: by fresh infection or exacerbation of a latent toxoplasmosis, encephalitis and meningoencephalitis are the main symptoms, without therapy often fatal in patients with AIDS.

Congenital toxoplasmosis: only when a pregnant woman is infected for the first time, in Germany about 6000 to 7000 first infections annually, in about 50 % of cases the pathogen infects the foetus, severe damage occurs in about 300 to 400 foetuses; severity of damage depends on the time of the first infection: during the first trimester frequent abortions, in the second and third trimesters in about 1 % of cases classical triad of hydrocephaly, intracerebral calcification, retinochoroiditis, in about 10 % of cases signs of inflammation of the heart, lungs, liver, eye, in about 90 % asymptomatic course with late manifestation of brain and eye damage during the first 20 years of life.

5   Special medical examination

Detection of infectious agent
Microscopy (limited success): in acute infections trophozoites in blood; lymph node aspirate, liquor, biopsy material; in congenital infections also detection of tissue cysts (placenta, foetus, newborn baby); in older children and adults mainly cysts in the muscles and brain as proof of a chronic persistent infection.

Detection of antibodies
To establish the susceptibility to infection and for diagnosis: indirect immunofluorescence test, double sandwich ELISA (DSIgM-ELISA), reverse enzyme immunoassay, immunosorbent agglutination assay, ELISA, complement fixation reaction, Sabin-Feldman dye test, direct agglutination test.

6   Specific medical advice

Before exposure
Exposure prophylaxis: general hygienic measures, especially when handling cats and when working outdoors; freeze raw meat, do not eat raw or insufficiently cooked meat (pork), wash raw vegetables and fruit before consumption; serological checks for pregnant women (antibody screening test, IgM antibody test, clarification procedure); monitoring of children at risk; oocysts extremely resistant to the effects of normal disinfectants, remain infectious for years in damp earth, killed by heating over 55°C and by drying out;
Disposition prophylaxis (vaccination) not available.

After exposure
Treat infected persons with pyrimethamin, sulfadiazine, folic acid, in persons with sulfonamide-intolerance with clindamycin, spiramycin instead; postnatal (florid) infection of immunocompetent persons without organ manifestations require no therapy; in cases with severe or persistent symptoms, during pregnancy (seroconversion) begin with spiramycin, from week 16 of pregnancy combination therapy; immunodeficient patients should be treated on suspicion of encephalitis, disseminated or cardiopulmonary manifestations; then maintenance therapy for life (HIV-positive patients).

7   Additional notes
Any national notification regulations are to be observed.

Treponema pallidum

1   Infectious agent

Treponema pallidum subspecies (ssp.) *pallidum*, the agent causing venereal syphilis/lues, Gram-negative bacterium, difficult to stain, saw-tooth-shaped, microaerophilic, obligate pathogen, characteristic motility, resistant to environmental factors; *T. pallidum* ssp. *endemicum* (bejel), *T. pallidum* ssp. *pertenue* (yaws), *T. carateum* (pinta); *in vitro:* pathogenic *T. vincentii* (Vincent's angina); family Spirochaetaceae; classification in group 2 as defined in the Directive 2000/54/EC.

2   Occurrence
General
Distributed worldwide, marked decrease in the number of cases reported between the end of the 1970s and the end of the 1990s in western industrial countries, incidence of cases currently increasing; in the year 2004 in Germany 3345 reported cases (incidence 4.1 per 100000 inhabitants); morbidity currently highest in the third to fourth decade of life; fresh infections twice as common in men as in women; 85 % to 90 % of infected men are homosexual; co-infection of persons infected with HIV is not uncommon.

Occupational
Research institutes, consulting laboratories, the health service: paediatrics (congenital syphilis), gynaecology (midwives), dermatology.

3   Transmission route, immunity
Man the only natural host (pathogen reservoir); transmission most often via apparently undamaged mucosa (microlesions), direct sexual contact, risk of infection during sexual intercourse with an infected person during the primary and secondary stages is 30 % to 60 %, in the late stage generally no risk of infection; accidental (rare) via contaminated objects, by blood transfusion, transplacental (foetal infection); *immunity:* during the primary stage some protection against reinfection, in the secondary stage reinfection practically excluded, in the latent stage immunity highest.

4   Symptoms

About 50 % of infections result in symptoms, spontaneous recovery 30 % (untreated cases); various forms (chronic cyclic infectious disease); incubation period 14–24 (90) days; *contagious* during primary and secondary syphilis (stages I, II), not during latent or late syphilis (from stage III).

Early syphilis (≤ 1 year after infection, highly contagious)
Primary syphilis: initial induration at the inoculation site, erythema, then formation of a papule which develops into a painless highly infectious ulcer with a hard centre and clearly raised edge, heals spontaneously (4–6 weeks) and leaves a scar (synonym primary lesion, hard ulcer, syphilitic ulcer, chancre): location depends on methods of sexual intercourse; the primary lesion together with regional lymphadenopathy, which is practically painless and can persist for months, comprise the so-called *primary complex.*
Secondary syphilis: 4–10 weeks after infection lymphohaematogenous dissemination with diverse symptoms: uncharacteristic symptoms, development of inflamed hardened lymph nodes, characteristic exanthema, enanthema (syphilid): not itching skin efflorescences especially on the trunk (*macular syphilid, roseola*), regress after 2–3 weeks (also without treatment), sometimes typical more papular recurrences during 1–3 weeks (*lichen syphiliticus*), in immunodeficient patients ulcers/necrotic foci (*lues maligna*); local hair loss (*alopecia areolaris specifica*), raspberry/cauliflower-like papillomas among the hair of the head or beard (*frambesiform syphilid*), post-inflammatory depigmentation (leukodermia in the neck region, collar of venus), furrowed opaque patches on the oral mucosa ("plaques muqueuses"), concomitant angina specifica, efflorescences on the palms of the hands and soles of the feet (*palmoplantar syphilid*), unusual formation of horny skin (*clavi syphilitici*), broad, flat, confluent, weeping papules (*condylomata lata*) in intertriginous body regions; all wet efflorescences (skin and mucosa) highly infectious.

Note: syphilis can imitate practically every other skin disorder!

Late syphilis
Tertiary syphilis (late syphilis): in cases of untreated early syphilis, sometimes after latent syphilis (asymptomatic not infectious phase which develops in about 30 % of cases after secondary syphilis); painless tuberonodular efflorescences with scab formation (*tubero-serpiginous syphilid*), mainly on the upper extremities, back and face; subcutaneous painless granulomas or ulcerating scarring tumours (*lues gummosa*) as possible late manifestations in all organs/bones; cardiovascular endarteritic changes (the dreaded mesoaortitis syphilitica), dilated aorta ascendens, aneurysm.
Neurosyphilis: CNS manifestation of late syphilis; increasing in importance because of co-infection with HIV; intrathecal synthesis of specific anti-*Treponema pallidum* antibodies (sometimes without symptoms); tabes dorsalis: degeneration of the posterior funiculus of the spinal cord 20 years after the initial infection, loss of sensitivity, lightening pains in the lower abdomen and legs, atactic gait disorders, hyporeflexia, areflexia, atrophy of the optic nerve (progressive loss of sight, reduced field of vision),

impotence, incontinence; syphilitic (aseptic) meningitis: brain nerve paresis, increased intracranial pressure, specific antibodies (liquor, blood); chronic form: meningovascular syphilis of the vertebral canal (paresthesia, hemiparesis, focal/ generalized seizures); untreated after 15–20 years progressive paralysis/parenchymatous syphilis (nerve cell degeneration and even brain atrophy): psychiatric defects, Argyll Robertson pupil sign (slow reaction to light, normal convergence reaction), speech disorders, transient paresis, manifest organic psychosyndrome with hallucinations, progressive loss of intellectual ability (memory and personality disorders, e.g. delusions of grandeur, paralytic dementia); if untreated fatal within 4–5 years.

G 42

Congenital syphilis
Rare in Germany (prenatal care); from the fourth month of pregnancy transplacental infection, depending on the stage of the disease, intrauterine foetal death or postpartum congenital syphilis; congenital syphilis: syphilitic rhinitis, syphilitic pemphigus (highly contagious), furrows on the lips which heal leaving scars, epiphysiolysis on the ulna, generalized hardening of the lymph nodes, interstitial hepatitis; late congenital syphilis (from age 3 years): like the tertiary stage of adult syphilis, not contagious, furrows around the mouth, Hutschinson's triad (parenchymatous keratitis, inner ear deafness, tooth and bone deformations: saber shin, saddle nose); if the pregnant mother had late syphilis, 70 % of the children are born healthy.

5   Special medical examination

Detection of infectious agent
Only during the highly infectious phase, directly in secretions (primary lesion, condylomata lata) by dark field microscopy, in tissues by silver staining; direct immunofluorescence test, PCR.

Detection of antibodies
Combination of an unspecific test (e.g. cardiolipin cholesterol lecithin antigen) with a specific test for *Treponoma pallidum:* in routine testing the VDRL (Venereal Disease Research Laboratory) test and/or the TPHA (Treponema pallidum haemagglutination) test (screening test) and FTA-ABS (fluorescent treponemal antibody-absorption) test (confirmation test).
Unspecific screening test (VDRL test): detects so-called reagins (reaginic antibodies) directed against phospholipids (tissue destruction), seropositive results 4–6 weeks after infection (titration steps 1:4), 0.2 % false positive results; not suitable on its own for the demonstration of fresh infections but good for monitoring course of the disease (quantitative test).
Treponema pallidum haemagglutination (TPHA) test or *Treponema pallidum* particle agglutination (TPPA) test: specific screening tests, detect anti-*Treponema pallidum* antibodies; seropositive results from 3–5 weeks after infection, generally for life, not suitable for monitoring therapy.

Evaluation of test results (according to Hof, Dörris, Müller)

VDRL test	TPHA test	FTA-ABS test	Evaluation of test results
negative	negative	negative	no syphilis or a very early stage; given clinical indication repeat after 3 weeks, then the TPHA and FTA-ABS tests could be positive (earliest positive results 3 weeks after infection)
negative	positive	positive	treated syphilis (syphilitic scar), fresh infection cannot be excluded completely; given clinical indication repeat after 3 weeks, then the VDRL test could yield positive results (earliest positive result 6 weeks after infection)
positive	positive	positive	syphilis requiring treatment

Fluorescent treponemal antibody absorption (FTA-ABS) test: improved specific confirmatory test, positive results from 3–4 weeks after infection, detects anti-*Treponema pallidum* antibodies, confirms diagnosis given positive results in the TPHA test (see Table).

Detection of IgM antibodies (early phase): serological tests (e.g. IgM FTA-ABS test, IgM enzyme immunoassay, FTA-ABS 19S IgM test, IgM Western blot) for first infections before the other tests yield positive results; in cases of *neurosyphilis* the results of the VDRL test correlate with the activity of the disease, intrathecal anti-*Treponema pallidum* antibody index (ITPA index) documents intrathecal synthesis of specific antibodies but not always indication for therapy.

Every case of syphilis requires detection or exclusion of other sexually transmissible diseases including a test for HIV – also for the sexual partner!

6   Specific medical advice

Before exposure

Exposure prophylaxis: information about safe sexual intercourse, screening for syphilis (maternity care, blood transfusion service); hygienic and disinfection measures, technical and organizational measures for handling the pathogen in special laboratories (handling live pathogens).

Disposition prophylaxis (vaccination) not available.

After exposure
Medicinal therapy: penicillin G drug of choice (for all stages); see the guidelines provided by the societies for internal medicine; serological checks (VDRL test, quantitative TPHA test) 3, 6, 9 and 12 months after therapy; consider post-exposure prophylaxis with single dose of benzathine penicillin; serological check-up after 12 weeks without symptoms.

Note: syphilis sleeps – but it does not die!

7   Additional notes

Any national notification regulations are to be observed.

Trypanosoma cruzi

1   Infectious agent
Trypanosoma (T.) cruzi, parasitic protozoan (chagas disease), flagellated, non-proliferating form in peripheral blood (trypomastigote), unflagellated, oval, proliferating form in tissues (amastigote) with pseudocyst formation; family Trypanosomatidae; classification in group 3 as defined in the Directive 2000/54/EC.

2   Occurrence
General
Endemic especially in country areas: southern states of North America, Mexico, large parts of Latin America (Venezuela, Brazil, northern Chile, Argentina); the WHO has estimated that there are about 20 million persons infected with the disease and 200000 fresh infections annually, dissemination occurs via contact with contaminated parts of buildings (palm leaves, cracks, walls) or animals.

Occupational
Research institutes, laboratories, reference centres, the health service, work in areas where the pathogen is endemic.

3   Transmission route, immunity
Pathogen reservoir: man, 150 species of animals (pets, wild animals, warm-blooded animals); in the host *T. cruzi* exists in two forms: the amastigote in the tissues and the trypomastigote in the bloodstream; infection via blood-sucking, flying triatomid bugs; developmental cycle in the bug, excretion with the faeces as the infectious trypomastigote; penetration of the skin or mucosa of a warm-blooded animal by scratch-

ing the infectious faeces (indirect infection); transmission via blood transfusion, via injection needles, transplantation, transplacental, amniotic fluid, mother's milk, infection through intact skin has not been described; no immunity, the antibodies formed offer no protection.

4 Symptoms

Acute phase
Primary reaction at the site of entry, duration ≥8 weeks (intracellular proliferation), local oedematous inflammation (chagoma), local lymph node swelling; rarely parasitaemia.

Incubation period: 5–40 days; *contagious* as long as the pathogen is present in the blood, in adults the infection is mostly subclinical: persistent or remittent raised temperature ("flu"-like infection), occasionally with general symptoms, generalized lymphadenopathy, urticarial exanthema mainly on the trunk, subcutaneous painful nodules (lipochagoma), hepatosplenomegaly; complications (frequent in children <10 years old) acute/diffuse myocarditis, meningoencephalitis; spontaneous regression after weeks or months is possible, otherwise progression to chronic phase after an intermediate phase which can last years or even decades (10 % to 30 % of infections).

Chronic phase
Often asymptomatic, trypomastigotes not detectable in blood; chronic myocarditis with cardiac insufficiency, cardiomyopathy, megacor, aneurysm of the apex of the heart, arrhythmia (50 %), sudden death from cardiac failure; infection of the nervous system of the intestinal wall: chronic loss of tonus, motility, dilation of visceral hollow organs (mega organ formation, typically oesophagus, colon), volvulus, strangulation ileus; often fatal, normal life expectancy in 10 % of persons with inapparent infection.

5 Special medical examination

Detection of infectious agent
Acute phase: direct microscopic detection of motile trypomastigotes in the blood (from 1–2 weeks after infection); thick blood smear for staining (Pappenheim, Giemsa stain); peak parasitaemia in months 2 to 3 of the illness; low pathogen count makes enrichment procedures necessary.

Chronic phase: direct microscopic detection of pathogen not possible; microhaematocrit method, xenodiagnosis successful in 50 % of cases: feeding sterile triatomid bugs with heparinized blood from infected persons or persons suspected of having the disease, detection of trypomastigotes in the bug faeces (30, 60, 90 days); *histological detection* of amastigotes: skeletal muscle, myocardium, intestine.

Detection of antibodies
Often the only evidence of infection: indirect immunofluorescence test, indirect haemagglutination, ELISA routine methods; otherwise direct agglutination test, radio-

immunoassay, PCR; cross reactions with *Leishmania donovani* (visceral leishmaniasis).

6   Specific medical advice

Before exposure
Exposure prophylaxis: bug control, insecticide-containing paints; improved living conditions; protection from bug bites; screening of blood donors;
Disposition prophylaxis (vaccination) not available (vaccines are being tested).

G 42

After exposure
Medicinal therapy: only successful during acute phase, nifurtimox daily for 3–4 months; benznidazole daily for 60 days; perhaps with additional administration of recombinant immune interferon-gamma; damage caused by the infection (chronic phase) cannot be treated.

7   Additional notes

Any national notification regulations are to be observed.

Varicella-zoster virus (VZV)

1   Infectious agent

Varicella-zoster virus (VZV), human alpha-herpesvirus 3 (HHV-3), DNA virus, family Herpetoviridae; classification in group 2 as defined in the Directive 2000/54/EC.

2   Occurrence

General
Worldwide endemic, man and primates the only pathogen reservoirs, varicella most common in winter and spring (temperate climatic zones); in Germany most common of the vaccinable infectious diseases (in children), annually about 700000 cases; level of endemic infection in 1-year-olds 7 %, 88 % (in the age group 6 to 7 years), ≥95 % (16 to 17 years), not until ≥40 years old almost 100 % (source: Robert Koch Institute, 2000); annual incidence of herpes zoster infections 10/10000 children (<10 years old), currently >8000 persons treated in hospital each year.

Occupational
Facilities for medical examination, treatment and nursing of children and for care of preschool children, research institutes, laboratories, the health service (gynaecology, obstetrics).

3   Transmission route, immunity

Contagiousness of varicella high, of herpes zoster low; droplet infection (aerogenic), over great distances (up to 20 m) via contents of vesicles, contact infection, indirect infection (scabs), transmission ratio among siblings 90 %, in institutions 10 %–35 %; transplacental T cell-mediated life-long immunity.

4   Symptoms

Varicella (chickenpox)
Incubation period 14–16 days (but can be as short as 8 or as long as 28 days); *contagious* generally from 2 days before appearance of the rash until the last vesicle has scabbed (about 7 days); clinically apparent manifestation in 95 % of cases: uncharacteristic prodromes (1–2 days), temperature up to 39°C, enanthema, itching maculopapular exanthema; polymorphic syndrome; rash spreads centripetally over the face (sometimes also over the scalp), trunk, extremities (apart from palms of the hands and soles of the feet), generally recovery without sequelae; sometimes afebrile, mild form of the infection; varicella in pregnant women is rare (0.1–0.7 ‰); severe course in immunodeficient persons, during high dose glucocorticoid therapy, in newborn babies.

Complications
Varicella pneumonia: 3–5 days after appearance of the illness (20 % of cases are adults);
CNS manifestations (0.1 % of cases): acute cerebellar ataxia with good prognosis, aseptic meningitis, encephalitis (fatal in 15 % of cases), polyradiculoneuropathy (Guillain-Barré syndrome), acute encephalopathy (Reye syndrome), together fatal in 30 % of cases; *occasionally:* arthritis, acute glomerulonephritis, hepatitis, myocarditis, corneal lesions.

Congenital varicella syndrome (varicella embryopathy)
Embryopathy in 0.4 % of children whose mothers were infected with varicella during weeks 1–20 of pregnancy, from week 21 of pregnancy no embryopathy in spite of increasing proportion of foetal infections; fully developed disease with severe skin changes, hypoplastic extremities, cataract, microphthalmos, chorioretinitis.

Neonatal varicella
Neonatal infection (up to 7 days before, 2 days after birth), often severe, life-threatening course (in up to 30 % of cases).

Herpes zoster (shingles)
Endogenous recurrent varicella (years/decades), most important late complication, virus persists in neuroglial cells of sensory brain nerves and lumbosacral ganglia; recurrent neural virus dissemination in efferent innervation areas (dermatomes T3 to L3, trigeminal area); painful polyradiculoneuritis (hyperaesthesia); in 10 %–15 % of cases postzoster neuralgia, severe and sometimes even life-long; mostly unilateral

itching vesicular exanthema in a single dermatome, heals without scarring in 2–3 weeks, reactivation after latent phase especially when immunity decreases or is disturbed, herpes zoster unproblematic in pregnant women (VZV antibodies), spontaneous occurrence possible.

Other zoster manifestations
Zoster generalisatus: disseminated, severe zoster infection not limited to single dermatomes (in 30 %–50 % of cases), with a varicella-like clinical picture, pneumonia (fatal in 3 %–5 % of cases); infection of the brain nerves III–VIII (z. ophthalmicus, z. maxillaris, z. oticus); meningoencephalitis, granulomatous angiitis with contralateral hemiplegia; ascending myelitis (sometimes with motor paralysis).

G 42

5   Special medical examination

Detection of infectious agent
Microscopy: smear (blister contents) with monoclonal antibodies (direct immunofluorescence test); *culture:* virus culture often successful during the first 3 days of the illness; *molecular biology:* detection of DNA (PCR) in cases of varicella embryopathy, in liquor (meningoencephalitic forms), aqueous humor (retinitis), tears (facial paralysis), in the acute phase of herpes zoster also in blood.

Detection of antibodies
To establish vaccination status/susceptibility to infection, anamnesis of illnesses and vaccinations is not sufficient, inspection of vaccination documents required; ELISA (method of choice); paradoxically IgG antibodies appear earlier (!) than IgM antibodies; fluorescent-antibody-to-membrane-antigen (FAMA) test for clarification or confirmation; VZV infection: significant increase in IgG titre (two samples during the first week of illness); then always specific anti-VZV IgA antibodies, IgM antibodies regularly detectable only for varicella.

6   Specific medical advice

Before exposure
Exposure prophylaxis ineffective; personal protective equipment: particle filtering half mask (FFP3);
Disposition prophylaxis (vaccination): live VZV vaccine, seroconversion in 95 % of cases, 85 % protection from varicella infection, post-vaccination infections milder. Note: vaccine virus-associated varicella (8 % after vaccination), potentially transmissible, latent persistent infection possible, reactivated vaccination virus can cause mild herpes zoster infection; indicated for unvaccinated 12 to 15-year-olds without varicella anamnesis and for seronegative women who wish to have children, before immunosuppressive therapy or organ transplantation, in persons over 60 years old, persons working in the health service (VZV risk areas, nursing immunodeficient patients), new appointments in institutions for pre-school children; general varicella vaccination no longer considered to be justified: the necessary vaccination level of

>95 % currently not achievable; seroprevalence ratios for women of child-bearing age reveal up to 7 % with no immunity.

After exposure
Disposition prophylaxis (vaccination): it makes sense to carry out active immunization during varicella outbreaks (paediatrics, institutions), vaccination indicated within 5 days after exposure or up to 3 days after appearance of the rash. Passive immunization (post-exposure prophylaxis): anti-varicella-zoster immunoglobulin (VZIG) within 96 h of exposure for contact persons (after 1 h face-to-face contact, household contact) or persons at risk; unvaccinated pregnant women without varicella anamnesis; newborn babies after perinatal infection.
Virustatic medicinal therapy (perhaps in combination with interferon/VZIG): aciclovir, valaciclovir famciclovir; also brivudin, foscarnet (reserve medication) in cases with resistance against DNA-nucleoside analogues. *Symptomatic therapy* (immunocompetence): skin care, topical bandages, drying antipruritic medications (ointments, pastes); isolation necessary in hospital but not at home.

7   Additional notes
Any national notification regulations and restrictions on activities and employment are to be observed.

Vibrio cholerae

1   Infectious agent
Vibrio (V.) cholerae, Gram-negative, comma-shaped rods; facultative anaerobes, motile, *serovar O1:* biovar cholerae (classical cholera) and biovar eltor (El Tor cholera); *serovar O139* (Bengal strain): related to serovar O1/biovar eltor (pandemic strain); *virulence factors* e.g. heat-labile cytotonic AB enterotoxin (choleragenic), mucinase, neuraminidase; alkali-tolerant, sensitive to drying out, UV irradiation; family Vibrionaceae; classification in group 2 as defined in the Directive 2000/54/EC.
Has been placed in category B on the list of potential bioterrorism agents by the US Center for Disease Control and Prevention (CDC).

2   Occurrence
General
The pathogen is a classical cause of epidemics with pandemic dissemination; endemic mainly in Southeast Asia, Southern Asia, the Near East, South America, Africa, but also in Europe, Australia, America; in coastal bodies of fresh and brackish

water and river mud, infects water animals and birds; since 1961 *V. cholerae* (bio-var eltor) has spread in waves over almost all continents (apart from Europe and Antarctica); serovar O139 first isolated in 1993, continual spread over Southeast Asia, conceivably a new pandemic serovar; coexistence of serovar O1 and serovar O139 in India and Bangladesh, typical for low socio-economic standards and hygiene; last extensive epidemic in Germany in the year 1892 (Hamburg) with about 17000 infected persons, in recent times 1–3 infections annually (El Tor cholera) imported from India, Pakistan, Thailand, Nigeria, Tunisia.

Occupational
Research institutes, the health service, work in areas where the pathogen is endemic.

3   Transmission route, immunity

Man is the only pathogen reservoir: asymptomatic carriers play a greater role in dissemination than persons with apparent disease; transmission entirely faecal-oral; infectious dose thought to be 100 to 1000 vibrios, nosocomial infections (paediatrics) have been described; *immunity* for 6 months after an infection, in areas where the pathogen is endemic relatively more protection because of repeated infections.

4   Symptoms

Asymptomatic/mild course in 20 % to 30 % of infected persons, during cholera outbreaks in 60 % to 75 %.

Cholera gravis
Incubation period 12–72 hours; *contagious* from person to person as long as the pathogen is excreted (2–3 weeks after diarrhoea ends, rarely up to 7 weeks); without prodromes diarrhoea, hoarseness (vox cholerae); later profuse watery, milky coffee-like or rice-water diarrhoea without tenesmus (500–1000 ml/h), uncontrollable vomiting; when water-loss reaches about 5 % of body weight severe illness with cardiac irregularity, dehydration, loss of electrolytes; scaphoid abdomen; excessively painful muscle cramps, hypovolaemic shock with metabolic acidosis, renal failure; patients often conscious until terminal stage; untreated fatal in about 60 % of cases (classical cholera), 15 % to 30 % (El Tor cholera); given adequate therapy fatal for less than 1 %; rare *cholera fulminans/siderans* with vomiting, diarrhoea and death with 2–3 hours; also rare is *cholera sicca* without gastroenteritic symptoms, death within a very short period.

5   Special medical examination

Detection of infectious agent
Microscopy: rapid screening test within 2 hours in native sample (stool, vomit, duodenal fluid) by means of dark field or light field microscopy, stained sample with Gram stain; *culture:* culture, enrichment from foodstuffs, water samples; biochemical

differentiation, detection of O1 or O139 antigen; otherwise diagnosis possible within 8 hours provided the organisms are preserved in the transport medium, e.g. in alkaline peptone water (pH 8.5–9.2) or Cary-Blair transport medium; *molecular biology* (cholera enterotoxin gene) with PCR, detection limit about 10^3 vibrios/g faeces. *Identification of toxin* (cholera enterotoxin) in serum by ELISA.

Detection of antibodies
Makes epidemiological sense but is otherwise not of significance: first detectable 3–4 weeks after infection.

6   Specific medical advice

Before exposure
Exposure prophylaxis: of prime importance is a proper water supply and sewage disposal in areas where the pathogen is endemic; strict avoidance of potentially contaminated liquids, "Boil it, cook it, peel it or forget it"; 5-day *medicinal prophylaxis* recommended at the start of outbreaks; appropriate technical and organizational protective measures;
Disposition prophylaxis (vaccination): not generally recommended, only when the foreign country requires it, in exceptional cases, there is no WHO recommendation; vaccination protects only for 6 months (50 % to 60 %); least protection provided by oral killed vaccines or genetically engineered oral live vaccines, the use of which is not permitted in Germany; better protection is provided by parenteral (i.m./s.c.) killed vaccines, two doses 1–2 (8) weeks apart.

After exposure
Quarantine for 5 days required (WHO); immediate water, glucose and electrolyte replacement therapy within the first 30 minutes; in addition 3-day *medicinal therapy* (doxycycline, erythromycin, trimethoprim/sulfamethoxazole, ciprofloxacin), do *not* wait for the results of the microbiological tests. Note: multiresistance in areas where the pathogen is endemic.

7   Additional notes

Any national notification regulations and restrictions on activities and employment are to be observed.

Yellow fever virus

1   Infectious agent

Yellow fever virus, enveloped icosahedral RNA virus (40–50 nm); variously virulent African/South American strains, not environmentally stable (drying out, cold), inactivation temperature 55°C; family Flaviviridae; classification in group 3 as defined in the Directive 2000/54/EC.

Has been placed in category A on the list of potential bioterrorism agents by the US Center for Disease Control and Prevention (CDC).

G 42

2   Occurrence

General

Worldwide, estimated 200000 cases per year (areas where the organism is endemic), 30000 deaths; endemic in tropical regions, yellow fever belt in Africa (latitude 15° north to 10° south) and South America (20° north to 40° south), the coastal regions to the west of the Andes are considered to be free of yellow fever as is the whole of Asia; at present the disease is rare among travellers in areas where the organism is endemic; in Germany the last imported fatal case of yellow fever was in an unvaccinated person in 1999.

Occupational

Research facilities, laboratories (regular work and contact with infected animals/ samples, samples and animals suspected of being infected, other contaminated objects or materials containing the infectious agent given a practicable route of transmission), work in areas where the disease is endemic, farming, timber industry.

3   Transmission route, immunity

Vectorial transmission via insect bites; *pathogen reservoir:* primates, mosquitoes (*Aedes* spp., *Haemagogus* spp.); transovarial transmission within the mosquito population, survive dry periods; epidemics of urban yellow fever possible, man as source of infection; man is only sporadically infected with jungle or sylvan yellow fever which is generally transmitted between primates and mosquitoes; *immunity* is lifelong (also after inapparent infections).

4   Symptoms

The illness can take various clinical courses: inapparent; abortive with mild symptoms and generally recovery without sequelae; severe illness with haemorrhagic manifestations, shock syndrome, multiorgan failure; typical biphasic course (fatal in 10 % to 20 % of cases): *incubation period* 3–6 days; *contagious* from person to person (rare) during the first week of the illness (viraemic phase), e.g. via blood donations; acute uncharacteristic begin with high temperature, general symptoms, epigastric lumbosacral pain, generalized myalgia, conjunctival injection, gingival haemorrhage, epistaxis; clinical chemistry (from day 4 of the illness): granulocytopenia, thrombocytopenia, lymphocytosis, monocytosis, proteinuria; remission of clinical symptoms after 3–4 days followed generally by recovery; in 15 % of cases after brief remission toxic fulminant relapse: temperature increases again with relative bradycardia, toxic damage to the cardiac muscle (Faget's law), abdominal pain, hepatitis, hepatic coma, aseptic meningitis, central nervous disorders, haemorrhagic diathesis (bleeding in the organs, e.g. respiratory tract, gastrointestinal tract, genital tract, skin), nephritis, renal failure; fatal in 50 % of cases; recovery (also from inapparent infections) results in life-long *immunity*.

5　　　　Special medical examination

Detection of infectious agent
Virus isolation in cell culture, baby mice; nucleic acid detection, e.g. reverse transcription PCR (method of choice), generally positive on day 1 of the illness; *detection of antigens:* e.g. direct immunofluorescence test (liver biopsy material), antigen capture ELISA (serum).

Detection of antibodies
IgG and IgM antibodies first detectable 5 to 10 days after the start of the illness: indirect immunofluorescence test, enzyme immunoassay (antibody ELISA), neutralization test; IgM antibodies disappear after 6–12 months, IgG antibodies persist for life (protect against reinfection). Note: cross-reacting antibodies (haemorrhagic dengue fever, Japanese B encephalitis, West Nile fever, FSME); *histopathological detection* possible.

6　　　　Specific medical advice

Before exposure
Exposure prophylaxis: vector control (mosquito breeding areas), clothing which covers the body, mosquito nets, repellents; appropriate technical/organizational preventive measures when handling the organism intentionally in laboratories and industry; wearing of personal protective clothing during therapy and nursing: gloves, protective clothing, particle-filtering half mask (FFP3), eye protection;
Disposition prophylaxis (vaccination): note vaccination anamnesis; highly immunogenic, well-tolerated attenuated live vaccine is available (at the latest 10 days before the journey); observe vaccination regulations of the destination and transit countries (tropical Africa, South America); entry restrictions for unvaccinated persons (WHO); vaccination at clinics authorized for yellow fever vaccination; single dose (s.c.), protection at the earliest from day 7 (10) after vaccination; booster at 10-year intervals.

After exposure
Given a febrile patient think in time of yellow fever (travel anamnesis!); if yellow fever is suspected transfer the patient to a hospital for tropical medicine; specific therapy

not available; treatment according to the symptoms; special measures not normally necessary for contact persons; control of outbreaks by vaccination campaign *(mass vaccination)*.

7   Additional notes
Any national notification regulations are to be observed.

G 42

Yersinia pestis

1   Infectious agent
Yersinia (Y.) pestis, Gram-negative, non-motile, aerobic bacterium; pathogenicity/virulence factors: protein capsule, V antigen, W antigen, yersiniabactin, plasminogen activator protein; resistant to environmental factors in sputum, flea faeces, soil (rodent nests); family Enterobacteriaceae; classification in group 3 as defined in the Directive 2000/54/EC.
Has been placed in category A on the list of potential bioterrorism agents by the US Center for Disease Control and Prevention (CDC).

2   Occurrence
General
Pathogen reservoir in animals: wild rodents in symbiosis with ectoparasites (ticks, fleas, mites, lice, bugs); when the population of wild rodents is reduced by plague the ectoparasites transfer their attention to brown rats and black rats; plague epidemics in man possible via rat fleas; endemic in limited areas of Russia, Kazakhstan, Middle East (Iran), India, China, Mongolia, Myanmar (Burma), Vietnam, Africa (Congo), Central and South America (Brazil, Bolivia, Ecuador, Peru), USA (southwest), Mexico, Madagascar; at the beginning of the 20th century the incidence of plague cases decreased, since 1960 tendency to increase: worldwide at present about 3000 cases annually.

Occupational
Research institutions, laboratories, consulting laboratories, veterinary medicine, hostels for asylum seekers, hunting, work in areas where the pathogen is endemic.

3   Transmission route, immunity
Without plague in rodents no plague in man; transmission from person to person rare; rat fleas, body lice transmit infection by stings and bites (bubonic plague); rarely transmitted via skin wounds (indirect infection) during handling of rodents,

rodent excrement (dissection); alimentary (rat flesh); from person to person (droplet infection) possible in cases of primary pneumonic plague; also during bioterrorism attacks; *immunity:* long-term but not absolute protection against reinfection.

4   Symptoms

Cyclic general infection; *incubation period* 2–7 days (bubonic plague), a few hours to 4 days (primary pneumonic plague); *contagious* as long as the pathogen is detectable in aspirate, sputum or blood; fatal nowadays (treated) in 10 % to 14 % of cases.

Bubonic plague (80 % to 90% of cases)
Initial symptoms uncharacteristic, in persons who have not been vaccinated or who are incompletely vaccinated a pathogen-containing blister/pustule (primary lesion) appears at the site of entry, within 1–2 days temperature raised to about 40°C, local painful swelling of the lymph nodes (bubo), mostly femoral/inguinal, less often axillary/cervical; occasionally spontaneous opening of haemorrhagic colliquative lymph nodes; untreated (rare) dissemination into the liver, spleen, meninges, lungs (secondary pneumonic plague); milder forms very rare (pestis minor).

Septicaemic plague (5 % to 10 %)
Primary septicaemia (not preceded by local lymphadenopathy), secondary to bubonic plague (mostly) as systemic infection with raised temperature, hepatosplenomegaly, arrhythmia, meningitis, delirium; disseminated intravascular coagulation, endotoxin shock, gangrenous skin necrosis, preterminal renal failure, ileus; the untreated disorder is almost always fatal (multiorgan failure).

Primary pneumonic plague (plague pneumonia)
Initially bronchitis, from day 2 of illness fulminant febrile disorder, severe bronchopneumonia: first slimy, later more liquid highly infectious sputum which is pale blood-red; gastrointestinal symptoms; the untreated disorder is almost always fatal (multiorgan failure).

Plague pharyngitis
Oropharyngitis, cervical lymphadenitis; the untreated disorder is almost always fatal (multiorgan failure).

5   Special medical examination

Detection of infectious agent
Blood, sputum, lymph node aspirate; *microscopy:* Gram stain or Wayson stain; *culture:* primary culture on blood agar, MacConcey agar, blood culture; biotype determination only in special laboratories; *detection of antigens:* direct immunofluorescence test, haemagglutination test, antigen capture ELISA, rapid F1 antigen test (dipstick); *molecular biology:* PCR.

Detection of antibodies
Anti-F1 IgG (enzyme immunoassay) not relevant for the acute disorder (positive results first obtained on or after day 10 of the illness), retrospective use for epidemiological purposes.

6   Specific medical advice

Before exposure
Exposure prophylaxis in areas where the pathogen is endemic: control of rodents, elimination of rats and vectors; in cases of pneumonic plague particle-filtering half mask (FFP3); *medicinal prophylaxis* when handling the pathogen, when unvaccinated persons have been in potentially infectious contact with the disease, for brief visits to areas where the pathogen is endemic; hygienic and disinfection measures, technical and organizational measures when *handling the pathogen* in (specialized) laboratories; waterproof protective clothing when contact with the pathogen is conceivable during handling of blood or other body fluids;
Disposition prophylaxis (vaccination): use of vaccine not permitted in Germany; use of killed vaccine (bubonic plague) permitted in USA/Canada, protection for only a limited period, revaccination at 6-month intervals: live vaccine: protection not certain, does not prevent pneumonic plague; during long-term exposures a combination of medicinal prophylaxis and vaccination is recommended, in Germany very critical analysis of the indications is recommended.

G 42

After exposure
Quarantine required (WHO); isolation of cases of pneumonic plague, perhaps in a special clinic for at least 48 hours after the start of effective therapy (resistance determination) and improvement of symptoms; *medicinal therapy* within 15 hours of first appearance of symptoms (duration 14 days); parenteral: streptomycin as drug of choice, *oral:* doxycycline, tetracycline; given high level exposure in a *bioterrorist attack* perhaps modified antibiotic dosing.
Measures for *outbreaks*, especially after intentional dissemination of the pathogen in *bioterrorist attacks:* cordoning off contaminated areas; for local task force and ambulance personnel respiratory protection with particle-filtering fine dust mask FFP2, medicinal prophylaxis for persons in direct contact with patients suspected of having pneumonic plague.

7   Additional notes

Any national notification regulations and restrictions on activities and employment are to be observed.
Persons with pneumonic plague and those thought to have it or to have been in contact with it are to be isolated immediately in an appropriate hospital (quarantine).

Abbreviations

ELISA   enzyme immunoassay (enzyme linked immunosorbent assay)
PCR   polymerase chain reaction

Definitions

Social or welfare work
establishments for care of handicapped persons, children's clinics, facilities for medical examination, treatment and nursing of children and for care of preschool children.

The health service
facilities for medical examination, treatment and nursing of persons, establishments for care of handicapped persons including supply and service areas of these institutions (e.g. cleaning), emergency and rescue services, pathology, research institutes, laboratories (regular activities involving potential contact with infected animals/samples, samples and animals suspected of being infected and objects or materials containing or contaminated with the pathogen, given a transmission route).

G 44   Hardwood dust

Committee for occupational medicine, working group "Hazardous substances", Berufsgenossenschaft der chemischen Industrie, Heidelberg

Preliminary remarks

The present guideline describes a scheme for occupational medical prophylaxis which aims to prevent or ensure early diagnosis of adenocarcinomas of the nasal cavity which can develop in persons exposed to hardwood dust.

G 44

Schedule

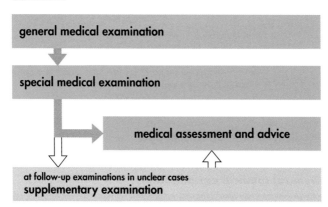

1   Medical examinations

Occupational medical examinations are to be carried out for persons at whose work-places exposure to hardwood dust could endanger health (e.g. the occupational exposure limit value is exceeded).

1.1   Examinations, intervals between examinations

initial examination	before taking up the job
first follow-up examination	until age 45 years: within 60 months from age 45 years: within 18 months (provided that the beginning of exposure was more than 15 years previously)
further follow-up examinations	until age 45 years: within 60 months from age 45 years: within 18 months (provided that the beginning of exposure was more than 15 years previously) and when leaving the job
premature follow-up examination	• after a serious or prolonged illness which could cause concern as to whether the activity should be continued • in individual cases when the physician considers it necessary, e.g. when there is short-term concern about the person's health • when requested by an employee who suspects a causal association between his or her illness and work

1.2   Medical examination schedule

1.2.1   General medical examination

Initial examination

• review of past history (general anamnesis, work anamnesis, symptoms)
Particular attention is to be given to:
• obstruction of nasal breathing
• increased nasal discharge
• nose bleeding
• previous disorders of the nose and nasal sinuses

Follow-up examination

interim anamnesis (including work anamnesis).

1.2.2   Special medical examination

Follow-up examination

• inspection of the nasal cavity with the speculum
For persons aged 45 years or more also:
• endoscopy of the nasal cavity with a rigid or, if necessary, flexible endoscope
Also helpful:
• photographic documentation of the findings if they are abnormal or unclear

1.2.3   Supplementary examination

Follow-up examination

G 44

In unclear cases: e.g. if a tumour is suspected, further examination by an ENT specialist is necessary (e.g. repeated endoscopy, biopsy for histological examination). The further examination by a specialist is intended to clarify any tissue changes observed in endoscopy by means of biopsy.

1.3   Requirements for the medical examinations

• competent doctor or occupational health professional
• a nasal speculum and a nasal endoscope
• either cooperation with an ENT specialist or a minimum number of 50 endoscopic examinations of the nasal cavity carried out per year

2   Occupational medical assessment and advice

An assessment is only possible when the workplace situation and the exposure of the individual are known. For this purpose a risk assessment as defined in Article 4 Council directive 98/24/EC must have been carried out; it must specify which technical, organizational and individual protective measures have been applied.

2.1   Assessment criteria

2.1.1   Long-term concern about health

Initial examination

Previous malignant tumours of the nasal cavity or nasal sinuses.

Follow-up examination

Manifest malignant tumours of the nasal cavity or nasal sinuses for persons in whom dysplastic changes have been confirmed by biopsy: shorter intervals between follow-up examinations.

2.1.2   Short-term concern about health

not applicable

2.1.3   No concern about health under certain conditions

not applicable

2.1.4   No concern about health

Initial examination   **Follow-up examination**

All other persons, provided there are no restrictions on their employment.

2.2   Medical advice

The advice in an individual case should be commensurate with the workplace situation and the results of the medical examinations.

The observance of general hygienic measures should be recommended.

The employees should be told of the carcinogenic effects of beech and oak wood dust.

If the results of occupational medical examinations indicate focal cumulation of health risks, the physician, while observing medical confidentiality, is to inform and advise the employer.

3   Supplementary notes

3.1   External and internal exposure

3.1.1   Occurrence, sources of hazards

Dust is produced during work with hardwoods in processes such as sawing, boring and sanding. Protective measures are required when large amounts of hardwood are processed. Workplaces involving such high levels of dust exposure include:

- cabinetmakers' workshops
- parquet flooring workshops
- staircase production
- mould making (foundries)
- production and processing of wood dust (sawdust)
- production of wood pellets
- cartwrights' workshops

G 44

3.1.2   Physicochemical properties and classification

Dusts consist of particles of solid matter which have been produced in mechanical processes or have been stirred up and dispersed in gases. The information system on hazardous substances (GESTIS) provides details of classification, evaluation and other substance-specific information (see Section 4).

Beech dust
ZVG-No.[1]   530159

Oak dust
ZVG-No.[1]   530158

Additional information is to be found in the recommendations of the DFG Commission for the Investigation of Health Hazards of Chemical Compounds in the Work Area (List of MAK and BAT Values).

---

[1] The Zentrale-Vergabe-Nummer (ZVG-No.) is the unambiguous identification number of a substance in the GESTIS substance database.

3.1.3   Uptake

The dust is taken up via the airways.

3.2   Functional disorders, symptoms

The adenocarcinomas of the nasal cavity are relatively slow-growing tumours. From their site of origin in the region of the middle nasal turbinate, in the middle nasal meatus near the boundary with the ethmoid bone, they invade and destroy surrounding tissues, mainly the ethmoid bone, the eye socket and the front part of the base of the skull from where they can also infiltrate the meninges and forebrain. Lymphogenic metastases in the cervical lymph notes and disseminated haematogenic metastases first develop in a very late irreversible stadium of the disorder. Histologically, the tumour is a special type of adenocarcinoma which has similarities with gastrointestinal tumours and therefore is described as "intestinal type" or "colonic type".

3.2.1   Mode of action

The dust is deposited from the main air stream in the inner nose especially in the area of the middle turbinate. Well-founded statements as to the nature and intensity of its carcinogenic effects cannot be made at present.

The carcinogenic principle is not known. Hypotheses being discussed at present suggest that the cancer is induced at the site of deposition by

- natural wood components or
- chemicals which were applied to the wood during wood preparation and which are attached to the dust particles or
- chemicals used separately from the wood which are inhaled in the form of aerosols and deposited as well as the dust or
- a combination of these mechanisms.

Tumours are mainly observed in patients who worked with chemically treated hardwoods or who were exposed to chemicals such as wood preservatives during or after exposure to wood dust.

4   References

Commission Recommendation 2003/670/EC concerning the European schedule of occupational diseases. Annex I

Council Directive 67/548/EEC on the approximation of the laws, regulations and administrative provisions relating to the classification, packaging and labelling of dangerous substances

Council Directive 98/24/EC on the protection of the health and safety of workers from the risks related to chemical agents at work

Deutsche Forschungsgemeinschaft (German Research Foundation, DFG) (ed) List of MAK and BAT Values 2007. Maximum Concentrations and Biological Tolerance Values at the workplace. Wiley-VCH, Weinheim

Deutsche Forschungsgemeinschaft (German Research Foundation, DFG) (ed) The MAK-Collection for Occupational Health and Safety. Wiley-VCH
at: www.mrw.interscience.wiley.com/makbat

GESTIS-database on hazardous substances. BGIA
at: www.dguv.de/bgia/gestis-database

Kleinsasser O, Schroeder HG (1988) Adenocarcinomas of the inner nose after exposure to wood dust. Morphological findings and relationships between histopathology and clinical behavior in 79 cases. Arch Otorhinolaryngol 245: 1–15

G 44

G 45 Styrene

Committee for occupational medicine, working group "Hazardous substances", Berufsgenossenschaft der chemischen Industrie, Heidelberg

Preliminary remarks

The present guideline describes a scheme for occupational medical prophylaxis which aims to prevent or ensure early diagnosis of disorders which can be caused by styrene.

G 45

Schedule

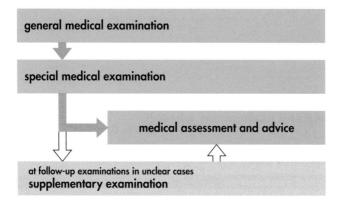

1   Medical examinations

Occupational medical examinations are to be carried out for persons exposed at work to levels of styrene which could have adverse effects on health (e.g. when the occupational exposure limit value is exceeded) or for whom dermal absorption could endanger health.

1.1   Examinations, intervals between examinations

initial examination	before taking up the job
first follow-up examination	after 24 months
further follow-up examinations	after 24 months and when leaving the job
premature follow-up examination	• after an illness lasting for several weeks or when a physical handicap gives cause for concern about whether the work should be continued • in individual cases when the physician considers it necessary, e.g. when there is short-term concern about the person's health • when requested by an employee who suspects a causal association between his or her illness and work

1.2   Medical examination schedule

1.2.1   General medical examination

Initial examination

• review of past history (general anamnesis, work anamnesis)
• urinalysis (multiple test strips)

Follow-up examination

• interim anamnesis (including work anamnesis)
• urinalysis (multiple test strips)

1.2.2   Special medical examination

Initial examination   **Follow-up examination**

- neurological screening (motor system, reflexes, sensitivity, co-ordination)
- checking for irritative or neurotoxic effects of styrene

In addition to reviewing the person's past history, particular attention should be paid to:

- disorders of attention, concentration and memory (short-term memory)
- unusual fatigue, repeated headaches, dizziness and feeling dazed
- irritation of skin and mucous membranes (eyes, nose, throat, airways)

especially if the occurrence of these complaints or symptoms (at follow-up examinations) is associated temporally with the exposure to styrene

- biomonitoring (see Section 3.1.4) – but not at the initial examination

Also helpful:

- γ-GT, SGPT (ALT), SGOT (AST)
- full blood count
- blood sugar
- spirometry
- checking the vibratory sensitivity on the ankle (malleolus medialis) by pallaesthesiometry
- checking for neurotoxic effects of styrene by means of a questionnaire (see Sections 3.3.1 and 3.3.2)

G 45

If the occupational exposure limit value for styrene is not observed, biomonitoring should be carried out at shorter intervals.

1.2.3   Supplementary examination

Follow-up examination

In unclear cases further examination by a specialist should be considered.

1.3   Requirements for the medical examinations

- competent doctor or occupational health professional
- laboratory analyses carried out with appropriate quality control (Good Laboratory Practice)

2   Occupational medical assessment and advice

An assessment is only possible when the workplace situation and the exposure of the individual are known. For this purpose a risk assessment as defined in Article 4 Council directive 98/24/EC must have been carried out; it must specify which technical, organizational and individual protective measures have been applied.

2.1   Assessment criteria

2.1.1   Long-term concern about health

Initial examination	Follow-up examination

Persons with
- chronic skin disorders if these could be aggravated by styrene because of where they are localized (e.g. on the hands and arms)
- marked neurological and psychiatric disorders (polyneuropathy, Korsakoff syndrome, recurrent seizures, severe endogenous psychosis)
- addiction to alcohol, drugs or medication
- diabetes mellitus which is difficult to control
- chronic obstructive airway disorders

2.1.2   Short-term concern about health

Initial examination	Follow-up examination

Persons with the disorders mentioned in Section 2.1.1, provided recovery is to be expected.

2.1.3   No concern about health under certain conditions

Initial examination	Follow-up examination

Persons with chronic skin disorders provided that their localizations ensure that they cannot be aggravated by styrene (e.g. facial acne)
If the illnesses or functional disorders mentioned in Section 2.1.1 are less severe, the doctor should establish whether or not it is possible for the person to return to work or go on working under certain conditions. Such conditions could include
- technical protective measures
- organizational protective measures, e.g., limitation of exposure periods
- transfer to workplaces known to involve lower levels of exposure
- personal protective equipment which takes the individual's state of health into account
- more frequent follow-up examinations

2.1.4   No concern about health

Initial examination	Follow-up examination

All other persons, provided there are no restrictions on their employment.

2.2   Medical advice

The advice in an individual case should be commensurate with the workplace situation and the results of the medical examinations.

Employees are to be informed about the biomonitoring results.

Employees should be informed about general hygienic measures and personal protective equipment. Substance-specific protective measures are documented in the information system on hazardous substances (GESTIS) in the section "Handling and usage" (see Section 4).

The employees are to be advised that alcohol consumption potentiates the effects of the substance.

If during the course of his work in the company the occupational physician finds indications that the risk assessment should be brought up to date to improve health and safety standards, he is to inform the employer. When this is necessary, the interests of the employee are to be protected (medical confidentiality).

G 45

3   Supplementary notes

3.1   External and internal exposure

3.1.1   Occurrence, sources of hazards

Occurrence and hazards for specific substances are documented in the information system on hazardous substances (GESTIS) (see Section 4).

Styrene is used mainly in the production of polymers. Examples of the large number of styrene-based thermoplastics, thermosetting resins, elastomers and dispersions include polystyrene, copolymers with acrylonitrile, butadiene and acrylonitrile, and polyester resins.

There is a risk of exceeding the occupational exposure limit value when handling styrene-containing reaction resins (unsaturated polyester resins: UP resins, vinylester resins: VE resins).

Especially during manual work and then particularly during open processing of large surfaces, e.g. laminating processes in boat building, production of rotors for wind turbines, installation of acid-resistant coatings, winding jobs on large objects, the occupational exposure limit value can be exceeded markedly.

Even when mechanical methods and air extraction systems are used, in some areas exposures above the threshold limit value must be expected.

In the production and processing of styrene, a variety of technologies are used and the exposure levels vary accordingly in the different work areas. Because of the processes involved, the workers are often simultaneously exposed to other solvents, dust, etc.

3.1.2   Physicochemical properties and classification

Styrene is a colourless, highly refractive, inflammable liquid which is very sparingly soluble in water and has a characteristic sweetish smell at low concentrations. The odour threshold (0.05–0.08 ml/m3) is very much lower than the occupational exposure limit value. But it should be remembered that an acclimatization process affects the sense of smell. Styrene is not very volatile. Its vapour, which is formed particularly at higher temperatures, is very much heavier than air and accumulates at floor level.

Styrene
Formula C_8H_8
CAS number   100-42-5
MAK value[1]   20 ml/m^3, 86 mg/m^3

The information system on hazardous substances (GESTIS) provides details of classification, evaluation and other substance-specific information (see Section 4).

3.1.3   Uptake

Styrene is taken up mainly via the airways. If large areas of skin come into contact with styrene, it is conceivable that the substance be absorbed in quantities which cause relevant internal exposure.

3.1.4   Biomonitoring

Information about biomonitoring may be found in Appendix I "Biomonitoring". Consumed alcohol can affect the metabolism of styrene and delay the excretion of metabolites. This should be taken into account when evaluating the biomonitoring results.

---

[1] Maximale Arbeitsplatz-Konzentration = maximum workplace concentration

Biological tolerance value for occupational exposures from the List of MAK and BAT values

Substance	Parameter	BAT[2]	Assay material	Sampling time
styrene	mandelic acid plus phenyl-glyoxylic acid	600 mg/g creatinine	urine	end of exposure or end of shift; for long-term exposures: after several shifts

Biomonitoring should be carried out with reliable methods and meet quality control requirements.

3.2   Functional disorders, symptoms

G 45

3.2.1   Mode of action

The main symptoms of styrene poisoning are neurotoxic effects on the central nervous system. Irritation of the skin and mucous membranes (eyes, respiratory tract) appears early and is not strictly dependent on the exposure concentration. Attention should be paid to the individual disposition.

Styrene is rapidly distributed in the organism. In the liver styrene is metabolized mainly to mandelic acid (about 85 %) and phenylglyoxylic acid (about 10 %); these metabolites are excreted in the urine. Hippuric acid is also formed but in much smaller quantities (about 5 %).

3.2.2   Acute and subacute effects on health

Irritation of the mucosa of the eyes and upper airways and the first effects on the central nervous system appear after exposure to concentrations from about 50 ml/m^3 (ppm), which is markedly higher than the occupational exposure limit value.

At even higher concentrations the following especially prenarcotic symptoms have been described: disorders of attention, concentration and memory (short-term memory), unusual fatigability, frequent headaches, dizziness, nausea, feeling of inebriation, a dazed feeling and even unconsciousness.

---

[2] Biologischer Arbeitsstoff-Toleranzwert (BAT) = biological tolerance value for occupational exposures

3.2.3   Chronic effects on health

Mainly effects on the central nervous system have been described. Predominant are psychomotor and cognitive functional disorders (slower reaction times, reduced memory performance).

In scientific publications, acquired disorders of colour vision (blue to yellow), vestibular disorders and effects on the peripheral nervous system with reduced nerve conduction velocity have been described.

Exposure to liquid styrene and to high concentrations of the substance in the air can cause severe irritation of skin and mucous membranes and, after repeated contact, inflammation and toxic-degenerative alterations.

3.3   Comments

3.3.1   Questionnaire "Q 18" (for the special medical examination, Section 1.2.2)

A special questionnaire (modified "Q 16"), an anamnestic tool for the examining physician (see Section 1.2.2), is to be found below. Under no circumstances should the sum of the questions answered with "yes" be used as an occupational medical criterion for evaluation of the results of the medical examination. It is important for observing the course of any changes that the questionnaire be filled in and reconsidered at every follow-up examination.

3.3.2   Questionnaire PNF I or PNF II

The working group "styrene" has decided to recommend that the occupational physician makes use of the modified form of the questionnaire "Q 16". Of course, other questionnaires such as PNF I or PNF II can equally well be used.

Details of PNF I
Seeber A, Schneider H, Zeller H-J (1978) Ein Psychologisch-Neurologischer Fragebogen (PNF) als Screeningmethode zur Beschwerdenerfassung bei neurotoxisch Exponierten. (A neuropsychological questionnaire for use in screening persons exposed to neurotoxic substances.) Probl Erg Psychol 65: 23–43

Details of PNF II
Sietmann B, Kiesswetter E, Zeller H-J, Seeber A (1996) Untersuchung neurotoxisch verursachter Beschwerden. Die Standardisierung des Psychologisch-Neurologischen Fragebogens, "PNF II". (Examination of persons with neurotoxic symptoms. Standardization of the psychological.neurological questionnaire "PNF II".) Verh Deutsch Ges Arbeitsmed Umweltmed: 36

Details of PNF I + II
Seeber A, Golka K, Bolt H M (1990) Arbeitsmedizinische und psychologische As-
pekte des chronischen organischen Psychosyndroms. (Occupational and psychological aspects of the chronic organic neuropsychologic disorder.) Erstes Heidelberger
Arbeitsmedizinisches Kolloquium, Schriftenreihe des Hauptverbandes der gewerb-
lichen Berufsgenossenschaften, 1990, 83–95, Polyneuropathie oder Enzephalopa-
thie durch organische Lösungsmittel oder deren Gemische. (Polyneuropathy or encephalopathy caused by organic solvents or mixtures of organic solvents.)

4   References

Commission Recommendation 2003/670/EC concerning the European schedule of
    occupational diseases. Annex I
Council Directive 98/24/EC on the protection of the health and safety of workers
    from the risks related to chemical agents at work
Deutsche Forschungsgemeinschaft (German Research Foundation, DFG) (ed) List of
    MAK and BAT Values 2007. Maximum Concentrations and Biological Tolerance
    Values at the workplace. Wiley-VCH, Weinheim
Deutsche Forschungsgemeinschaft (German Research Foundation, DFG) (ed) The
    MAK-Collection for Occupational Health and Safety. Wiley-VCH
    at: www.mrw.interscience.wiley.com/makbat
GESTIS-database on hazardous substances. BGIA
    at: www.dguv.de/bgia/gestis-database
GESTIS-international limit values for chemical agents. BGIA
    at: www.dguv.de/bgia/gestis-limit-values

G 45

5 Use of the special occupational medical questionnaire "Q 18"
see Sections 1.2.2 and 3.3

5.1 Objective

The questionnaire is a German version of the "questionnaire for neuropsychiatric symptoms, Q 16", of Hogstedt et al. (1980). It is used in the slightly modified form of Triebig (see Ihrig et al, 2001). This questionnaire is a procedure for diagnosis of symptoms which have been shown in scientific studies to be potentially indicative of neurotoxic effects of exposure to solvents (including styrene).

An abnormal finding can therefore be an indication of unwanted effects of exposure to concentrations of hazardous substances relevant for occupational medicine.

The interpretation of the results, however, must always be made in the context of the other information and results obtained in the medical examination. Only together with other evidence or more detailed examinations, for example in the form of cognitive performance diagnostics, can early neurotoxic effects be diagnosed.

5.2 Procedure

As an instrument for recording a person's sense of well-being, the special questionnaire is subject to a large number of potential confounders such as time of day, motivation, private stress, age, education, etc. When using the questionnaire, therefore, such confounders should be avoided as far as possible or made note of.

To this end, the person should be allowed to fill in the questionnaire in a quiet place and without pressure of time. A third person is not permitted to observe or influence the participant during the filling in of the questionnaire. To promote motivation, it should be made clear to the participant that the answers to the questions are subject to medical discretion and will not be passed on to a third person. In addition, the participant should not be under the influence of alcohol, drugs or medication.

The questionnaire is to be filled in by the employee. No further instructions are necessary.

- If questions arise as to the time period to which the questions apply, these should be answered with "recently" or "in the last weeks and months".
- If a person cannot decide between "yes" and "no", he or she should be asked to mark the answer which more often applies.
- A person who claims to drink no alcohol should mark the answer "no" for question 18.

Once an employee has filled in the questionnaire, it should be checked for completeness by the examiner. If a question has not been answered or the answer is not clear, the questionnaire should be given back to the participant with the request that they decide on an answer. The processing time is only a few minutes.

Because it is possible to evaluate the filled-in questionnaire with a glance, if the result is abnormal a short discussion of the reasons the person gives for the disorders in his or her sense of well-being should follow immediately after the test.

5.3   Evaluation and interpretation

To evaluate the special questionnaire, the sum of the "yes" answers is calculated.
If the sum is greater than or equal to 4 (for persons under 28 years old) or 6 (for persons over 28 years old) the result is considered to be abnormal.
An abnormal result is not always caused by neurotoxic effects of occupational exposures. None the less, an abnormal result should be considered to be potential evidence of neurotoxic effects especially when no other cause of the reported symptoms is to be found in the discussion following the test.
In the discussion the examiner should ask the participant for his opinion of the origin of the symptoms. An abnormal result always requires further steps.
In the discussion the following important points should be covered:

- current situation: does the person suffer from private or occupational stress?
- physical state: is the participant over-tired or ill? Has he or she consumed medication, alcohol or other drugs?
- motivation: is the participant over-motivated or bored?
- expectations: what expectations does the person have as to the consequences of the test (e.g. improvement of working conditions, loss of the job, retirement with a pension)?
- exposure to neurotoxic substances: to which? Is there an association between exposure times and symptoms? Are the symptoms better after work-free intervals (e.g. holidays)?

The concluding discussion may very well yield only relatively vague evidence of an aetiology of the symptoms. In such cases an evaluation of the course of the disorder is required. The reproducibility of the reported symptoms may be determined using the same method at shorter intervals.

G 45

5.4   References

Hogstedt C, Hane M, Axelson O (1980) Diagnostic and Health Care Aspects of Workers Exposed to Solvents. In: Zenz C (ed) Developments in Occupational Medicine. Medical Publishers Chicago, pp 249–258

Ihrig A, Triebig G, Dietz MC (2001) Evaluation of a modified German version of the Q16 questionnaire for neurotoxic symptoms in workers exposed to solvents. Occup Environ Med 58(1):19–23

Special occupational medical questionnaire
modified by Triebig (1989)

Please answer the following questions about your state of health.
Your answers are subject to medical discretion and will not be passed on to any third party.
(Please mark the answer which applies to you with a cross)

1. Do you have a short memory? — yes ☐ no ☐

2. Have your relatives told you that you have a short memory? — yes ☐ no ☐

3. Do you often have to make notes about what you must remember? — yes ☐ no ☐

4. Do you generally find it hard to get the meaning from reading newspapers and books? — yes ☐ no ☐

5. Do you often have problems with concentrating? — yes ☐ no ☐

6. Do you often feel irritated without any particular reason? — yes ☐ no ☐

7. Do you often feel depressed without any particular reason? — yes ☐ no ☐

8. Are you abnormally tired? — yes ☐ no ☐

9. Do you have palpitations even when you don't exert yourself? — yes ☐ no ☐

10. Do you sometimes feel an oppression in your chest? — yes ☐ no ☐

11. Do you perspire without particular reason? — yes ☐ no ☐

12. Have you had frequent headaches recently (at least once a week)? — yes ☐ no ☐

13. Are you less interested in sex than you think is normal? — yes ☐ no ☐

14. Do you often feel nauseous? — yes ☐ no ☐

15. Do your hands or feet feel numb? — yes ☐ no ☐

16. Do you notice a lack of strength in your arms or legs? — yes ☐ no ☐

17. Do your hands tremble? — yes ☐ no ☐

18. Do you tolerate alcohol badly? — yes ☐ no ☐

G 46   Strain on the musculoskeletal system (including vibration)

Committee for occupational medicine, working group "Strain on the musculoskeletal system", Berufsgenossenschaft Metall Nord Süd, Mainz

Preliminary remarks

This guideline describes a scheme for occupational medical prophylaxis for persons whose work puts strain on the musculoskeletal system.

The objective is to prevent or ensure early diagnosis of disorders which can be caused by physical strain at work (see Section 3.1) and to enable employees with musculoskeletal disorders to return to work.

These disorders can also be caused by non-occupational conditions, factors and effects, but they can be made worse or can appear earlier or more often as a result of certain kinds of undue or misplaced effort at the workplace.

The first main section of the guideline is a general part which describes the medical examinations, the occupational medical assessment criteria, the kind of advice which can be given, and other information. This part covers strain on the musculoskeletal system including whole body vibration. In addition, the second main section of the guideline deals with hand-arm-vibration and contains a questionnaire for the specific anamnesis required in the supplementary examination.

Schedule

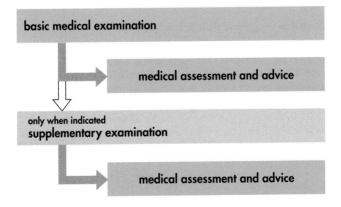

General part

1   Medical examinations

Occupational medical examinations are to be carried out for persons whose work-place activities involve health risks for the musculoskeletal system.

Workers exposed to mechanical vibration in excess of the exposure action values stated in the Directive 2002/44/EC shall be entitled to appropriate health surveil-lance. The daily exposure action value standardized to an eight-hour reference peri-od is 5 m/s^2 for hand-arm-vibration and 1.15 m/s^2 for whole-body vibration.

1.1   Examinations, intervals between examinations

initial examination	before starting work at a workplace whre strain on the musculoskeletal system can be expected and where the selection criteria are fulfilled
follow-up examinations	after 60 months; after 36 months for persons aged 40 years or more; when leaving the job
premature follow-up examination	• when as a result of a medical examination the physician considers it necessary to recommend a shorter interval between examinations • when requested by an employee who suspects a causal association between his or her illness and work • for an assessment of the individual physical capacity, e.g. for a person returning to work after a prolonged illness or operation

1.2   Medical examination schedule

The use of a tried and tested anamnesis and examination procedure which includes documentation is recommended (see Appendix 2 "Diagnosis of musculoskeletal dis-orders in occupational medical examinations"). Imaging diagnostics are not carried out or instigated regularly during these medical examinations.

1.2.1   Basic examination

| Initial examination | Follow-up examination |

- Anamnesis (see anamnesis questionnaires 1 and 2 and Appendix 2)
  - review of past history (general anamnesis, work anamnesis, symptoms)
  - identification of the locality and severity of work-related musculoskeletal symptoms
  - recording of any medical or physiotherapeutic treatment of the musculoskeletal system, especially during the previous 12 months,
  - of work-related activities which make the symptoms much worse
  - and any resolution of the symptoms when the strain is relieved
- clinical examination
  - inspection of the musculoskeletal system during standing and walking
  - screening for mobility and functionality

G 46

Schedule and assessment scheme for the basic examination

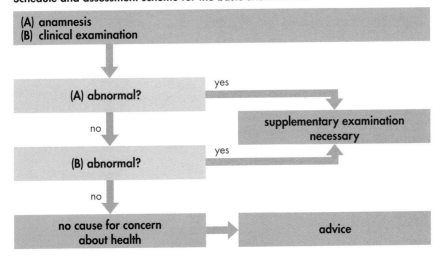

1.2.2   Supplementary examination

Initial examination   Follow-up examination

Supplementary examinations should be carried out when indicated by the results of the basic examination (see Section 1.2.1). If indicated by the diagnosis or symptoms, the supplementary examination can concentrate on the parts of the body affected by the person's work. The use of a tried and tested examination procedure is recommended (see Appendix II "Diagnosis of musculoskeletal disorders in occupational medical examinations").

At the initial examination it can be expedient to carry out the supplementary examination even when there are no abnormal findings or symptoms if the intended work makes this seem necessary. This procedure makes it possible to assess the course of any changes detected in follow-up examinations.

Schedule and assessment scheme for the supplementary examination

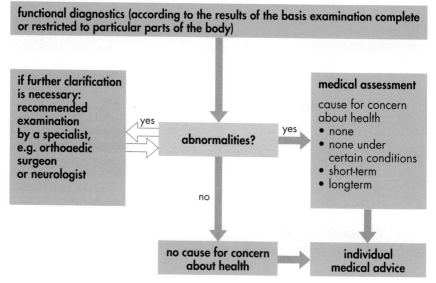

1.3   Requirements for the medical examinations

The basic and supplementary examinations and the consultation are to be carried out by a competent doctor or occupational health professional. The supplementary examination requires specialized knowledge which may be obtained in courses in occupational medical orthopaedics.

Abnormal findings in the supplementary examination generally have diagnostic and therapeutic consequences.

2   Occupational medical assessment and advice

The occupational medical assessment and advice requires knowledge of the kind and extent of physical strain involved in the employee's work and of the appropriate preventative and rehabilitative measures for maintenance and restoration of working and earning ability.

For this purpose a risk assessment as defined in Article 9 Council directive 89/391/EEC must have been carried out.

2.1   Assessment criteria

The assessment of the person's fitness for work in cases with functional disorders and diseases of the musculoskeletal system must take the individual health risk into account in relation to

- the concrete requirements of the workplace and the possibilities for adaptation
- any possible treatment to restore or stabilize fitness and work capacity
- compensating measures which make it possible to meet the work requirements in the short term or permanently
- the period remaining before the person retires

Because physical strain has complex effects, disorders of other organ systems (e.g. cardiocirculatory and neurological disorders) should also be taken into account in the assessment.

G 46

2.1.1   Long-term concern about health

| Initial examination | Follow-up examination |

Long-term concern about whether the person should take up or continue the work is generally only to be expressed if, from an occupational medical point of view, the person is not able or no longer able to do the work in the long-term. See the comments in Section 2.1.3.

2.1.2   Short-term concern about health

| Initial examination | Follow-up examination |

Short-term concern about whether a person should take up or continue the work should be expressed when, from the occupational medical point of view, the person is currently not able to do the work but when an improvement in fitness or work capacity or a restoration of the functions is to be expected within a reasonable period because of therapy, training, recovery or healing.

2.1.3   No concern about health under certain conditions

Initial examination	Follow-up examination

Most persons with disorders or diseases of the musculoskeletal system still have a chance of taking up or continuing a job. The works physician is to examine and advise the person about the necessary conditions (e.g. restrictions on the time under strain, ergonomic organization of the workplace, individual measures). This applies particularly to disorders which result from chronic degenerative changes and which usually develop over a period of many years (see Section 2.2).

2.1.4   No concern about health

Initial examination	Follow-up examination

All other persons, provided there are no restrictions on their employment.

2.2   Medical advice

2.2.1   Advising the employee

Degenerative and other structural damage, slight musculoskeletal malformations and especially functional disorders of the musculoskeletal system often have only slight effects on the fitness of persons at the beginning or in the middle of their working lives, provided that they have well-developed and well-trained musculature. They are readily compensated and do not necessarily result in long-term restrictions in physical capacity.

Employees can counteract functional disorders actively and in good time by maintaining appropriate levels of physical exercise during and after work and by compensating functional deficits with appropriate exercises and training procedures. Temporary classification of a person as unfit for work is therefore to be limited to the therapy required to overcome acute problems. Secondary preventive measures should begin before the fitness for work is reduced by illness and early enough to avoid the development of chronic disorders.

The main objective of occupational medical advice is to maintain or improve the fitness of the employees for work. The consultation should cover:

- changing the workplace, task and behaviour at the workplace within the possibilities of the employee:
  - equipping the workplace to reduce undue and misplaced effort
  - learning to cope with the task without excessive strain by taking part in ergonomic training
  - using ergonomic tools and any available aids and transport equipment
  - avoiding very monotonous work or extreme strain (e.g. by organizational measures)

- personal behaviour for the maintenance of physical fitness:
  - individual measures for promoting health and physical fitness according to the localization and severity of health problems (e.g. fitness training, back exercise programs)
  - recommendation of a differential diagnostic clarification of the symptoms by, e.g., an orthopaedic surgeon or neurologist
  - learning procedures for coping with symptoms which return frequently
  - introduction to an outpatient pain clinic for persons with chronic severe pain (> 3 months)
- general change in lifestyle with an increase in physical exercise during free time and avoiding of days with little physical activity

2.2.2   Advising the employer

The employer should be convinced of the general usefulness of preventive measures for the maintenance of working and earning capacity in the form of ergonomic and organizational solutions. The consultation can be aimed at

G 46

- the general situation at the workplace when the causes of symptoms described by employees and the physician's own occupational medical experience suggest that certain activities or conditions under which the persons are working are the reasons for persistent symptoms
- the individual employee when he or she is already known in the company for complaints and illness and the works physician is expected to contribute to the solving of the problem in an individual case.

In the consultation with the employer the physician is subject to the rules of medical discretion.

In co-operation with the specialists for safety at work and other members of the company, technical and organizational solutions for the problem of undue and misplaced effort at work should be sought. In this process, the protection of health, technical safety measures, trouble-free work processes and medium-term economic success should all be taken into consideration.

The consultation should cover especially:

- reduction of work-related strain (see Section 3.1)
- content of the general occupational medical advice given to employees about health risks associated with musculoskeletal strain
- provision and use of specific aids and transport equipment
- selection and provision of machines and tools according to ergonomic considerations
- furnishing the workplace
- work organization, e.g. short breaks and opportunities for movement and change of activity when strain is unavoidable, e.g. when the job requires long periods of work in awkward positions
- use of devices and machines with low vibration magnitudes
- reduction of sources of psychomental strain such as pressure of time

If during the course of his work in the company the occupational physician finds indications that the risk assessment should be brought up to date to improve health and safety standards, he is to inform the employer. When this is necessary, the interests of the employee are to be protected (medical confidentiality).

3   Supplementary notes

3.1   Exposure

Work-related strain on the musculoskeletal system is caused especially by:
- *manual handling of loads*
  - lifting, holding, carrying
  - pulling, pushing
- *forced body positions*
  - sitting
  - standing
  - bending the body forward
  - squatting, kneeling, lying
  - arms above shoulder level
- *work involving increased effort and/or force*
  - workplaces accessible with difficulty (mounting stairs, climbing)
  - use of the hand/arm system as a tool (knocking, hammering, twisting, pressing)
  - use of effort/force to operate equipment
- *repetitive tasks with high hand activity levels*
- *whole body vibration*
- *hand-arm vibration*

3.2   Functional disorders, symptoms

Work in the situations listed in Section 3.1 can cause acute and/or chronic functional disorders and diseases of the musculoskeletal system. In addition, particular attention should be paid to other illnesses and dispositions which impair musculoskeletal fitness and so the ability to work (e.g. diseases of the rheumatic type).

For the occupational physician the following musculoskeletal syndromes are of particular importance because of their functional effects:

Disorders of the vertebral column:
- intervertebral disk lesions with persistent radicular symptoms
- marked degenerative changes in the vertebral column
- inherited or acquired severe changes in the bones or vertebral column, sometimes with neurological effects (e.g. vertebral canal stenosis, severe spondylolisthesis, osteoporosis, marked scoliosis, Bekhterev syndrome, malformations and variations of the vertebral column)
- marked postoperative or posttraumatic disorders (e.g. postdiscotomy syndrome)
- tumours of the vertebral column or osteomyelitis

Disorders of the shoulder-arm region
- functional disorders in the shoulder joint with temporarily reduced load-bearing capacity (e.g. impingement syndrome, frozen shoulder, habitual dislocation of the shoulder, condition after traumatic shoulder dislocation)
- diseased and irritated tendons, tendon sheaths, tendon attachment points (styloiditis) and synovial bursa
- degenerative changes in the shoulder, elbow, hand, wrist, metacarpal and finger joints
- disorders of the shoulder joint leading to reduced stability and load-bearing capacity (e.g. rotator cuff rupture, biceps tendon rupture)
- compression syndromes (e.g. nervus subscapularis, thoracic outlet syndrome, scalenus syndrome, hyperabduction syndrome, carpal tunnel syndrome)
- transient condition after fracture or dislocation
- disorders of the wrist bones (e.g. lunatomalacia, bone necrosis, pseudoarthrosis)
- circulatory disorders/Raynaud's phenomenon/hand-arm vibration syndrome
- tumours or osteomyelitis

G 46

Disorders of the hip, knee, ankle and foot regions
- meniscus disorders until full functional recovery is achieved
- degenerative changes in the hip, iliosacral, knee, ankle, tarsal, metatarsal and toe joints
- diseased and irritated tendons, tendon sheaths, tendon attachment points and synovial bursa
- chondropathy of the patella
- sequelae of fractures and soft tissue lesions (e.g. condition after a broken ankle, or rupture of the Achilles tendon or genicular ligament)
- symptomatic calcaneal spur, Haglund's deformity
- marked malformations of the foot (e.g. club foot, tip foot)
- necrosis of the head of the femur
- hip dysplasia
- deformations of the head of the femur as in Perthes disease
- tumours or osteomyelitis

Cause-effect relationships have been demonstrated for a number of occupational activities. Most musculoskeletal damage has, however, not been demonstrated unambiguously to result from the kinds of exposures and work situations listed in Section 3.1.

The assessment is made more difficult by the fact that a large number of other parameters may be seen as cofactors or even as independent causes.

In addition to the specifically orthopaedic disorders of the musculoskeletal system, when estimating fitness and prognosis in a given work situation other performance-limiting disorders should also be taken into account, disorders which can develop at the same time as the musculoskeletal disorders as a result of ageing processes and which can increase the performance deficits. These include especially:

- high blood pressure which cannot be regulated medicinally
- ischaemic heart disease
- arrhythmia which cannot be sufficiently compensated therapeutically
- arteriosclerosis leading to functional deficits, e.g. of the leg musculature
- chronic obstructive respiratory disorders leading to severe functional deficits
- bronchial asthma with a high frequency of attacks or attacks induced by physical exertion
- insulin-dependent diabetes mellitus
- kidney disorders with functional deficits

4   References

Commission Recommendation 2003/670/EC concerning the European schedule of occupational diseases

Council Directive 89/391/EEC on the introduction of measures to encourage improvements in the safety and health of workers at work

Council Directive 90/269/EEC on the minimum health and safety requirements for the manual handling of loads where there is a risk particularly of back injury to workers

Council Directive 2002/44/EC on the minimum health and safety requirements regarding the exposure of workers to the risks arising from physical agents (vibration)

5   Recommended forms

Anamnesis questionnaires:
1   Self-reported musculoskeletal disorders,
    and
2   Medical anamnesis of musculoskeletal disorders and hand-arm vibration exposure

G 46   Self-reported musculoskeletal disorders (anamnesis questionnaire 1)

Name .... First name .... Date ....

1. Have you ever had disorders, operations or severe accidents affecting the spinal column, the arms or legs?

   | no | yes |

   If yes, which? _____

2. Have you **during the last 12 months** had symptoms in the spinal column, the arms or the legs?
   (aches or pains, a burning feeling, weakness, numbness, coldness, skin changes, etc.)

   | no | yes |

   If yes, please mark the two figures with crosses (x) to show exactly where the symptoms were.

G 46

3. Have you been to a doctor at any time during the last 12 months because of these symptoms?

   | no | yes |

   If yes, what did the doctor diagnose? _____

4. Have you been unfit to work at any time during the last 12 months because of these symptoms?

   | no | yes |

   If yes, how often? _____ x   and how many weeks in all? _____ weeks

5. Have you any symptoms in the spinal column, the arms or legs **today**?

   | no | yes |

   If yes, where? _____

6. What kind of strain is involved in your work and causes pain or other symptoms?

Strain caused by	This kind of strain is involved in my work		This kind of strain has caused pain or symptoms or made them worse	
	yes	no	yes	no
handling heavy loads	O	O	O	O
working bent over or with the body twisted	O	O	O	O
kneeling or squatting	O	O	O	O
standing for long periods	O	O	O	O
working with the hands above the shoulders	O	O	O	O
vibration from tools	O	O	O	O
sitting on motor vehicles or machines	O	O	O	O
sitting in the office	O	O	O	O
other unnamed activities				

G 46 Medical anamnesis of musculoskeletal disorders (anamnesis questionnaire 2)

Name	First name	Date

1. *Character of the pain*: how would you describe the pain or symptoms which you have had in the arms and legs, muscles or spinal column?

None ○   Yes ○, the pain or symptoms can be described as follows:

dull pain	○	aching muscles	○ ....
where?		weak muscles	○ ....
shooting pains	○	other symptoms	○ ....
burning sensation	○	prickling sensation/paresthesia*	○ ....
ache	○	numbness*	○ ....
stabbing pain	○	Raynaud's phenomenon*	○ ....
stiffness	○		(* see page 2)
cramp	○		
tenseness	○		

2. *Shooting pains*: do the pains shoot from one part of the body to another and, if yes, where to?

No ○   Yes ○, the pains shoot into the following parts of the body:

neck, cervical spine	○	hip joint, thigh	○ left ○ right	shoulder, upper arm	○ left ○ right
thoracic spine	○	knee, lower leg	○ left ○ right	elbow, forearm	○ left ○ right
lumbar spine	○	foot, ankle	○ left ○ right	hand, wrist, fingers	○ left ○ right

3. *Provokability*: can the pain be provoked (e.g. by coughing, straining, certain movements, work with vibrating tools, work in the cold)?

No ○   Yes ○, by: ....

4. Do the symptoms get better away from work (at night, over the weekend, on holiday)?

No ○   Yes ○, when I: ....

5. *Intensity of pain*: how bad was the worst pain of this kind that you have had in the last 30 days? Give the symptoms a score between 0 (no symptoms) and 10 (the worst you can imagine)

no symptoms ○ ○ ○ ○ ○ ○ ○ ○ ○ ○ ○   the worst pain
             0   1   2   3   4   5   6   7   8   9 10

6. *Weekly prevalence*: have you today or have you had in the last 7 days (in the last week?) pain or symptoms in the arms, legs, muscles or spine?

No ○   Yes ○, in the following parts of the body:

neck, cervical spine	○	hip joint, thigh	○ left ○ right	shoulder, upper arm	○ left ○ right
thoracic spine	○	knee, lower leg	○ left ○ right	elbow, forearm	○ left ○ right
lumbar spine	○	foot, ankle	○ left ○ right	hand, wrist, fingers	○ left ○ right

7. Further anamnestic information (pain characteristics, provokability, course, functional disorders, disabilities, previous treatment, previous diagnoses, evidence of systemic disorders, medication abuse, smoking):

....

....

....

....

....

....

....

Date, physician's signature..

Medical anamnesis for hand-arm vibration exposure

1. Have you during the last 12 months noticed that your fingers feel numb or that they go white and dead?

never	several times per year	several times per month	several times per week	several times daily
○	○	○	○	○

If such changes were noticed

2. Which fingers were affected by this feeling of numbness or going white and how much finger was affected (please mark the area exactly)?

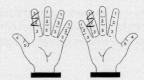

Example

G 46

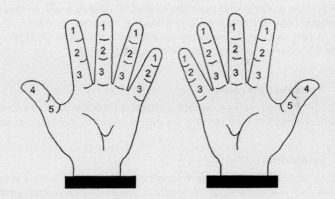

Comments:

....

....

....

....

Disorders caused by hand-arm vibration

During work with hand-held or hand-guided devices or with stationary machines, mechanical vibrations are transmitted to the hand-arm system. The result can be damage to the bones and joints or to vessels and nerves of the arms and hands.

1   Damage to bones and joints of the arms and hands

1.1   Cause

Exposure of the arms and hands to predominantly low frequency mechanical vibration (< 50 Hz) can cause attrition of the articular surfaces in the joints and critical reduction of the blood supply with consequent trophic disorders or even fatigue fractures.

1.2   Occurrence

At risk are persons working with machines or devices operated with compressed air (e.g. pneumatic hammers and chisels, construction hammers) or electrically driven tools such as percussion drills, electrical construction hammers or percussion screwdrivers (see the table in the special anamnesis questionnaire).

1.3   Transmission route

Decisive for the damaging effects is that the vibration is transmitted to the forearm via the mechanical contact of the hand with the device (gripping, holding and pressing).

1.4   Symptoms

The traumatic effect of vibrations results from the prolonged mechanical stress exerted on bones and joint surfaces which results in progressive destruction of the cartilage in the joints. The damage appears clinically as degenerative changes which are not different from those with other causes. In order of decreasing prevalence, arthrosis develops in the elbow joint, wrist bones, distal radioulnar articulation, and acromioclavicular articulation. In addition, there are isolated cases of lunatomalacia, fatigue fracture of the scaphoid bone, sometimes followed by pseudarthrosis, and circumscribed osteochondrosis dissecans in the elbow joint. The symptoms can be associated with peripheral nerve damage. The predominant joint symptoms are lack of strength, pain at the start of work and at rest (at night!) and painful restrictions on movement.

Conspicuous during the examination are circumscribed swellings, local reductions in muscle mass, bone and joint deformities and tenderness to pressure in muscle and tendon attachment areas. Sidedness is to be noted because the limb which exerts more pressure on the working device is generally more severely affected. For differential diagnosis, arthrosis and chondromatosis of other genesis, e.g. as sequelae of earlier injuries to bones, joints and nerves of the arms and hands, must be considered. Progression of the degenerative changes is to be expected even after the end of vibration exposure.

1.5   Special medical examination

The radiogram of vibration-induced bone and joint damage presents a general picture of arthrosis deformans or osteochondrosis dissecans. Given appropriate indications, specialized examination procedures for early diagnosis of lunate bone or scaphoid bone damage may be necessary (special radiographic procedures, bone scan or MRI).

1.6   Advising the employee

The real danger depends on the intensity and duration of vibration exposure. The form in which the damage is manifested suggests, however, that constitutional joint weakness predisposes to the disorder.

G 46

2   Hand-arm vibration syndrome (vibration-induced white finger)

2.1   Cause

Hand-arm vibration syndrome (a vasospastic syndrome) is caused by predominantly high frequency vibrations (> 50 Hz) which produce attacks of local sensitivity and circulatory disorders in the hands; the latter appear clinically as Raynaud's phenomenon.

2.2   Occurrence

At risk are persons working with, e.g., high speed drills, chisels, milling cutters, machines for cutting, sanding and polishing, power-driven chain saws and also compressed air-driven tools which produce high frequency vibrations, e.g., the lettering chisel of the stonemason (see the table in the special anamnesis questionnaire).

2.3   Transmission route

The danger depends on the pressure of the hands on the handles and on the intensity and duration of the vibration exposure.

2.4   Symptoms

Especially in the cold, there is a drastic reduction in blood supply to the fingers (predominantly II-V, rarely also the thumb and palm of the hand) with the feeling of numbness/cold, going white, impairment of fine motor ability, stiffness and paraesthesia. Cyanotic discoloration and later redness with feeling of warmth occur frequently but not in all cases. Unlike in Raynaud's disease, trophic disorders hardly ever develop. The cause is a vasospasm which is associated with damage to the pacinian corpuscles. The symptoms appear and spread proximally from the finger tips within a few minutes. Regression is very variable and can take from a few minutes up to an hour. The frequency of attacks varies between occasional and several times daily.

Hand-arm vibration syndrome develops after several months or years of vibration exposure, depending on the duration and intensity of exposure. The prevalence of milder forms of the disorder is relatively high. Between 50 % and 80 % of exposed persons have typical symptoms, but in only few cases are they so severe that the person must give up the work (occupational disease). Initially the symptoms appear in winter shortly after starting work; in the advanced stages of the disorder the symptoms also appear away from the workplace (e.g. when cycling without gloves, washing the car). Between attacks the affected persons have no symptoms and are without clinical manifestations. Early diagnosis of hand-arm vibration syndrome is based on the work anamnesis and reports of the typical symptoms.

For differential diagnosis other peripheral circulatory disorders should be considered (e.g. Raynaud's disease, cold-provokable vasospasm in cases of acrocyanosis and livedo reticularis, constitutional predisposition to cold hands). The consumption of certain medicines (e.g. ergotamine, β-blockers), nicotine abuse, Raynaud's phenomenon as a concomitant symptom of systemic disorders or occupational exposure to chemicals such as vinyl chloride, solvents (n-hexane, ketones, carbon disulfide), metals (lead, arsenic, thallium, mercury), pesticides (carbamates, organic phosphorus compounds), nitrates or acrylamide should also be considered.

For assessment of the symptoms of hand-arm vibration syndrome, the Stockholm Scale is very helpful.

Classification of the sensorineural symptoms on the fingers (Stockholm Scale)

Mark stage with a cross	Sensorineural symptoms
0 SN	exposed to vibration, but no symptoms
1 SN	attacks of numbness with or without a prickling sensation
2 SN	attacks of numbness or persistent numbness, reduced sensitivity
3 SN	attacks of numbness or persistent numbness, reduced sense of touch and/or reduced dexterity

Classification of the vascular symptoms on the fingers (Stockholm Scale)

Mark stage with a cross	Vascular symptoms
0	no vasospastic attacks
1	occasional vasospastic attacks which affect only the tips of one or more fingers
2	occasional vasospastic attacks which affect only the distal and middle phalanxes of one or more fingers (very rarely also the proximal phalanx)
3	frequent vasospastic attacks which affect the phalanxes of most fingers
4	like stage 3, with trophic disorders of the finger tips

2.5   Special medical examination

G 46

As a criterion for vessel function a cold provocation test can be carried out with determination of the skin temperature and the recovery time. Pallanesthesiometric procedures are appropriate for determining the sensitivity of the finger tips for vibration.

2.6   Advising the employee

Especially persons working in the cold should be advised about appropriate behaviour, e.g., that it is particularly important to wear suitable warm clothing and special gloves, to rub the hands together and slap oneself on the back, to drink hot drinks and to abstain from smoking. Heated handles on motorized chain saws have proved particularly helpful. Generally the frequency of the vasospastic attacks decreases markedly in summer. The prognosis depends on how long the person has suffered from such attacks and on the severity of the symptoms.

2.7   Supplementary notes

The diagnosis of hand-arm vibration syndrome is based on reports of cold-induced circumscribed sensitivity disorders or white fingers. Therefore anamnesis is the best diagnostic method. If the anamnesis is indicative of hand-arm vibration syndrome, it should be followed up with a supplementary examination in which the employee fills in a more extensive questionnaire (see below). The answers should be validated by the physician in conversation with the employee. The first symptoms are exposure-related, that is, there is no reason to suspect other causes: it is clear that the first vasospastic attacks appeared after starting work with vibrating tools.

3 References

Bovenzi M (1998) Exposure-response relationship in the hand-arm vibration syndrome: an overview of current epidemiology research. Int Arch Occup Environ Health 71: 509–519

Council Directive 2002/44/EC on the minimum health and safety requirements regarding the exposure of workers to the risks arising from physical agents (vibration)

Gemne G, Pyykko I, Taylor W, Pelmear PL (1987) The Stockholm workshop scale for the classification of cold-induced Raynaud's phenomenon in the hand-arm vibration syndrome (revision of the Taylor-Pelmear scale) Scand J Work Environ Health 13: 275–278

Griffin MJ, Bovenzi M (2002) The diagnosis of disorders caused by hand-transmitted vibration: Southampton Workshop 2000. Int Arch Occup Environ Health 75: 1–5

Griffin MJ, Bovenzi M, Nelson CM (2003) Dose-response patterns for vibration-induced white finger. Occup Environ Med 60: 16–26

ISO/DIS 14835-1 (2003) Mechanical vibration and shock – Cold provocation tests for the assessment of peripheral vascular function – Part 1: Measurement and evaluation of finger skin temperature. Part 2: Measurement and evaluation of finger systolic blood pressure

Kurozawa Y, Nasu Y, Hosoda, Nose T (2002) Longterm follow-up study on patients with vibration-induced white finger (VWF). J Occup Environ Med 44: 1203–1206

Lindsell CJ, Griffin MJ (1998): Standardised diagnostic methods for assessing components of the hand-arm vibration syndrome. Contract Research Report 197, Health and Safety Executive Books, Sudbury, Suffolk

N. N.: Research Network on Detection and Prevention of Injuries due to Occupational Vibration Exposures. EC Biomed II project no. BMH4-CT98-3251. At: www.humanvibration.com/EU/VINET/

Olsen N (2002) Diagnostic aspects of vibration-induced white finger. Int Arch Occup Environ Health 75: 6–13

Palmer KT, Griffin MJ, Syddall H, Cooper C, Coggon D (2002) The clinical grading of Raynaud's phenomenon and vibration-induced white finger: relationship between finger blanching and difficulties in using the upper limb. Int Arch Occup Environ Health 75: 29–36

4 Recommended questionnaire

Questionnaire for the supplementary examination of persons exposed to hand-arm vibration

G 46   Supplementary examination of persons exposed to hand-arm vibration

| Name .... | First name .... | Date |

1.   Are you

right-handed   O | left-handed   O | ambidextrous   O

2.   Do you work with devices or machines which cause vibrations that are transmitted to your hands?
(e.g. sanding machines, chainsaws, construction hammers, compressed air hammers; see list of devices)

No, I do not work with such devices   O   if the answer is no, the anamnesis ends here.
Yes   O   since when?.......................

3.   How often do you work with vibrating devices?

hours per day   .... | days per week   .... | weeks per year   ....

4.   Are your hands cold?

| | (spasmodically) | (spasmodically) | (spasmodically) | (persistently) |
| never   O | rarely   O | sometimes   O | often   O | always   O |

5.   Do your fingers ever prickle or feel numb?

| | several times | several times | several times | several times |
| never   O | per year   O | per month   O | per week   O | per day   O |

6.   Do your fingers ever go white and feel dead?

| | several times | several times | several times | several times |
| never   O | per year   O | per month   O | per week   O | per day   O |

7.   When do your fingers go white or feel numb or prickle?

more often | more often | independent
in the **cold** season of the year   O | in the **warm** season of the year   O | of the season   O

8.   When did you notice that one or more fingers felt dead, prickled or had gone white?

for the **first time** | for the last time | for the last time | for the last time
in the year .... | ....days ago | ....months ago | ....years ago

9.   In which situations do your fingers prickle or go dead?

mainly in the cold   O   after a break   O
when touching cold objects   O   at night   O
after working for several hours with vibrating tools   O   when swimming   O
when cycling or driving a moped or motor cycle   O

in other situations ....

10.   Do you have such symptoms on your toes too?

no   O | yes   O

11.   Do you have problems doing fiddly jobs?
(e.g. doing up buttons, pressing switches, picking up coins, sorting nails or such)

no   O | yes   O, with ....

12.   Do you take medication regularly?

no   O | yes   O, I take ....

....
....
....

Date, physician's signature

G 46

Examples of devices which are known to be able to cause hazard via hand-arm vibration

- Ballast tampers in mines: railway construction (underground in black coal mines)
- Blacksmith's hammers
- Chainsaws (with AV-handle)
- Chainsaws (without AV-handle)
- Chainsaws, power saws
- Combi-hammers (electrical percussion drills)
- Compactors (vibration tampers, vibration cylinders, rammers (general purpose), rammers (building sites), compacting rams, levelling harrows)
- Cutters (trimmers, lawn mowers, sheet metal shears, electric cutters, scythe mowers, shears with a mechanical drive, pneumatic cutters, vertical knife cutting machines)
- Demolition hammers and breakers
- Drills, rock drills
- Drop hammers (air hammer, spring hammer)
- Floor-mounted or bench-mounted drills
- Foam rubber cutters, reciprocating saws
- Frog rammers
- Garden vacuum cleaners (hand-held)
- Grinding machines (concrete grinding machines, grinders/bench grinders, articulated arm grinders (with stand and swing arm))
- Hammers (ballast tampers, rust removing tools)
- Hedge trimmers with petrol motor
- Impact drills, percussion drills
- Impact drills, rotary hammers, combi-hammers
- Impact wrenches

- Jigsaws
- Needle descalers
- Nibblers (bevelling machines), nibbling machines
- Percussion drills/combi-hammers
- Percussion hammers (spade chisels, chisel hammers, breakers, demolition hammers)
- Planers (filers, scrapers), floor-mounted
- Portable circular saws
- Powder-actuated tools, "nail guns"
- Power planers
- Power routers (hand-held), hand routers, spindle moulders/shapers, universal milling machines, pin routers
- Riveting hammers
- Riveting tools (riveting hammer, dolly, clinching tool)
- Rotary screwdrivers
- Sanders (vertical sanders, angle grinders, cutting grinders, straight grinders, hand-held belt sanders, oscillating spindle sanders, 3-D sanders)
- Sanding machines
- Sewing machines
- Staple guns
- Stonemason's hammers (deadblow)
- Surface cleaning machines (needle descalers, surface cleaners, shot blasting cabinets, high pressure cleaners)
- Tree pruning pole saws with petrol motors
- Trimmers, brush cutters
- Vibration cylinders, hand-held
- Vibration tampers

Appendices

3

3

Appendices

Appendix 1   Biomonitoring

K.H. Schaller and J. Angerer (Universität Erlangen-Nürnberg) for the working group "Hazardous substances" of the Committee for occupational medicine

Definition of Biomonitoring

Biomonitoring is the analysis of biological material obtained from employees for the presence of hazardous substances, their metabolites or parameters of their biochemical or biological effects. The objective is to determine the internal exposure of the employees, to compare the analytical results with threshold values and to suggest appropriate measures to reduce exposure.

There are two kinds of biomonitoring: internal exposure monitoring and biological and biochemical effect monitoring. In internal exposure monitoring, the levels of the hazardous substances and their metabolites in biological material are determined. Biological effect monitoring determines the biological reactions at cellular level (e.g. mutations, cytogenetic and cytotoxic effects). The monitored effects themselves need not have adverse consequences for the organism. Biochemical effect monitoring is generally understood to mean the quantification of reaction products of mutagenic substances which are bound covalently to macromolecules such as protein and DNA (e.g. DNA adducts and protein adducts).

A 1

Use and purpose of biomonitoring

Biomonitoring is a tool for the assessment of working conditions, is used in association with the occupational medical examination as a part of occupational medical prophylaxis. The necessity for biomonitoring is given by legal regulations or specific conditions which may be a result of the workplace situation or of specific properties of a substance. The occupational physician determines whether biomonitoring is necessary and advises the employer.

Biomonitoring makes it possible to determine
- the amounts of hazardous substances taken up by employees by inhalation, through the skin or by swallowing
- specific biochemical and biological effects of exposure to a hazardous substance
- individual differences in the metabolism of hazardous substances
- individual hygiene in handling hazardous substances
- the effectiveness of protective measures at the workplace

and so makes it possible to assess health risks.

Requirements for toxicological assessment in occupational medicine

An occupational medical assessment involving biomonitoring requires
* formulation of the occupational medical question
* assessment of the workplace situation
* selection of the assay parameter and the biological material to be analysed
* collection of the sample of biological material
* analytical determination and quality control
* occupational medical assessment of the results.

With the exception of the analytical determination and the associated quality control, these tasks are the responsibility of the occupational physician.

Requirements in practice

* Appropriate biological material must be available for the analysis; sample collection must be acceptable for the employee and practicable for the physician.
* Appropriate analytical parameters – specific and sensitive biomarkers – must be known.
* Quantitative determination of the biomarkers requires reliable analytical methods and adequate quality control.
* The assessment of the results of biomonitoring must be based on toxicological threshold values, taking any modifying factors and confounders into account, and on medical experience.

Biomonitoring is a part of medical practice and so is subject to the statutory regulations of the medical profession.

Biological material for analysis

In the context of occupational medical examinations, biological material for analysis is whole blood, plasma and/or urine in which the assay of the required parameter is carried out. In occupational medical practice 24-h pooled urine samples cannot be used, the analyses must make use of spontaneous urine samples. To take diuresis-induced variation into account, the analytical results should be expressed in terms of the creatinine level or this should be determined as an exclusion criterion. Spontaneous urine samples are not suitable for analysis if they are – for reasons of diuresis – very concentrated or very dilute. In practice, the creatinine levels in the urine samples are used for orientation. Representative exclusion criteria: samples with creatinine concentrations below 0.5 g/l or above 2.5 g/l should not be used.

Biological materials such as hair, sweat, saliva and alveolar air are not used for biomonitoring in occupational medical prophylaxis.

Assay parameters – biomarkers

The assay parameter is the chemical substance or biological indicator for which the level in biological material is determined. Required of an assay parameter is that it indicates the internal exposure or the effects of the hazardous substance reliably, sensitively and specifically. The choice of appropriate assay parameters requires specialist occupational medical knowledge. Some information is provided in the *Guidelines for Occupational Medical Examinations*.

Tables 1 and 2 indicate for which hazardous substances biological monitoring makes sense.

Table 1: Biomonitoring parameters in occupational medical prophylaxis carried out according to the *Guidelines for Occupational Medical Examinations*

Guideline G short title	Parameter	Material	Sampling time
2 Lead	lead	whole blood	a
3 Alkyllead compounds	lead	urine	b
4 Skin cancer (PAH)	1-hydroxypyrene	urine	b, c
5 Ethylene glycol dinitrate or glycerol trinitrate	ethylene glycol dinitrate 1,2-glyceryl dinitrate or 1,3-glyceryl dinitrate	whole blood plasma	b b
6 Carbon disulfide	2-thio-4-thiazolidine carboxylic acid (TTCA)	urine	b
7 Carbon monoxide	CO-Hb	whole blood	b
8 Benzene	benzene trans,trans-muconic acid S-phenylmercapturic acid	whole blood urine urine	b b b
9 Mercury	mercury	urine	a
10 Methanol	methanol	urine	b, c
14 Trichloroethene and other chlorinated hydrocarbon solvents dichloromethane	trichloroacetic acid (TCA) dichloromethane CO-Hb	urine whole blood whole blood	b, c b b
tetrachloroethene 1,1,1-trichloroethane	tetrachloroethene trichloroethane	whole blood whole blood	d c, d
15 Chromium(VI) compounds	chromium chromium	urine erythrocytes	b b

A 1

Table 1 continued

Guideline G short title	Parameter	Material	Sampling time
16 Arsenic	arsenic[1]	urine	b
19 Dimethylformamide	N-methylformamide	urine	b
27 Isocyanates			
diphenylmethane-4,4'-diisocyanate (MDI)	4,4'-diaminodiphenyl-methane (MDA)	urine	b
hexamethylene-1,6-diisocyanate (HDI)	hexamethylene diamine (HDA)	urine	b
isophorone diisocyanate (IPDI)	isophorone diamine (IPDA)	urine	b
1,5-naphthylene diisocyanate (NDI)	1,5-diaminonaphthalene (1,5-naphthalenediamine)	urine	b
toluene diisocyanate (TDI)	toluenediamine	urine	b
29 Benzene homologues	toluene	whole blood	b
	o-cresol	urine	b, c
	xylene	whole blood	b
	methylhippuric (toluric) acid	urine	b
	ethylbenzene	urine	b, c
	mandelic acid + phenyl-glyoxylic acid (MA + PGA)	urine	b, c
	2-ethylphenol, 4-ethylphenol	urine	b, c
32 Cadmium	cadmium	whole blood	a
	cadmium	urine	a
33 Aromatic nitro and amino compounds (e.g. aniline, nitro-benzene)	aniline, free	urine	b, c
	aniline, released from aniline-haemoglobin conjugate	whole blood	b, c
	nitrobenzene	whole blood	b, c
	aniline, released from aniline-haemoglobin conjugate		
34 Fluorine	fluoride	urine	b
	fluoride	urine	d
36 Vinyl chloride	thiodiglycolic acid	daytime urine	b
38 Nickel	nickel	urine	b

Table 1 continued

Guideline G short title	Parameter	Material	Sampling time
39 Welding fumes	chromium^2	urine	b
	chromium^2	erythrocytes	b
	nickel^2	whole blood	b
	nickel^2	urine	b
	aluminium^2	urine	b
45 Styrene	mandelic acid + phenyl- glyoxylic acid (MA + PGA)	urine	b, c

a   not fixed
b   end of exposure or end of shift
c   for long-term exposures: after several shifts
d   at the beginning of the next shift

[1]   volatile arsenic compounds determined by direct hydrogenation
[2]   methods apply only for welding with materials containing Cr/Ni or welding of aluminium and aluminium alloys

A 1

Table 2: Biomonitoring parameters to be used for persons exposed to hazardous substances which are not included in the *Guidelines for Occupational Medical Examinations*

Metals

Substance	Parameter	Material	Sampling time
aluminium	aluminium	urine plasma	b b
antimony	antimony	urine	b, c
barium	barium	urine	b, c
beryllium	beryllium	urine	b, c
cobalt	cobalt	urine	a
copper	copper	urine	b
manganese	manganese	whole blood	b, c
molybdenum	molybdenum	urine	b
palladium	palladium	urine	b
platinum	platinum	urine	b
selenium	selenium	urine plasma	b, c b, c
tellurium	tellurium	urine	b, c
thallium	thallium	urine	b
vanadium	vanadium	urine	b, c
zinc	zinc	urine	b

a   not fixed
b   end of exposure or end of shift
c   for long-term exposures: after several shifts
d   at the beginning of the next shift

Organic solvents and their metabolites

Substance	Parameter	Material	Sampling time
acetone	acetone	urine	b
aliphatic hydrocarbons: screening	aliphatic hydrocarbons	whole blood	b
aromatic hydrocarbons: screening	aromatic hydrocarbons	whole blood	b
butanol isomers	butanol isomers	urine	b
2-butanone (methyl ethyl ketone)	2-butanone	urine	b
butyl acetate	butanol	whole blood	b
chlorobenzenes	chlorobenzenes	whole blood	b
	chlorophenols	urine	b, c
chloroform (trichloromethane)	chloroform	whole blood	b
cyclohexanone	1,2-cyclohexanediol	urine	b
1,1-dichloroethane and 1,2-dichloroethane	dichloroethane	whole blood	b
1,1-dichloroethene and 1,2-dichloroethene	dichloroethene	whole blood	b
dioxane	β-hydroxyethoxyacetic acid	urine	b
glycol ethers 2-butoxyethanol	2-butoxyacetic acid	urine	b, c
2-ethoxyethanol	2-ethoxyacetic acid	urine	b, c
2-methoxyethanol	2-methoxyacetic acid	urine	b, c
2-methoxy-1-propanol	2-methoxypropionic acid	urine	b, c
1-methoxy-2-propanol	1-methoxy-2-propanol	urine	b, c
halogenated hydrocarbons: screening	halogenated hydrocarbons	whole blood	b
heptanone	heptanone	whole blood	b
n-hexane	2,5-hexanedione	urine	b
hexanol	hexanol, 1,2-cyclohexanediol	urine	b
2-hexanone (methyl butyl ketone)	2,5-hexanedione	urine	b

A 1

Organic solvents and their metabolites (continued)

Substance	Parameter	Material	Sampling time
methanol	methanol	urine	b, c
methyl isobutyl ketone (hexone)	methyl isobutyl ketone	urine	b
chlorobenzene	total 4-chlorocatechol	urine	d
	total 4-chlorocatechol	urine	b
monochloromethane (methyl chloride)	monochloromethane	whole blood	b
pentachloroethane	pentachloroethane	whole blood	b
2-propanol	acetone	urine	b
		whole blood	b
styrene	mandelic acid (MA)	urine	b
	phenylglyoxylic acid (PGA)	urine	b
tetrahydrofuran	tetrahydrofuran	urine	b
tetrachloroethane	tetrachloroethane	whole blood	b
tetrachloromethane (carbon tetrachloride)	tetrachloromethane	blood	b, c

a   not fixed
b   end of exposure or end of shift
c   for long-term exposures: after several shifts
d   at the beginning of the next shift

Pesticides and their metabolites

Substance	Parameter	Material	Sampling time
chlorophenols	chlorophenols	urine	b, c
DDT (dichlorodiphenyl-trichloroethane)	p,p'-DDE (1,1-dichloro-2,2-bis(p-chlorophenyl)-ethylene)	whole blood	a
hexachlorobenzene	hexachlorobenzene	whole blood	a
hexachlorocyclohexanes α-hexachlorocyclohexane β-hexachlorocyclohexane γ-hexachlorocyclohexane (lindane)	α-HCH β-HCH γ-HCH	plasma, whole blood	b
organophosphates	DMP (dimethyl phosphate), DEP (diethylphosphate), DMTP (dimethylthio-phosphate), DETP (diethylthiophosphate), DMDTP (dimethyldithio-phosphate), DEDTP (diethyldithio-phosphate)	urine	b, c
parathion	p-nitrophenol acetylcholine esterase	urine erythrocytes	b, c b, c
pentachlorophenol	pentachlorophenol pentachlorophenol	urine plasma	a a
polychlorinated biphenyls (chlorinated biphenyls)	*polychlorinated biphenyls*	plasma, a whole blood	
pyrethroids	Cl$_2$CA (3-(2,2-dichloro-vinyl)-2,2-dimethylcyclo-propane-carboxylic acid) 3-PBA (3-phenoxybenzoic acid) Br$_2$CA (3-(2,2-dibromo-vinyl)-2,2-dimethylcyclo-propane carboxylic acid) F-PBA (4-fluoro-3-phenoxy-benzoic acid)	urine	b, c
pyrethrum	chrysanthemum-dicarboxylic acid	urine	b, c

A 1

Other hazardous substances

Substance	Parameter	Material	Sampling time
acrylonitrile	N-cyanoethylvaline	erythrocytes	a
1,3-butadiene	N-acetyl-S-(3,4-di-hydroxy-butyl)-L-cysteine	urine	b
bisphenol A (4,4'-isopropylidenediphenol)	bisphenol A released by hydrolysis	urine	b
4,4'-diaminodiphenyl-methane (MDA)	4,4'-diaminodiphenyl-methane	urine	b
dimethyl sulfate (DMS)	N-methylvaline	erythrocytes	a
diphenylmethane-4,4'-diisocyanate	4,4'-diaminodiphenyl-methane	urine	b
ethylene	hydroxyethylvaline	erythrocytes	a
ethylene oxide	hydroxyethylvaline	erythrocytes	a
nitroaromatics	nitroaromatics	whole blood	b, c
nitrobenzene	aniline released from aniline-haemoglobin conjugate	whole blood	b, c
perfluorooctanoic acid and its inorganic salts	perfluorooctanoic acid	serum	a
phenol and cresol isomers	phenol and cresol isomers	urine	b
phthalates	2-ethyl-5-hydroxyhexyl-phthalate 2-ethyl-5-oxohexyl-phthalate	urine	b

a   not fixed
b   end of exposure or end of shift
c   for long-term exposures: after several shifts
d   at the beginning of the next shift

Sampling time

Samples for biomonitoring must be taken at the times specified in Tables 1 and 2. In cases where such information is not available, samples should be taken at a time when the internal exposure of the person is in equilibrium with the external exposure. Information about toxicokinetics may be found, for example, in the GESTIS database on hazardous substances (see References). Equilibrium cannot be expected if a job does not take long to carry out (repair jobs, servicing, etc.). In such cases the sample should be taken when the job is finished. Generally the materials for analysis are collected at the end of a shift, if possible after 3 days at work.

Sampling

It is important that sampling is carried out without contamination and without losses. It is recommended that the physician take advantage of the service generally offered by analytical laboratories to supply sampling equipment, vessels for transport of samples and information about sample collection. For the transport of biological samples the regulations for infectious, human biological material must be observed; that means that the vessels must be packaged to ensure containment of the material. Blood and urine samples should be dispatched immediately after taking the samples. If this is not possible, the samples may be stored in a refrigerator at 4°C for a maximum of 5 days. Longer storage is generally possible in the deep frozen state. Separation of plasma and erythrocytes must take place before freezing the samples.

A 1

Collecting urine samples

For urine samples, disposable plastic containers (about 50–100 ml, wide-necked) are normally used. The sample is urinated directly into the container. For analysis of metals it is important that the person is no longer wearing working clothes and has cleaned his or her hands before taking the sample. Contamination by dust, gases or vapours from the workplace must be avoided. The urine volume should be at least 20 ml.

For the determination of volatile organic substances (e.g. acetone, methanol) about 2 ml of a freshly collected spontaneous urine sample is transferred to a sealed (rubber septum) glass ampoule with a disposable syringe. The ampoules serve as storage and transport vessels and are provided by the laboratory.

Collecting whole blood and plasma samples

For the analysis of whole blood and plasma, venous blood samples with added anticoagulant are required. Coagulation must be prevented by thorough shaking of the sample in the container. Suitable for taking the sample is a disposable syringe or disposable cannula, e.g., Monovette® or Vacutainer®. The Monovette® and Vacutainer® vessels contain the appropriate quantity of anticoagulant (e.g. K-EDTA). They serve simultaneously as transport and storage containers. For most analyses, 5 ml whole blood is sufficient.

For the determination of volatile organic substances (halogenated and aromatic/aliphatic hydrocarbons) about 2 ml whole blood must be transferred into a sealed ampoule immediately after collection. The use of disinfectants containing solvents for disinfection of the skin to be punctured should be avoided; the skin can instead be disinfected with, e.g., a 3 % aqueous solution of hydrogen peroxide. The sealed ampoules serve as storage and transport vessels. These special containers are provided by the analytical laboratory.
Monovette® and Vacutainer® vessels with K-EDTA are also suitable for collecting plasma samples. After centrifugation without haemolysis, the plasma is drawn off and transferred to a plastic tube with a lid.
Storage and transport of the biological material is to be carried out so that factors which could alter the analytical results *in vitro* are kept to a minimum. Here too, the occupational physician should seek the advice of the analytical laboratory.

Choice of an analytical laboratory

The laboratory must
- offer specialist advice and support for sampling and for transport and storage of the samples
- make use of up-to-date analytical methods
- carry out regular internal and external quality control
- support the occupational physician in the interpretation of the analytical results.
Sampling, analysis and evaluation are part of medical care and so are subject to medical quality control. Fundamentally, if in the course of biomonitoring an occupational physician makes use of an external analytical laboratory, he is required to ensure that the laboratory involved has appropriate expertise and apparatus and makes use of reliable analytical methods.

Reliable methods

In the guidelines which allow for biological monitoring, it is pointed out that reliable (analytical) methods are to be used to determine the relevant biomonitoring parameters in blood and urine. Such analytical methods are developed and published by the DFG Commission for the Investigation of Health Hazards of Chemical Compounds in the Work Area (see References). The analytical reliability and reproducibility of these methods has been tested.

Quality control for toxicological examinations in occupational medicine

The occupational physician who commissions toxicological analyses (e.g. the determination of lead in blood) and includes the laboratory results in his occupational medical assessment should be aware that, by so doing, he accepts responsibility for the correctness of the analytical results. In this context he must make sure that the laboratory which he uses carries out laboratory internal and laboratory external quality control. This quality control tests the correctness and exactness of the laboratory results. Without being in a position to or having to check these procedures individually, the physician has fulfilled his responsibilities if he makes sure that the laboratory which he uses takes part regularly and successfully in intercomparison programmes for occupational medical toxicological analyses. Such laboratory intercomparison programmes with international participation are carried out, for example, for the German Society of Occupational and Environmental Medicine (Schaller et al 2002). For the successful participation in such programmes the participants receive a certificate which is valid for one year. This certificate should be inspected by the physician before he commissions analyses. The certificate stipulates the analytical parameters (e.g. the determination of lead in blood) for which the laboratory involved took place successfully in the intercomparison programme.

Interpretation of the analytical results by the works physician

The works physician evaluates the analytical results by comparison with occupational medical and environmental threshold values. Threshold values may be found in the List of MAK and BAT Values (see References).

For this evaluation the working conditions (intense physical activity), the characteristics of the hazardous substance (toxicokinetics) and individual features (medication, alcohol intake, smoking) should be taken into account as potential modifying factors. In some cases background exposures from sources not related to the workplace must be taken into account (mercury, arsenic).

That a threshold value is exceeded does not generally result in a ban on working. It is necessary to decide in each individual case whether health risks speak against further employment at that workplace.

A 1

Strategy and procedure of biomonitoring

During biomonitoring the generally accepted rules of occupational medicine, as described for example in the *Guidelines for Occupational Medical Examinations*, must be observed. The intervals between determinations of the parameter in question are established as a function of the job and the specific properties of the hazardous substance. The results of the risk assessment and previous biomonitoring results are to be taken into account. The intervals between examinations for occupational medical prophylaxis can serve as orientation.

Because a single analysis of a parameter is not always sufficient for an assessment, repeat determinations may be necessary to confirm the results.

It is recommended that the biomonitoring results be applied as follows:

- the works physician discusses his assessment of the biomonitoring results with the employee involved;
- the results of biomonitoring are included in the documentation of the occupational medical examinations;
- the biomonitoring results are taken into account in the risk assessment as stipulated in the Council Directive 98/24/EC, while observing the rules of medical confidentiality; if necessary, protective measures are introduced.

Biological monitoring at initial examinations

Substances taken up at work are eliminated from the blood and via the urine with elimination half times which generally do not exceed a few weeks. The amount of information about any previous uptake of hazardous substances which may be obtained from analyses of biological material sinks rapidly *post expositionem*. For this reason biological monitoring in initial examinations is not planned in the guidelines. However, under certain conditions the physician may consider that it makes sense to carry out an objective determination of a known or suspected previous exposure of an employee. In such cases the procedure described for biological monitoring in follow-up examinations is to be followed.

References

Angerer J, Greim H (eds) The MAK-Collection for Occupational Health and Safety. Part IV: Biomonitoring Methods, Vol 1–10. Wiley-VCH

Council Directive 98/24/EC on the protection of the health and safety of workers from the risks related to chemical agents at work

Deutsche Forschungsgemeinschaft (German Research Foundation, DFG) (ed) List of MAK and BAT Values 2007. Maximum Concentrations and Biological Tolerance Values at the workplace. Wiley-VCH, Weinheim

Deutsche Forschungsgemeinschaft (German Research Foundation, DFG) (ed) The MAK-Collection for Occupational Health and Safety. Wiley-VCH at: www.mrw.interscience.wiley.com/makbat

Drexler H, Greim H (eds) The MAK-Collection for Occupational Health and Safety. Part II: BAT Value Documentations, Vol 1–4. Wiley-VCH

Fiserova-Bergerova V, Mraz J (2000) Biological Monitoring of Exposure to Industrial Chemicals. In: Harris RL (ed) Patty's Industrial Hygiene, Volume 3, pp 2001–2060, John Wiley & Sons

GESTIS-database on hazardous substances. BGIA at: www.dguv.de/bgia/gestis-database

Schaller KH, Angerer J, Drexler H (2002) Quality assurance of biological monitoring in occupational and environmental medicine. Journal of Chromatography B, 778:403–417

World Health Organization (1996) Biological Monitoring of Chemical Exposure in the Workplace. Guidelines. WHO, Geneva

Appendix 2   Diagnosis of musculoskeletal disorders in occupational medical examinations

B. Hartmann (BG Bau, Hamburg), M. Spallek (VW Nutzfahrzeuge Hannover), F. Liebers (Bundesanstalt für Arbeitsschutz und Arbeitsmedizin, Berlin), S. Schwarze (Institut für Arbeitsmedizin der Universität Düsseldorf), O. Linhardt (Orthopädische Klinik Regensburg)
for the working group "Strain on the musculoskeletal system" of the Committee for occupational medicine

Background

Workplace activities make a wide spectrum of specific demands on the physical capabilities of the employee and involve various kinds of musculoskeletal work which should be recorded during the risk assessment of the workplace. For the employee to fulfil these demands and to cope with the work, not only are certain motor capabilities such as strength and stamina necessary but also functional abilities such as coordination and mobility of the joints. The kind, extent and duration of physical activity at the workplace and the characteristics of the individual employee result in different levels of work for the musculoskeletal system and in some cases even strain. The questions raised in this context for occupational medical examinations include:

- How may the musculoskeletal effects of the physical work associated with certain activities or jobs be evaluated?
- Which physical characteristics must an employee possess if he or she is to cope with the physical work at a certain workplace?
- Which health risks for the employee could result from this physical work?
- Has the physical work already caused musculoskeletal symptoms, functional deficits or damage?
- Which individual or workplace-related measures could prevent further progression of symptoms or functional disorders and should therefore be included in any occupational medical advice or intervention?

Methods

The diagnosis of musculoskeletal disorders in occupational medicine must be fitted into a firm's system of occupational medical prophylaxis. It generally involves persons who are able to work and who come to the medical examination from the workplace during working time. Generally, acute symptoms are present only by chance. Instead, the main medical findings are often enduring symptoms of subacute or chronic defects or disorders.

Essential requirements for the occupational medical examination are
- detailed knowledge of the concrete dangers at the employee's workplace given by a risk assessment
- a targeted anamnesis which records current and recent symptoms and disorders and their relationship with the workload
- a clinical examination to detect job-relevant functional deficits and potential disorders

The object of the occupational medical prophylaxis is an overall evaluation and assessment of symptoms and findings from the examination with respect to
- current functional ability and fitness
- the extent to which work has caused the symptoms and findings
- any health risk associated with continuing to do the work
- any therapeutic or rehabilitative treatment necessary to maintain fitness for work

The results of the examination make it clear whether the employee requires advice about behaviour at the workplace and away from work, about therapy or rehabilitation measures and about work organization but also whether the employer should be advised about any generally applicable results of the medical examinations in the form of suggestions as to modification of the risk assessment, recommendations for ergonomic organization of the workplace and work organization in general.

Anamnesis

As in any medical examination, in the recognition and assessment of musculoskeletal disorders a thorough general and special anamnesis is of great importance. Often the anamnestic findings suggest the diagnosis and form the basis for the assessment of functional deficits.

A standardized and reproducible system for documentation of anamnesis data, especially for use in occupational epidemiology, should make use of tested and standardized tools. For the effective and standardized documentation of the relevant information, it is recommended (Hartmann et al. 2005a) that the anamnesis be divided into parts which are used consecutively or, in the case of hand-arm vibration, as necessary.

Anamnesis questionnaire 1: "Self-reported musculoskeletal disorders"
This anamnestic questionnaire (at the end of G 46) documents systematically the occurrence and localization of musculoskeletal symptoms. The questionnaire is filled in independently by the employee before the medical examination.
The questionnaire covers the following points:
- previous disorders and operations including serious accidents which, given the current state of the musculoskeletal system, could have adverse effects on function and prognosis
- particular symptoms associated with work, outlined as examples from the previous 12 months
- localization of symptoms on sketches of the back and front of the body and the extremities

- a question as to whether the person has seen a doctor about the symptoms is intended to establish their importance for the employee
- medical diagnoses, as information from any earlier detailed examinations, are included for purposes of confirmation and functional assessment
- frequency and total duration of periods of inability to work during the previous 12 months are intended to document the real effects of any musculoskeletal disorders or damage on work
- work which causes pain or other symptoms (lifting/carrying heavy loads, bent or twisted posture, kneeling or squatting, prolonged standing, work with the arms above shoulder level, vibrations in the hand-arm system from tools or vibrating machines, vibrations in the whole body when sitting on vehicles or machines) is recorded in detail

Anamnesis questionnaire 2: "Medical anamnesis of musculoskeletal disorders"
If an employee describes relevant symptoms, a medical anamnesis of musculoskeletal disorders is required (questionnaire at the end of G 46). Its objective is to obtain more information about the reported symptoms.
This questionnaire, to be filled in by the physician, covers the following points:

- The patient is questioned about quality and character of pain felt during the previous 12 months. In addition, unspecific pains and other complaints, e.g. of psychosocial origin, are differentiated.
- The discussion of acute pain radiating from the backbone serves to associate radicular pain with specific spinal nerves and to differentiate pseudoradicular symptoms. Symptoms resulting from excessive strain, from joint diseases and irritation of nerves and vessels in cases of outlet syndrome (e.g. shoulder) are also documented.
- Questions as to pain provocation by certain movements or loads provide information as to the level of strain involved. This helps in the assessment of occupational relevance.
- Work-related pain is felt initially while working and disappears or is much less severe during work-free periods. If the pain does not become less severe at night, at the weekends or on holiday, the development of chronic pain which is not work-related must be considered.
- The severity of the dominant pain is documented semi-quantitatively on a 10-point scale (visual analogue scale, VAS).
- The prevalence of the symptoms over the week documents again their relevance for the current examination interval.
- Additional anamnestic details which are obtained for the diagnosis and assessment of musculoskeletal disorders in an individual case can be documented in free form.

"Medical anamnesis for hand-arm vibration exposure"
In this additional section of the questionnaire for employees exposed to hand-arm vibration characteristic anamnestic information such as numbness and circulation disorders in the hands is documented. They can be marked on a sketch of a hand.

A 2

For the specific anamnesis required in the supplementary examination the question-naire *"Supplementary examination of persons exposed to hand-arm vibration"* at the end of the second main section "Disorders caused by hand-arm vibration" of the G 46 can be used. This questionnaire contains a list of devices which are known to be able to cause hazard via hand-arm vibration.

The suggested documentation sheets summarize the targeted anamnestic data and explain the details. The fact that jobs involving high levels of strain for the muscu-loskeletal system are more frequently carried out by persons with little education or who come from abroad and speak a foreign language can make it necessary to record the sense of an anamnesis expressed in simplified language. The content and structure of the anamnesis should, however, not be altered.

Clinical examination

The clinical examination of the musculoskeletal system should be modular. This makes it possible, on the one hand, to work efficiently and save time by restricting the examination to the particularly affected regions of the body. On the other hand, it is possible to include all modules and so carry out a total examination of the mus-culoskeletal system. The examination of the musculoskeletal system is generally car-ried out as part of a general clinical examination. Abnormalities are sought by in-spection, tests for mobility, and palpation. If abnormalities are found, then individual regions of the musculoskeletal system are examined more closely with special func-tional tests. However, because local disorders in single regions can affect wider areas (e.g. in a series of joints) or even the whole musculoskeletal system, it is recom-mended that the clinical status of the whole system be examined, at least at the initial examination.

Medical examination programmes in occupational medicine
The clinical examination of the musculoskeletal system can be carried out most effi-ciently if it is carried out in steps:
a) a *basic examination* seeks functional abnormalities or relevant findings associat-ed with subjective symptoms
b) a *supplementary examination* seeks the reason for any abnormalities and per-haps any other more general causes.
It is recommended that the course of the examination and documentation is oriented on the following regions:
- inspection of the various regions
  - general inspection (gait pattern, posture, mobility when bending and stand-ing up)
  - inspection of the upper extremities, the back and the lower extremities
- examination of the cervical spine and the upper extremities, perhaps including neurological problems in the areas:
  - cervical spine
  - shoulder-upper arm
  - forearm-hand

- examination of the spine of the trunk and the lower extremities, perhaps including neurological problems in the areas:
  - lumbar spine and iliosacral articulations
  - hip joints
  - knee joints
  - foot and ankle joints

Inspection
The physical examination begins with the inspection of the whole musculoskeletal system and the assessment of general condition and nutritional state. Unusual gait, posture and mobility (e.g. bending to take the shoes off) and any use of orthopaedic aids (e.g. orthopaedic insoles) are to be documented. Difficulties in taking off clothes can give the first hint of functional disorders.
During the inspection particular attention is to be paid to:
- external changes (swelling, atrophy)
- asymmetry (different leg lengths)
- deformities (angulation)
- skin changes (e.g. calluses)
- assessment of the harmony of movement (e.g. gait pattern).

Mobility tests
In tests for the range of movement of joints, which are first carried out actively (by the patient alone) and then passively (the movements guided by the physician), both restricted movement (hypomobility) and increased capacity for movement (hypermobility) can be recognized.
Because interindividual differences can be large, it is important to compare the two sides of the person's body. Documentation of the capacity for joint movement can be qualitative (physiological, restricted, highly restricted, etc.) or quantitative (according to the neutral-zero method). The recommended examination sheets assume use of this procedure and contain the values for normal mobility. If it is planned to follow the course of any changes, the girth of the extremities at fixed points should be recorded for both sides.

Clinical functional tests
If the patient reports pain and in cases with functional impairment, in addition to testing the mobility of joints palpation of the affected regions should be carried out. Particular attention should be paid to
- provocation of pain by active movement, at the end of the range in passive joint movement and during isometric tensioning of muscles
- changes of the contours and in the tissues around joints, muscles, tendons, ligaments and other structures (oedema, swelling, effusion, myogelosis, hyperthermia)
- friction phenomena (snapping hip, arthrotic friction, crepitation of the tendons in tendosynovitis, sounds)

Restriction of the examination to certain parts of the musculoskeletal system can be problematical: symptoms are often projected into other regions of the body. In a separate examination of, e.g., the lumbar spine, changes in the iliosacral articulations, hip and knee joints and deformities of the feet which can be responsible for several symptoms can be missed. Therefore, on the one hand, it is recommended that all the joints of a region of the body be examined. On the other hand, because of the circumstances of occupational medical practice, the examination should be kept to the minimum which is medically and practically justifiable.

To achieve a rational and ergonomic course of the examination, frequent changes in the position of the employee and the examining physician should be avoided. Tests which can be carried out standing should be carried out in series, likewise those carried out while the patient is seated, prone or prostrate.

The procedure for clinical examination of the musculoskeletal system is described in detail in standard orthopaedic text books (e.g. Hoppenfeld 1976, Brinker 1999, Kaufer et al. 2002, McRae 2004). Presented are a large number of alternative tests which provide the same or similar information. In general, these descriptions contain no statements as to the value of the test results for prophylaxis. For occupational medical practice, tests must be chosen which permit statements as to the health, function and fitness of the person for the job and which make it possible to recognize impaired function and fitness caused by defects or disorders which require further action.

For these special requirements of occupational medical examinations (efficient use of time, concentration on relevant defects and functional deficits) various systems for orthopaedic examinations on occupational medicine have been developed and tested and brief examination procedures published (Hartmann & Hartmann 1996, Kuhn et al. 1998).

The detailed schemes with step-wise examination procedures include
* a programme for step-wise diagnosis of musculoskeletal disorders in occupational medical practice (Grifka et al. 2006)
* the function-oriented system fokus[®] (Funktions-Orientierte Körperliche Untersuchungs Systematik) for physical examination of the locomotor system in occupational medicine (Spallek et al. 2005, 2007).

For details of these two programmes the reader is referred to the above sources.

Neurological and angiological assessment
If there are indications of vascular or sensorineural functional disorders in the fingers in persons exposed to hand-arm vibration from high frequency (from about 50 Hz) tools, the vascular status should be evaluated clinically and an orientating neurological examination carried out for differential diagnostic purposes. Simple clinical tests such as Allen's test or Adson's test can yield evidence of vascular disorders of other genesis (Bovenzi 2004). In the neurological examination, central, radicular and peripheral neurological disorders may be distinguished by demonstrating appropriate sensorimotor defects or increased, reduced or absent reflex amplitudes. Here too simple clinical tests such as the Roos test, Tinel test or Phalen sign can help to differentiate between neurological symptoms of various genesis.

Special medical examination
The clinical functional examination carried out by the works physician does not necessarily aim to yield a differential diagnosis of suspected syndromes. Therefore specific diagnostic and invasive methods (radiography, arthroscopy, etc). can be dispensed with. These are not required for occupational medical prophylaxis. If such questions arise, the patient should be recommended to see a specialist for orthopaedics or emergency medicine or a neurologist for further clarification of the clinical symptoms. The results of such examinations can then be used by the occupational physician when establishing the person's fitness for a new job or for a return to work.
Any effects of vibration exposure during work with compressed air tools are seen mainly in the bone structures and joints of the hand-arm system. These require an examination based on the methods for functional assessment recommended in G 46. The hand-arm vibration exposure caused by higher frequency (> 50 Hz) tools affects mainly the vascular and nervous systems. A carefully recorded anamnesis of the times of occurrence of specific patterns of symptoms, e.g., in the cold, is the main diagnostic tool for occupational medical prophylaxis. It is recommended that the criteria of the Stockholm Workshop Scale be used (Gemne et al. 1987). Vibration damage is very likely if the classical symptoms are described (Bovenzi 2004). The most important method for documentation and confirmation of the diagnosis of vibration-induced vascular or sensorineural damage is a cold provocation test with determination of restitution of the circulation in the fingers (ISO/DIS 14835-1). Pallaesthetic measurements may also be used. These methods require appropriate equipment and are generally part of the specialist assessment after notification of occupational diseases.

A 2

Assessment of the results of the medical examination

Occupational medical diagnosis, assessment and advice is a complex process of evaluation of the individual risk for an employee presented by his job and the conditions at an actual workplace or in a field of activity. This assessment of interrelationships is the core task of occupational medicine. The programmes of medical examinations and their documentation provide important aids and the basis for assessment, but they in no way replace the occupational medical knowledge and experience required for the final evaluation. Taking the diagnostic procedure together with the questions formulated above, the content of the complex of occupational medical diagnosis and assessment may be given as follows:

- Function: "Under what conditions can the particular job be carried out by a person with the detected functional deficits?"
- Nosology: "Does the person suffer from a musculoskeletal disorder which requires special treatment before advice about a return to work and the conditions of such a return can be given?"
- Prevention and therapy: "Which health improvement measures or which primary, secondary or tertiary preventive measures are necessary and sensible in the actual case? Are therapeutic or rehabilitative measures necessary?"

- Aetiology: "What is the probable cause of the disorder and what role is played by the working conditions?"
- Prognosis: "Can the defect or disorder be made worse if the work is continued without changes?"

For the occupational medical assessment, the results of the examination and any functional abnormalities are to be taken together with the anamnestic information to produce a presumption diagnosis. Diagnoses for medical documentation should be classified according to ICD 10, even when all its details cannot be used in the absence of a differential diagnosis commissioned by the occupational physician. Also pain syndromes without precise aetiology can be classified according to ICD 10. The works physician must decide whether further clarification and medical treatment is necessary for the comparatively rare individual cases of manifest musculoskeletal disorders.

For subsequent medical assessment and advice, use of the social model of disease results is recommended. A theoretical basis is provided by the ICF classification developed for rehabilitation medicine (ICF 2004 = International Classification of Functioning, Disability and Health) which provides suggestions for a systematic function-related assessment. Also from the occupational medical point of view, several levels of assessment of the results of disease can be differentiated:

- *Function:* this generic term covers all bodily functions and activities. Most important are the functional effects of defective physiological functions or structural damage.
- *Fitness:* the presumed ability to cope with certain forms of physical work at the workplace (handling loads, forced postures, holding objects, repetitive work, vibration exposure) is to be assessed here. The functionality is to be assessed in terms of potential limitations in working life. When advising the patient, suggestions for improvement or stabilization should be derived.
- *Health risk:* as well as the current abilities and fitness, expected development of the state of health should be included in the assessment. The estimated probability and severity of any potential damage determines the health prognosis or the risk for the person under the given conditions.
- *Earning capacity:* the possibility of maintaining the fitness for work and earning capacity of the person under the current workplace conditions or under alternative conditions in another job are to be assessed. This is not the same as an expert opinion on "reduced earning capacity".

More information about objectives and assessment of occupational medical prophylaxis for persons exposed to musculoskeletal strain has been published by Hartmann et al. (2005b).

Advising the employee and employer

The advice given to the employee and employer in practice demonstrates the preventive character of occupational medicine, in comparison with the curative care of the family doctor. Detailed advice should bring about, at various levels of behaviour

and workplace conditions, preventive changes which involve both the employee and the employer or the whole organization. It has the following objectives:
- proper weighing up of the relationships between medical findings and specific effects of various kinds of physical work at the workplace with respect to
- the kind of work (dynamic, static, vibration)
  - the part of the musculoskeletal system affected by the work
  - the probability of the situation arising or the frequency in that job
  - the duration of the exposure
- the possibility of affecting – in general or for the individual – the strain caused by work, something which differs enormously in the various branches of industry, kinds of technology, sizes and structures of businesses
- advice about the current work both with respect to the life perspectives of the employee, taking age and remaining working years into account and the real alternative occupations, but also including the person's private life ("work/life balance").
- influencing the willingness of the individual employee to cooperate in preventive measures especially when they are not yet motivated by suffering or when they do not see that it can help.

Advising the employee
Working life and private life have a great influence on each other in the long term. A health-conscious way of life with a physically active private life and avoidance of days with little activity as well as a healthy diet is variously well developed among employees of the various branches of industry. Employees who do a lot of physical work and for whom occupational medical prophylaxis of the musculoskeletal system is indicated often feel so tired out by their work that they do not seek physical activity in their free time. However, work involving physical strain does not affect all parts of the body or all motor abilities and a lack of stamina is often an important limiting factor. When the physical strain at work is one-sided, the result is often muscular imbalance and general deficits in endurance which should be compensated.
When advising the employee, therefore, the following points are important:
a) information about and explanation of the individual findings in the musculoskeletal system
b) additional findings in other organ systems which affect fitness for work (coronary heart disease, chronic obstructive bronchitis, pulmonary emphysema, etc.)
c) evaluation of functional deficits, reduced fitness and prognosis of the health risk and future work capacity
d) conceivable risks associated with the questions of whether it is possible to stay at the old workplace, whether ergonomic or organizational changes are necessary and possible there or whether a change of workplace is necessary
e) recommendations for efficient secondary prevention, therapy or rehabilitation
f) the possibilities for making a personal contribution to a reduction of the physical effort required at the workplace by acquiring and applying basic ergonomic knowledge
g) recommendations for changes in life style (e.g. exercise, diet, weight, stress)

A 2

h) suggestions for health-improving measures (sport clubs, health insurance schemes, pension insurance schemes, fitness studios, etc).

Individual health-promoting measures to increase physical stamina are part of the advice offered to employees by the works physician. Recommended health-promoting sports and fitness training should take into account the criteria for quality developed by the various organizations for

- *health-promoting sport*
- *exercising in health or fitness studios* according to the recommendations of a doctor qualified in sports medicine
- *"workhardening"*: exercise, coordination training, behavioural ergonomics (back exercise programmes) and direct practising of everyday jobs for persons with restricted ability (Kaiser et al. 2000)
- *multimodal procedure* for reducing musculoskeletal pain by physical activity, relaxation, psychic coping strategies, etc.
- *back exercise programmes*
- *rehabilitation sport* for persons with disabilities or persons threatened with disability, on prescription and with medical supervision

Taking part in health-promoting sport in a sports club is the cheapest kind of sport activity for the employee. It is also available in small towns and villages close to home. In general, the sport programmes should be multimodal. Endurance training should be combined with general and specific strength training (e.g. of the back muscles), coordination exercises, ergonomic components and relaxation techniques for coping with the psychomotor component.

To what extent it is possible to differentiate performance deficits in the course of an occupational medical examination and so provide the basis for a specific training programme depends on the experience and qualification of the occupational physician. For the works physician to be competent in this field requires further education in the fields of diagnosis and rehabilitation.

Special demands are involved in planning the stepwise return to work of employees who have been unfit to work for a long period when the employee seeks out the works physician to obtain advice as to the possibility of returning to work.

The medical examination and advice can then finally be the cause of initiating rehabilitation measures.

Advising the employer

The main points involved in advising the employer are appropriate preventive measures for reducing undue and misplaced effort at the workplace. The objective is the maintenance of fitness for work and earning capacity of the employees.

The advice, based on the results of the medical examinations, can be aimed at the general working conditions. This applies when the medical examinations and data from risk assessments suggest that certain work or working conditions could be a cause of persistent symptoms. However, medical confidentiality is to be maintained. Therefore in small businesses it can be difficult to refer directly to the results of medical examinations.

On the other hand, the physician's advice can involve an individual case when the employer has been told of the physical symptoms and disorders of an employee or when the works physician is actually expected to be involved in the solution of an individual problem. In some cases, success in the introduction of ergonomic, organizational and other person-related measures at the workplace is more readily achieved when the discussion with the employer involves an actual case and the employee is also present than it is when the recommendations remain abstract.

References

Bovenzi M (2004) Guidelines for hand-transmitted vibration health surveillance. Proceedings of 9th International Conference on Hand-Arm Vibration, INRS, France

Brinker MR (1999) Fundamentals of Orthopaedics. WB Saunders

Gemne G, Pyykko I, Taylor W, Pelmear PL (1987) The Stockholm workshop scale for the classification of cold-induced Raynaud's phenomenon in the hand-arm vibration syndrome (revision of the Taylor-Pelmear scale). Scand J Work Environ Health 13: 275–278

Grifka J, Peters Th, Linhardt O, Bär H, Liebers F (2001) Mehrstufendiagnostik von Muskel-Skelett-Erkrankungen in der arbeitsmedizinischen Praxis. (Step-by-step Diagnosis of Musculo-Skeletal Diseases in Occupational Health Practice. Publication Series from the Federal Institute for Occupational Safety and Health). Wirtschaftsverlag NW, Bremerhaven. Schriftenreihe der Bundesanstalt für Arbeitsschutz und Arbeitsmedizin

Hartmann B, Schwarze S, Liebers F, Spallek M, Kuhn W, Caffier G (2005a) Arbeitsmedizinische Vorsorge bei Belastungen des Muskel-Skelett-Systems. Teil 1 : Zielstellungen, Konzeption und Anamnese. (Occupational medical prophylaxis for the musculoskeletal system. Part 1: objectives, concepts and anamnesis). Arbeitsmed Sozialmed Umweltmed Präventivmed 40(2): 60–68

Hartmann B, Spallek M, Kuhn W, Liebers F, Schwarze S (2005b) Arbeitsmedizinische Vorsorge bei Belastungen des Muskel-Skelett-Systems. Teil 3: Die Beratung als Teil der arbeitsmedizinischen Vorsorge. (Occupational medical prophylaxis for the musculoskeletal system. Part 3: the consultation in occupational medical prophylaxis). Arbeitsmed Sozialmed Umweltmed Präventivmed 40(5): 288–296

Hartmann B (2000) Prävention arbeitsbedingter Rücken- und Gelenkerkrankungen: Ergonomie und arbeitsmedizinische Praxis. (Prevention of work-related disorders of the back and joints: ergonomics and occupational medical practice). ecomed, Landsberg

Hoppenfeld S (1976) Physical Examination of the Spine and Extremities. Prentice Hall

ICD 10 – International Statistical Classification of Diseases and Related Health Problems, Chapter XIII "Diseases of the musculoskeletal system and connective tissue (M00–M99)". WHO at: www.who.int/classifications/apps/icd/icd10online/

A 2

ICF – International Classification of Functioning, Disability and Health. At: www3.who.int/icf/icftemplate.cfm

ISO/DIS 14835-1 (2004) Mechanical vibration and shock – Cold provocation tests for the assessment of peripheral vascular function – Part 1: Measurement and evaluation of finger skin temperature

Kaiser H, Kersting M, Schian H-M, Jacobs A, Kasprowski D (2000) Der Stellenwert des EFL-Verfahrens nach Susan Isernhagen in der medizinischen und beruflichen Rehabilitation. (The role of functional capacity evaluation by the method of Susan Isernhagen in medical and occupational rehabilitation). Rehabilitation 39: 297–306

Kaufer, H, Fitzgerald, RH (2002) Orthopaedics. CV Mosby

Krämer J, Grifka J (2001) Orthopädie. (Orthopaedics) 6th edition. Springer

McRae, R (2004) Clinical Orthopaedic Examination. Churchill Livingstone

BAuA (2003) Mehrstufendiagnostik von Muskel-Skelett-Erkrankungen in der arbeitsmedizinischen Praxis – Datenbankanwendung und multimediale Untersuchungsanleitung. (Step-by-step diagnosis of musculoskeletal diseases in occupational health practice – the use of the database and multimedia guide to medical examination procedures.) Wirtschaftsverlag NW, Bremerhaven, Sonderschrift S77 der BAuA, CD-ROM Version 2.0

Morris CE (2005) Low Back Syndromes. McGraw

Spallek M, Kuhn W, Schwarze S, Hartmann B (2005) Arbeitsmedizinische Vorsorge bei Belastungen des Muskel-Skelettsystems. Teil 2: Funktionsorientierte körperliche Untersuchungssystematik (fokus®) des Bewegungsapparates in der Arbeitsmedizin. (Occupational medical prophylaxis for the musculoskeletal system. Part 2: Function-oriented system (fokus®) for physical examination of the musculoskeletal system in occupational medicine). Arbeitsmed Sozialmed Umweltmed 40(4): 244–250

Spallek M, Kuhn W, Schwarze S, Hartmann B (2007) Occupational medical prophylaxis for the musculoskeletal system: A function-oriented system for physical examination of the locomotor system in occupational medicine (fokus®). J Occup Med Toxicol 2: 12, at: www.occup-med.com